D0536742

Pediatric Oncology Imaging

Guest Editor

ERIC N. FAERBER, MD, FACR

RADIOLOGIC CLINICS
OF NORTH AMERICA

www.radiologic.theclinics.com

Consulting Editor
FRANK H. MILLER, MD

July 2011 • Volume 49 • Number 4

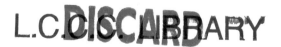
SAUNDERS an imprint of ELSEVIER, Inc.

W.B. SAUNDERS COMPANY
A Division of Elsevier Inc.

1600 John F. Kennedy Boulevard • Suite 1800 • Philadelphia, Pennsylvania 19103-2899

http://www.theclinics.com

RADIOLOGIC CLINICS OF NORTH AMERICA Volume 49, Number 4
July 2011 ISSN 0033-8389, ISBN 13: 978-1-4557-1150-5

Editor: Barton Dudlick
Developmental Editor: Donald E. Mumford

Radiologic Clinics of North America (ISSN 0033-8389) is published bimonthly by Elsevier Inc., 360 Park Avenue South, New York, NY 10010-1710. Months of issue are January, March, May, July, September, and November. Periodicals postage paid at New York, NY and additional mailing offices. Subscription prices are USD 386 per year for US individuals, USD 610 per year for US institutions, USD 185 per year for US students and residents, USD 450 per year for Canadian individuals, USD 766 per year for Canadian institutions, USD 556 per year for international individuals, USD 766 per year for international institutions, and USD 266 per year for Canadian and foreign students/residents. To receive student and resident rate, orders must be accompanied by name of affiliated institution, date of term and the signature of program/residency coordinatior on institution letterhead. Orders will be billed at individual rate until proof of status is received. Foreign air speed delivery is included in all *Clinics* subscription prices. All prices are subject to change without notice. **POSTMASTER:** Send address changes to *Radiologic Clinics of North America*, Elsevier Health Sciences Division, Subscription Customer Service, 3251 Riverport Lane, Maryland Heights, MO63043. **Customer Service: Telephone: 1-800-654-2452** (U.S. and Canada); **1-314-447-8871** (outside U.S. and Canada). **Fax: 1-314-447-8029. E-mail: journalscustomerservice-usa@ elsevier.com** (for print support); **journalsonlinesupport-usa@elsevier.com** (for online support).

Reprints. For copies of 100 or more of articles in this publication, please contact the Commercial Reprints Department, Elsevier Inc., 360 Park Avenue South, New York, New York 10010-1710. Tel.: (+1) 212-633-3812; Fax: (+1) 212-462-1935; E-mail: reprints@elsevier.com.

Radiologic Clinics of North America also published in Greek Paschalidis Medical Publications, Athens, Greece.

Radiologic Clinics of North America is covered in *MEDLINE/PubMed (Index Medicus), EMBASE/Excerpta Medica, Current Contents/Life Sciences, Current Contents/Clinical Medicine, RSNA Index to Imaging Literature, BIOSIS, Science Citation Index,* and *ISI/BIOMED*.

Printed in the United States of America.

Contributors

CONSULTING EDITOR

FRANK H. MILLER, MD
Professor of Radiology; Chief, Body Imaging
Section and Fellowship Program and GI
Radiology, Medical Director MRI, Department
of Radiology, Northwestern University
Feinberg School of Medicine, Chicago, Illinois

GUEST EDITOR

ERIC N. FAERBER, MD, FACR
Professor of Radiology and Pediatrics, Drexel
University College of Medicine; Chief, Section
of Neuroradiology; Director, Department of
Radiology, St Christopher's Hospital for
Children, Philadelphia, Pennsylvania

AUTHORS

PEDRO A.B. ALBUQUERQUE, MD
Assistant Professor, Department of Medical
Imaging, Montreal Children's Hospital, McGill
University, Montreal, Quebec, Canada

CSILLA BALASSY, MD
Department of Diagnostic Imaging, The
Hospital for Sick Children; Clinical Fellow,
Department of Medical Imaging, University of
Toronto, Toronto, Ontario, Canada; Staff
Radiologist, Department of Radiology, Vienna
General Hospital, Medical University of Vienna,
Vienna, Austria

LUCIA CARPINETA, MD
Assistant Professor, Department of Medical
Imaging, Montreal Children's Hospital, McGill
University, Montreal, Quebec, Canada

ALAN DANEMAN, MD
Department of Diagnostic Imaging, The
Hospital for Sick Children; Professor,
Department of Medical Imaging, University of
Toronto, Toronto, Ontario, Canada

ERIC N. FAERBER, MD, FACR
Professor of Radiology and Pediatrics, Drexel
University College of Medicine; Chief, Section
of Neuroradiology; Director, Department of
Radiology, St Christopher's Hospital for
Children, Philadelphia, Pennsylvania

RICARDO FAINGOLD, MD
Assistant Professor; Program Director of
Pediatric Radiology, Department of Medical
Imaging, Montreal Children's Hospital, McGill
University, Montreal, Quebec, Canada

KRISTIN A. FICKENSCHER, MD
Assistant Professor, Department of Radiology,
Children's Mercy Hospital and Clinics,
University of Missouri Kansas City,
Kansas City, Missouri

ELLIOTT R. FRIEDMAN, MD
Assistant Professor of Radiology, Department
of Diagnostic and Interventional Imaging,
University of Texas Health Science Center at
Houston, Houston, Texas

EVAN GELLER, MD
Department of Radiology, St Christopher's Hospital for Children; Assistant Professor of Radiology and Pediatrics, Drexel University College of Medicine, Philadelphia, Pennsylvania

R. PAUL GUILLERMAN, MD
Associate Professor of Radiology, Department of Pediatric Radiology, Baylor College of Medicine, Texas Children's Hospital, Houston, Texas

SUSAN D. JOHN, MD, FACR
Professor of Radiology and Pediatrics, Department of Diagnostic and Interventional Imaging, University of Texas Health Science Center at Houston, Houston, Texas

SUE C. KASTE, DO
Member, Departments of Radiological Sciences and Oncology, St Jude Children's Research Hospital; Professor, Department of Radiology, University of Tennessee School of Health Science Center, Memphis, Tennessee

POLLY S. KOCHAN, MD
Department of Radiology, St Christopher's Hospital for Children; Clinical Associate Professor of Radiology and Pediatrics, Drexel University College of Medicine, Philadelphia, Pennsylvania

MARIA F. LADINO-TORRES, MD
Department of Radiology, C.S. Mott Children's Hospital, University of Michigan, Ann Arbor, Michigan

CHARLES LAWRENCE, MD
Assistant Professor, Department of Radiology, Children's Mercy Hospital and Clinics, University of Missouri Kansas City, Kansas City, Missouri

LISA H. LOWE, MD, FAAP
Assistant Professor, Department of Radiology, Children's Mercy Hospital and Clinics, University of Missouri Kansas City, Kansas City, Missouri

JAMES S. MEYER, MD
Associate Professor of Radiology and Associate-Radiologist-in-Chief, Department of Radiology, Children's Hospital of Philadelphia, Philadelphia, Pennsylvania

OSCAR M. NAVARRO, MD
Department of Diagnostic Imaging, The Hospital for Sick Children; Associate Professor, Department of Medical Imaging, University of Toronto, Toronto, Ontario, Canada

BEVERLEY NEWMAN, MB, BCh, FACR
Professor of Pediatric Radiology, Lucile Packard Children's Hospital at Stanford University School of Medicine, Department of Radiology, Stanford, California

MICHAEL J. PALDINO, MD
Fellow, Division of Neuroradiology, Department of Radiology, Children's Hospital Boston, Boston, Massachusetts

BRUCE R. PARKER, MD
Professor of Radiology, Department of Pediatric Radiology, Baylor College of Medicine, Texas Children's Hospital, Houston, Texas

TINA YOUNG POUSSAINT, MD
Staff Neuroradiologist; Associate Professor of Radiology, Department of Radiology, Children's Hospital Boston, Harvard Medical School, Boston, Massachusetts

RICKI U. SHAH, MD
Resident, Department of Internal Medicine, University of Missouri Kansas City, Kansas City, Missouri

LEI SHAO, MD
Associate Professor, Department of Pathology, Children's Mercy Hospital and Clinics, University of Missouri Kansas City, Kansas City, Missouri

LISA J. STATES, MD
Assistant Professor of Clinical Radiology and Director of Outpatient Satellite Imaging, Department of Radiology, Children's Hospital of Philadelphia, Philadelphia, Pennsylvania

PETER J. STROUSE, MD
Section of Pediatric Radiology, Department of Radiology, C.S. Mott Children's Hospital, University of Michigan Health System, University of Michigan, Ann Arbor, Michigan

STEPHAN D. VOSS, MD, PhD
Assistant Professor of Radiology, Department of Radiology, Children's Hospital Boston, Harvard Medical School, Boston, Massachusetts

Contents

uncommonly occurs as a result of imaging performed for trauma. Clinical and standard imaging characteristics of the various tumor types are evolving in concert with treatment advancements and clinical trial regimens. This article reviews the 3 most common pediatric bone sarcomas—osteosarcoma, Ewing sarcoma, and chondrosarcoma—and their imaging as applicable to contemporary disease staging and monitoring, and explores the roles of evolving imaging techniques.

Leukemia and lymphoma are the most common and third most common pediatric malignancies, respectively, and share cell lineages, but the clinical and imaging manifestations of these malignancies vary substantially. Along with providing pertinent details on classification, epidemiology, and treatment, this article reviews the current roles of imaging in the management of childhood leukemia and lymphoma, with attention to diagnosis, staging, risk stratification, therapy response assessment, and surveillance for disease relapse and adverse effects of therapy. Advances in functional imaging are also discussed to provide insights into future applications of imaging in the management of pediatric patients with leukemia and lymphoma.

GOAL STATEMENT

The goal of the *Radiologic Clinics of North America* is to keep practicing radiologists and radiology residents up to date with current clinical practice in radiology by providing timely articles reviewing the state of the art in patient care.

ACCREDITATION

The *Radiologic Clinics of North America* is planned and implemented in accordance with the Essential Areas and Policies of the Accreditation Council for Continuing Medical Education (ACCME) through the joint sponsorship of the University of Virginia School of Medicine and Elsevier. The University of Virginia School of Medicine is accredited by the ACCME to provide continuing medical education for physicians.

The University of Virginia School of Medicine designates this enduring material activity for a maximum of 15 *AMA PRA Category 1 Credit*(s)™ for each issue, 90 credits per year. Physicians should only claim credit commensurate with the extent of their participation in the activity.

The American Medical Association has determined that physicians not licensed in the US who participate in this CME enduring material activity are eligible for a maximum of 15 *AMA PRA Category 1 Credit*(s)™ for each issue, 90 credits per year.

Credit can be earned by reading the text material, taking the CME examination online at http://www.theclinics.com/home/cme, and completing the evaluation. After taking the test, you will be required to review any and all incorrect answers. Following completion of the test and evaluation, your credit will be awarded and you may print your certificate.

FACULTY DISCLOSURE/CONFLICT OF INTEREST

The University of Virginia School of Medicine, as an ACCME accredited provider, endorses and strives to comply with the Accreditation Council for Continuing Medical Education (ACCME) Standards of Commercial Support, Commonwealth of Virginia statutes, University of Virginia policies and procedures, and associated federal and private regulations and guidelines on the need for disclosure and monitoring of proprietary and financial interests that may affect the scientific integrity and balance of content delivered in continuing medical education activities under our auspices.

The University of Virginia School of Medicine requires that all CME activities accredited through this institution be developed independently and be scientifically rigorous, balanced and objective in the presentation/discussion of its content, theories and practices.

All authors/editors participating in an accredited CME activity are expected to disclose to the readers relevant financial relationships with commercial entities occurring within the past 12 months (such as grants or research support, employee, consultant, stock holder, member of speakers bureau, etc.). The University of Virginia School of Medicine will employ appropriate mechanisms to resolve potential conflicts of interest to maintain the standards of fair and balanced education to the reader. Questions about specific strategies can be directed to the Office of Continuing Medical Education, University of Virginia School of Medicine, Charlottesville, Virginia.

The faculty and staff of the University of Virginia Office of Continuing Medical Education have no financial affiliations to disclose.

The authors/editors listed below have identified no financial or professional relationships for themselves or their spouse/partner:

Pedro A.B. Albuquerque, MD; Csilla Balassy, MD; Lucia Carpineta, MD; Alan Daneman, MD; Barton Dudlick (Acquisitions Editor); Eric N. Faerber, MD (Guest Editor); Ricardo Faingold, MD; Kristin A. Fickenscher, MD; Elliott R. Friedman, MD; Evan Geller, MD; R. Paul Guillerman, MD; Susan D. John, MD; Polly S. Kochan, MD; Maria F. Ladino-Torres, MD; Charles Lawrence, MD; Lisa H. Lowe, MD; James S. Meyer, MD; Frank H. Miller, MD (Consulting Editor); Oscar M. Navarro, MD; Beverly Newman, MB, BCh; Michael J. Paldino, MD; Bruce R. Parker, MD; Tina Young Poussaint, MD; Ricki U. Shah, MD; Lei Shao, MD; Lisa J. States, MD; Peter J. Strouse, MD; and Stephan D. Voss, MD, PhD.

The authors/editors listed below have identified the following financial or professional relationships for themselves or their spouse/partner:

Klaus D. Hagspiel, MD (Test Author) is an industry funded research/investigator for Siemens Medical Solutions.
Sue C. Kaste, DO is an industry funded research/investigator for Mindway Software.

Disclosure of Discussion of Non-FDA Approved Uses for Pharmaceutical Products and/or Medical Devices

The University of Virginia School of Medicine, as an ACCME provider, requires that all faculty presenters identify and disclose any off-label uses for pharmaceutical and medical device products. The University of Virginia School of Medicine recommends that each physician fully review all the available data on new products or procedures prior to clinical use.

TO ENROLL

To enroll in the Radiologic Clinics of North America Continuing Medical Education program, call customer service at 1-800-654-2452 or sign up online at http://www.theclinics.com/home/cme. The CME program is available to subscribers for an additional annual fee USD 245.

Radiologic Clinics of North America

THE CLINICS ARE NOW AVAILABLE ONLINE!

Access your subscription at:
www.theclinics.com

Preface
Pediatric Oncology Imaging

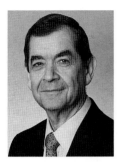

Eric N. Faerber, MD
Guest Editor

"Children are the world's best resource, and its best hope for the future."
—*President John F. Kennedy,*
UNICEF address, 1963

The imaging of pediatric oncology forms an important part of the duties of pediatric radiologists. When faced with the array of available imaging modalities, radiologists need to select the most appropriate imaging studies that are both time- and cost-effective and that deliver the least radiation to the patient. The ALARA and Imaging Gently Principles must be borne in mind.

This issue of *Radiologic Clinics of North America* devoted to pediatric oncology imaging is an update of a similar volume published many years ago. It covers the imaging of tumors in each organ system. It is once again intended to serve as a stand-alone volume for those physicians caring for children with tumors.

I am indebted to all the distinguished authors for their valued articles and to Barton Dudlick at Elsevier for his considerable assistance and patience during the preparation of this issue.

Eric N. Faerber, MD
Department of Radiology
St Christopher's Hospital for Children
3601 A Street
Philadelphia, PA 19134-1095, USA

E-mail address:
Eric.Faerber@tenethealth.com

Radiol Clin N Am 49 (2011) xi–xii
doi:10.1016/j.rcl.2011.05.012
0033-8389/11/$ – see front matter © 2011 Elsevier Inc. All rights reserved.

Dedication

To Esme, Jennifer, and Michael, for their unlimited support and encouragement. And to all the authors committed to the care and imaging of children everywhere.

Imaging Modalities in Pediatric Oncology

Lisa J. States, MD*, James S. Meyer, MD

KEYWORDS

- Pediatric oncology • Imaging • Malignancy

The incidence of childhood malignancy has remained relatively stable over the last 30 years. Fortunately, survival rates have improved.[1] Diagnostic imaging plays a central role in the evaluation of malignancy in children. This article reviews the roles of specific imaging modalities in the diagnosis and management of noncentral nervous system childhood cancer. Imaging modalities to be discussed include conventional radiography, ultrasound, computed tomography (CT), magnetic resonance imaging (MRI), and nuclear medicine, including positron emission tomography (PET). Emerging imaging techniques will also be discussed. Current literature will be referenced for more in-depth review.

RADIOGRAPHY

Conventional radiography plays an important role in the evaluation of cancer in children, not only as an initial screening tool, but also in the assessment of tumor response and recurrence. Conventional radiographs are fast, inexpensive, widely available, and often the initial imaging examination performed in a child with cancer. Conventional radiographs are useful in determining the aggressiveness of bone tumors, and they may identify calcifications in the soft tissues in the abdomen or pelvis or detect pathology in the chest and bones. Conventional radiographs, however, only provide a 1-dimensional representation of 3-dimensional structures, have relatively poor soft tissue contrast, and are often less sensitive and specific than more advanced imaging modalities.

Although conventional film-screen technology is still common, the digital modalities of computed radiography (CR) using a cassette-based system and direct radiography (DR) using a flat-panel based system are widely used. These technologies will likely gain further acceptance as a result of improvements in resolution and decreased radiation exposure in conjunction with more wide-spread use of picture archiving and communication systems (PACS).[2,3]

Chest

Conventional radiographs remain a necessary part of the imaging assessment for many tumors. Although chest CT is often performed due to the need for greater imaging detail and sensitivity, radiographs are often indicated for the detection of metastatic disease and the assessment of mediastinal tumors. In patients with known metastatic lung disease, chest radiographs can be used during therapy to assess response and may be preferred to CT due to the lower radiation dose during post-treatment surveillance. In lymphoproliferative disorders such as leukemia, Hodgkin disease and non-Hodgkin lymphoma, a 2-view chest radiograph is used to monitor treatment. In addition, for children with Hodgkin disease, posteroanterior and lateral chest radiographs are used for the determination of bulky mediastinal adenopathy, which is defined by the ratio of the transverse diameter of the mediastinal lymph node mass to the maximal measurement diameter of the chest cavity on an upright chest radiograph. A mediastinal-to-thoracic ratio of greater than or equal to 0.35 meets the criterion for bulky tumor and typically places the patient on a more aggressive treatment protocol (**Fig. 1**).[4]

Abdomen

Conventional radiography may reveal displacement of bowel gas, obliteration of fat planes,

Department of Radiology, Children's Hospital of Philadelphia, 34th Street and Civic Center Boulevard, Philadelphia, PA 19104, USA
* Corresponding author.
E-mail address: states@email.chop.edu

Radiol Clin N Am 49 (2011) 579–588
doi:10.1016/j.rcl.2011.05.008
0033-8389/11/$ – see front matter

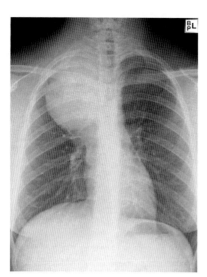

Fig. 1. Mediastinal mass in a patient with Hodgkin disease. An erect AP view of the chest reveals a right paratracheal mediastinal mass causing displacement of the trachea to the left. The mediastinal-to-thoracic ratio is 0.36.

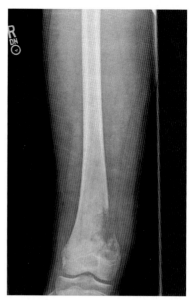

Fig. 2. Osteogenic sarcoma. An AP radiograph of the right femur demonstrates a poorly defined, destructive lesion in the medial distal femoral metaphysis consistent with an aggressive process.

distortion of muscle planes, or the presence of calcifications, suggesting the presence of a tumor. The identification of calcification in the abdomen raises the possibility of neuroblastoma, the most common tumor in children under the age of 5 years.[1] Although radiographically visible calcifications can occur in hepatoblastoma and Wilm tumor, the detection of calcification on radiograph in these tumors is much less common. Calcification in the form of a tooth can be diagnostic of a benign ovarian teratoma. Conventional radiographs of the abdomen, however, are relatively insensitive and are not useful for monitoring of therapy, surveillance, or recurrence.

Bones

Conventional radiographs are valuable tools to characterize and determine the aggressiveness of bone lesions. Specific plain radiographic features allow the identification of a classic benign cyst, fibrous or cartilaginous lesion, an osteoblastic process, or an aggressive destructive process. Radiographic signs of aggressive disease include: lamellated, interrupted, and sunburst periosteal reaction and poorly defined tumor margins (**Fig. 2**). The location of a lesion in the axial or appendicular skeleton or specific portions in the long bones (epiphysis, metaphysis, or diaphysis) and vertebra (body or posterior elements) further assists in providing diagnostic considerations and guiding the imaging required for treatment and staging. Conventional radiographs may also be used to

further assess abnormalities discovered on other imaging studies such as bone scintigraphy and MRI. In addition, conventional radiography may be used to assess complications and disease response or progression, especially in a patient with a metallic prosthesis, which can limit the accuracy of MRI.

Although conventional film-screen technology is still common, the digital modalities of CR using a cassette-based system and DR using a flat-panel based system are widely used. These technologies will likely gain further acceptance as a result of improvements in resolution and decreased radiation exposure in conjunction with more widespread use of PACS.[2,3]

ULTRASOUND

Ultrasound is an ideal imaging modality to screen for cancer in the abdomen and pelvis of neonates, children, and adolescents. Benefits include wide availability, lack of ionizing radiation, and the rare need for sedation. Tissue characterization is excellent. Ultrasound can detect lesions of varying etiology in the abdominal viscera, retroperitoneum, and pelvis. Ultrasound imaging characteristics can determine if a mass is cystic or solid, contains fat or calcification. Additionally, it can suggest a specific diagnosis such as in ovarian dermoid, teratoma, or neuroblastoma. Ultrasound can identify tissue planes by taking advantage of respiratory motion and organ movement. This is especially helpful in the evaluation of large abdominal tumors where organ of origin can be difficult to determine. Color Doppler imaging is helpful in distinguishing solid from cystic components of a mass (Fig. 3), and assessing tumor vascularity (Fig. 4), necrosis, and vascular thrombosis.

Ultrasound, with its lack of ionizing radiation and need for sedation, can be performed at short intervals, which is particularly useful when screening children with syndromes such as aniridia, hemihypertrophy, and Beckwith-Wiedemann syndrome. Children with these syndromes are at increased risk to develop Wilms tumor and typically undergo scanning every 3 months until the age of 8, after which time the Wilms tumor risk is considered low. Children with Beckwith-Wiedemann syndrome are also at risk for the development of pancreaticoblastoma, neuroblastoma, and hepatoblastoma and undergo total abdominal screening.

Ultrasound may also be used to guide tumor localization for percutaneous biopsy. Real-time imaging is used for needle placement, biopsy track embolization, and evaluation of postprocedural hemorrhage. The portability of ultrasound allows its use in combination with fluoroscopy, a clear benefit.

There is a limited role for ultrasound in abdominal imaging in the assessment of response to therapy primarily because it is highly operator dependent and has poor reproducibility for tumor measurements. Other limitations include inadequate evaluation of retroperitoneal tumors due to bowel gas and inability to assess spinal canal involvement in neuroblastoma.

CT

CT remains a keystone in the imaging of children with cancer. Multidetector CT technology (MDCT)

has allowed shorter scanning times while maintaining spatial and contrast resolution. Using the most advanced MDCT scanners, the abdomen and pelvis of many children can be obtained in less than 10 seconds. Images obtained using spiral technique provide a 3-dimensional volumetric dataset that allows for 2-dimensional reformatted images in the coronal and sagittal planes, providing more accurate measurements in the cephalocaudad dimension and often increasing the radiologist's confidence in the interpretation (Fig. 5). The shorter scan time has decreased the need for sedation, particularly in young children. Distraction techniques can also be very effective in helping a child participate in a CT scan without sedation. Some centers use projection systems to display a serene scene of moving images onto the walls, ceilings, or gantry of the CT imaging suite as a method of distraction.[5] In general, the combination of technologists, nurses, and child life specialists who are skilled in the care of children will not only decrease the need for sedation, but also improve the experience for the child and the parents of a child with cancer.

From 1980 to 2005, there was a 20-fold increase in the use of CT. As a result, there has been increasing concern for the development of radiation-induced cancers. It is accepted that the effects of ionizing radiation are greater in children than adults due to increased sensitivity of tissues secondary to increased growth and turnover, and the greater life span over which the child has to develop cancer. Infants and children are up to 10 times more susceptible to carcinogenesis from radiation exposure than adults.[6] When adult protocols are used on children, the radiation exposure is up to 6 times greater than is necessary to provide quality images.[7,8] CT scanning techniques in children should be modified by using a combination of factors (kVP, mA, scan time, pitch, table speed,

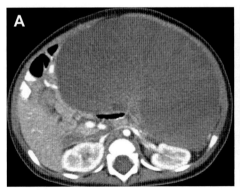
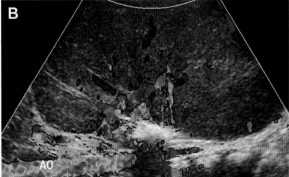

Fig. 3. Undifferentiated retroperitoneal sarcoma. (A) A contrast-enhanced abdominal computed tomography scan reveals a large central mass with low attenuation. The Hounsfield units ranged from 35 to 50. (B) An ultrasound shows central blood flow, confirming a solid mass.

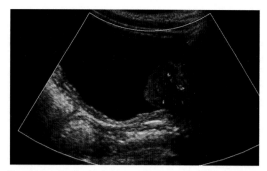

Fig. 4. Prostatic rhabdomyosarcoma. A sagittal ultrasound examination performed in a 4-year-old boy with gross hematuria reveals an intravesicle mass at the bladder base. Color Doppler examination shows increased blood flow within a mass, excluding an intravesical blood clot.

and rotation time) to maintain an acceptable level of image quality and diagnostic accuracy at the lowest possible radiation exposure. Furthermore, there are now vendor-specific techniques such as automatic exposure control that should be used to optimize dose reduction and preserve image quality.[1,9]

Optimizing these parameters for chest, abdomen, and pelvic imaging using a weight-based approach, the Broselow-Luten color scale has been developed to allow easy use while adhering to the ALARA (as low as reasonably achievable) principles.[10] Although the work by Frush and colleagues[10] is

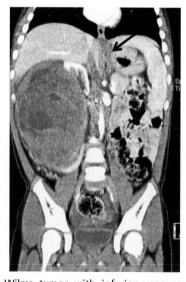

Fig. 5. Wilms tumor with inferior vena cava (IVC) tumor thrombus. A coronal reformatted image shows a heterogeneously enhancing, large right renal mass. Heterogeneous soft tissue representing tumor thrombus is seen within the IVC lumen (*arrow*).

vendor specific, it can be used as a guide to develop pediatric protocols. Breast shields made of bismuth provide an additional method to decrease radiation dose to breast tissue from both chest and abdominal scans without visibly compromising image quality.[11] Using proper protocols with breast shields, there is up to a 35% decrease in radiation exposure to breast tissue.[7,12]

Another simple way to decrease radiation exposure is to eliminate the routine practice of multiphase imaging. Multiphase imaging should be used on a case-by-case basis, as it can be helpful in the initial imaging assessment of a liver mass or in the evaluation of an atypical renal cyst. In addition, imaging of the chest and abdomen should be performed as a single run to avoid imaging breast tissue twice. The bismuth shields can also be used to decrease dose to the thyroid gland in head and neck imaging.[13]

Intravenous contrast is required for the CT evaluation of most tumors. Typically, pediatric imaging can be adequately performed by hand injection in young children. Rigsby and colleagues[14] found that hand injection provided adequate diagnostic quality in patients weighing less than 30 kg. Unfortunately, this approach leads to variability in enhancement and can confound the comparison of studies. It should also be remembered that appropriate training for hand injection is necessary, since catheter rupture can occur with hand injection.[15] Use of a power injector has become routine in many centers. Most published pediatric protocols using an antecubital peripheral line suggest an 18 G to 23 G intravenous catheter, with a volume of 2 cc/kg nonionic iodinated contrast and a power injector rate of 2 cc/s. The authors usually hand inject if the intravenous line is in the hand or foot, as these are typically 24 G or smaller. A uniformly common issue in this patient population is the presence of indwelling central venous access. As a general rule, the authors hand inject tunneled central venous catheters and implanted subcutaneous injection ports. The US Food and Drug Administration (FDA) has approved use of a power injector with specific peripherally inserted central catheters (PICCs) to assure that the catheter is designed to withstand high pressure. These PICCs have vendor-specific injection rates based on catheter lumen size, and the vendor's information should be consulted before injection.

In the chest, CT is superior to radiographs for the diagnosis of metastatic pulmonary disease. Current recommendations for most pediatric tumors including Wilms tumor, neuroblastoma, hepatoblastoma, Ewing sarcoma, and osteogenic sarcoma require CT for evaluation of pulmonary metastatic disease at diagnosis and during therapy (**Fig. 6**). CT of the chest generally does not require intravenous

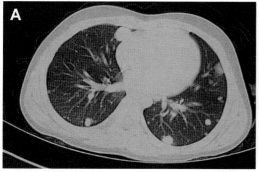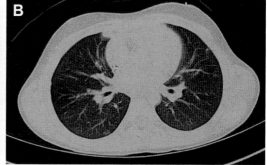

Fig. 6. Metastatic Ewing sarcoma. (*A*) An axial chest computed tomography (CT) scan at diagnosis shows multiple, peripheral metastatic nodules. (*B*) A repeat chest CT scan after therapy at 3 months shows a significant response to therapy.

contrast unless a palpable rib mass, mediastinal mass, or adenopathy is suspected or known to be present.

When imaging the abdomen and pelvis, oral contrast is extremely helpful at initial diagnosis, particularly in the evaluation of a retropitioneal mass or lymphadenopathy. The use of oral contrast during follow-up imaging may vary depending on tumor type, patterns of disease spread, and local preference. Some institutions have eliminated oral contrast from abdominal/pelvic imaging protocols to decrease the risk of aspiration if emesis occurs in a sedated patient.

An emerging CT technology includes 3-dimensional imaging to assist in radiation planning with intensity-modulated radiotherapy and proton therapy.[16]

MRI

The role of magnetic resonance in oncologic imaging continues to evolve with the development of faster scanning technique, improvements in coils, moving table platforms, and development of advanced post-processing techniques. MRI strengths are high soft tissue contrast and spatial resolution, lack of ionizing radiation, multiplanar capability, and excellent soft tissue characterization. MRI weaknesses include limited availability in some settings, relatively long examination time, physiologic motion artifact, suboptimal evaluation of the lungs, and high cost. Techniques used to assist in reduction of artifacts from physiologic bowel motion include keeping the patient from ingesting any food or liquids for at least 4 hours before an examination and the use of glucagon. Respiratory gating, navigator echo gating, and periodically rotated overlapping parallel lines with enhanced reconstruction (PROPELLER) imaging can reduce respiratory motion (**Fig. 7**). Breath

held sequences can be used in older children and adolescents. Distraction techniques such as video goggles used with a digital DVD system and MP3 audio systems can be used to decrease patient motion and avoid sedation in MRI. An additional concern when performing MRI is the recently recognized risk of nephrogenic systemic fibrosis (NSF) in patients receiving gadolinium-based contrast. NSF causes hardened skin with fibrotic nodules and plaques. Risk factors for the development of NSF include renal insufficiency, renal failure, and liver transplant.[17]

MRI is the primary advanced imaging modality used in the initial evaluation of musculoskeletal tumors. Children's Oncology Group (COG) Clinical Trials for Ewing sarcoma, osteogenic sarcoma, and soft tissue sarcomas use MRI for diagnosis, response to therapy, surveillance, and recurrence. MRI is used to define the tumor extent and its relationship to the neurovascular bundle. MRI is particularly useful in determining whether a tumor is amenable to limb salvage surgery and in planning the appropriate surgical procedure.[18,19]

MRI musculoskeletal tumor protocols should include short tau inversion recovery (STIR) and T1 weighted imaging in the sagittal or coronal planes that include the entire bone from joint to joint. The T1 sequence is used to estimate the length of involvement for prosthesis planning and to detect skip lesions or metastatic foci. The STIR sequence can be used to confirm T1 abnormalities but can overestimate tumor extent due to its high sensitivity in detection of water, which may represent peritumoral reactive edema rather than tumor. The rest of the MRI examination is focused on the tumor and the adjacent joint. The coil may be changed to improve signal characteristics. Axial T1, gradient echo, and T2 with fat saturation sequences will provide local detail. The gradient echo sequence is most useful for

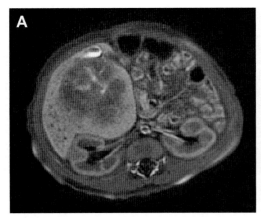
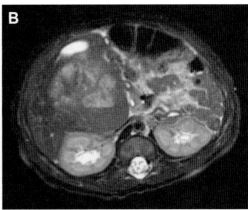

Fig. 7. Hepatoblastoma in a 1-week-old infant. Axial T1 (*A*) and axial T2 (*B*) magnetic resonance images of the abdomen were both performed using periodically rotated overlapping parallel lines with enhanced reconstruction (PROPELLER) technique. Note the mass in the right lobe of the liver. Artifact from multiple bowel loops is eliminated.

evaluating neurovascular bundle involvement. A sagittal or coronal T2 fat-saturated sequence at the joint adjacent to the tumor can help assess epiphyseal and joint involvement. Contrast-enhanced imaging can be performed with a dynamic sequence followed by axial and coronal or sagittal T1 sequence with fat saturation. A T1 sequence with fat saturation performed before contrast injection can be subtracted from the postcontrast-enhanced sequence T1 fat-saturated sequence to increase the conspicuity of contrast enhancement in a necrotic or hypovascular tumor and improve diagnostic confidence.

MRI is also very helpful is assessing the extent of intraspinal disease in children with neuroblastoma. Spinal canal involvement by neuroblastoma can present as a surgical emergency. MRI is used to assess mass effect on the spinal cord and roots, invasion in the paraspinal muscles, and marrow involvement in the spine (**Fig. 8**). In addition, MRI can be particularly useful in the evaluation of ovarian tumors to characterize the tumor, evaluate the contralateral ovary, and identify liver metastases and peritoneal seeding.[20] Preoperative assessment of liver tumors for determination of anatomic involvement and vascular invasion is another application of MRI. In these patients, a power injection can be helpful when performing dynamic vascular imaging.

A developing indication is the use of whole-body MRI (WBMRI) for tumor staging, response to therapy, and surveillance. The development of multichannel coils, a movable table, and parallel imaging have made this possible. This technology is available with both 1.5 and 3.0 Tesla magnets. Whole-body imaging is most useful in the evaluation of skeletal metastases, especially the bone

marrow. Protocols are based on coronal whole body imaging using fast T1 weighted and STIR sequences. Used together with axial fat-saturated fast spin echo T2 sequences that improve the visualization of rib lesions, the average MRI scan time for a total body MRI is in the range of 45 minutes. In a comparison of WBMRI with bone scintigraphy (BS) and [18]fluorodeoxyglucose (FDG) PET for the evaluation of skeletal metastases, WBMRI had a sensitivity of 97.5% and specificity of 99.4; BS had a sensitivity of 30% and specificity of 99.4%, and FDG PET/CT had a sensitivity 90.0% and specificity 100%. Both WBMRI and FDG PET/CT showed excellent agreement with the final diagnosis (**Fig. 9**).[21] Additional MRI techniques that are not in widespread use but have shown potential

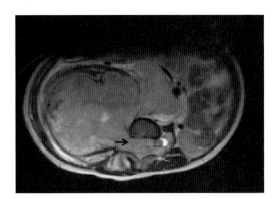

Fig. 8. Neuroblastoma with spinal involvement. An axial T2 weighted magnetic resonance image shows a large right retroperitoneal tumor invading the adjacent lumbar musculature and extending through the neural foramen into the spinal canal. There is significant displacement of the spinal cord (*arrow*) and thecal sac.

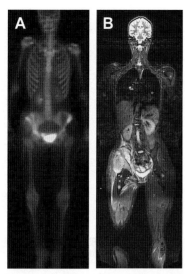

Fig. 9. Metastatic Ewing sarcoma. (*A*) Anterior view of a whole-body bone scan shows abnormal increased activity and photopenia in the right iliac wing corresponding to primary tumor. Faint, poorly defined activity is seen in the right proximal intertrochanteric region of the femur. (*B*) A whole-body magnetic resonance image demonstrates the primary tumor in the right iliac bone. Additional focal bull's eye lesions seen in the right proximal femur and left femoral neck are consistent with metastatic disease.

for application in children with cancer include: diffusion-weighted and dynamic contrast-enhanced MRI for the assessment of tumor response, and new intravenous contrast agents using iron particles to distinguish inflammatory from cancerous lymph nodes.[22–24]

NUCLEAR MEDICINE

Nuclear medicine techniques use targeted radiotracers to image specific organ system physiology or cellular processes and provide unique functional information. Technetium 99m- labeled- disphosphonate BS, [123]Iodine-labeled metaiodobenzylguanidine (123 IMIBG) scintigraphy and [18]Fluorodeoxyglucose positron emission tomography (FDG PET) are the most common nuclear medicine radiotracers used in the evaluation of children with cancer.

BS is currently the most cost effective and widely available whole-body imaging technique for the detection and monitoring of skeletal metastases. A positive study shows increased activity at sites of osteoblastic bone response. BS is highly sensitive for the detection of osteoblastic lesions but not specific for metastatic disease. Plain radiographs of abnormal or questionable scintigraphic findings increase the specificity of the bone scan, are used to confirm lesions, and are particularly

helpful in evaluating response to therapy. False-negative bone scans can occur before the development of an osteoblastic response in early stages of marrow metastases. In children, this occurrence is most common in metastatic neuroblastoma, with metastatic disease picked up by 123 IMIBG. In Ewing sarcoma, early marrow metastases may not be visible on BS but can be diagnosed with WBMRI or PET/CT. Scintigraphic findings of diffuse intense bone uptake associated with little or no renal activity, known as a super scan can be seen in patients with diffuse skeletal metastases. In addition, a false-positive bone scan can occur in a patient with known bone metastases that appear falsely increased in activity on follow-up. This flare phenomenon is seen after chemotherapy and can be misinterpreted as progression of disease. Plain radiographs can be helpful to confirm healing rather than progression in these patients.[25]

The 123 IMIBG scan is used extensively in the staging and assessment of tumor response and recurrence in children with neuroblastoma (NBL).[26,27] It is also the test of choice in the diagnostic evaluation of pheochromocytoma. The functional properties of MIBG, a norepinephrine analog, make it highly specific (**Fig. 10**). The main limitation of 123 IMIBG, however, is long examination performance time with delayed 24-hour imaging and high radiation dose. In addition, disease in the liver can be difficult to evaluate, since the background liver activity is high. Suspicious or nonuniform liver activity is best evaluated by MRI.

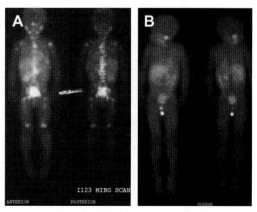

Fig. 10. Metastatic neuroblastoma. (*A*) Anterior and posterior views of a whole-body [123]iodine-labeled metaiodobenzylguanidine (I123 MIBG) scan reveal metastatic marrow disease in the spine, right pelvis, bilateral shoulders, and proximal and distal femurs. (*B*) Surveillance scan at 2 years after initial diagnosis and subsequent treatment demonstrates a normal physiologic distribution of 123 IMIBG activity and no evidence for recurrence.

Single photon emission tomography with CT (SPECT /CT) is an emerging hybrid technique that should increase the use of SPECT imaging as SPECT/CT scanners become more available The most promising application in pediatric oncology is the use of 123 IMIBG SPECT/CT.[28] In the evaluation of NBL, SPECT/CT can be particularly useful in distinguishing stasis of radiotracer in the renal pelvis from perirenal disease, adrenal activity from residual disease, nodal disease in the pelvis from marrow disease, and to identify low-grade activity in residual disease.

FDG PET is a molecular imaging tool used to identify hypermetabolic malignancy. The strengths of PET include imaging of the whole body and high sensitivity. The specificity of PET in lymph node staging is limited by the presence of uptake in inflammatory cells and macrophages in reactive or infected lymph nodes, which can be indistinguishable from malignancy. The clinical use of PET is best established in Hodgkin disease and includes staging, response to therapy, planning radiation therapy, restaging, and monitoring relapse.[29] PET has made a significant contribution in the assessment of tumors that have an increased fibrous stroma, such as nodular sclerosing Hodgkin diesease, which comprises 70% of Hodgkin disease in children. These tumors may respond completely to therapy as evidenced by loss of [18]FDG uptake while still showing a residual soft tissue mass on CT (Fig. 11). The role of PET in the evaluation of sarcomas such as rhabdomyosarcoma , Ewing sarcoma, and osteosarcoma is being studied. In addition, there may be a role for PET in the evaluation of neuroblastoma when the tumor is weakly or non-MIBG avid.[30]

When interpreting PET images, a metabolic response to therapy is considered to be present when the activity is equal to or less than background activity. Standardized uptake values (SUV), a semiquantitative analytical tool that is a measure of activity of radiotracer, can be used to confirm a visual metabolic response to therapy when comparing initial pretherapy scans to posttherapy scans. SUV cannot be used to reliably distinguish between malignant and benign lesions. A pitfall of [18]FDG uptake is the presence of activated brown fat, which is most common in the cervical region, supraclavicular region, and base of neck and can be confused with lymph node activity. The simplest method to diminish brown fat uptake is to keep the patient warm before and during the uptake phase, which is the time period between injection and scanning. Having the patient wear warm clothing and keeping the uptake room temperature over 75°Falso may be helpful. CT localization is also extremely helpful in distinguishing brown fat from

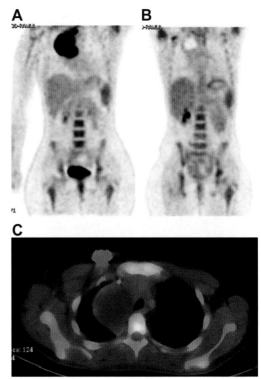

Fig. 11. Nodular sclerosing Hodgkin disease. (*A*) An FDG positron emission tomography scan at diagnosis reveals a large area of uptake in the mediastinal mass depicted on the CXR in **Fig. 1**. Increased activity in the spleen and bone marrow may be related to anemia or metastatic disease. (*B*) 3 weeks after therapy there is a complete metabolic response to therapy. Bone marrow and splenic activity have increased, likely in response to therapy. (*C*) The axial computed tomography low-dose noncontrast localization image demonstrates a large residual mass.

lymph nodes.[31] Another pitfall is the use of marrow stimulating agents, such as granulocyte colony-stimulating factor, which causes a hyperplastic marrow response that results in diffuse increased skeletal activity and increased splenic activity that can obscure metastatic disease. The effect wears off with time and resolves by 4 weeks after administration. Increased FDG activity can also be seen in infection, postsurgical granulation tissue, and post-radiation inflammatory changes.

In the evaluation of residual or recurrent disease in a patient with bone tumor treated surgically with a limb salvage procedure, PET/CT can be especially useful in the detection of recurrence at the site of a metallic prosthesis, which cannot be adequately evaluated by MRI or CT alone. If necessary, PET/CT can serve as a problem-solving tool in patients with suspected residual or recurrent disease. In patients requiring biopsy, identification of the hypermetabolic regions in a tumor mass can be used to guide biopsy. PET/CT is also used in the mapping and planning of radiation therapy fields for both intensity-modulated radiotherapy (IMRT) and proton therapy.[16] Currently, pediatric PET/CT protocols have not been standardized; however, Alessio and colleagues[32] offer a practical protocol using 11 weight categories, based on the Broselow-Luten color scale, which adheres to the ALARA principle.

Radiation and Cancer Risk

Medical radiation is very low dose, and statistical estimates have been used to predict the risk of developing a solid tumor from cumulative exposures. Using data from high-dose exposure from Nagasaki, Japan, one approach has been to use a linear fit extrapolating cancer incidence occurring at high-dose levels to estimate cancer incidence at low levels.

The "Image Gently" campaign was conceived in 2006 in the Society for Pediatric Radiology (SPR) by a committee designed to address radiation dose in children. This committee agreed it was important to include medical technologists, medical physicists, pediatricians, and CT vendors in this discussion on dose reduction and formed the Alliance for Radiation Safety in Pediatric Imaging. This was launched in 2008 and initially consisted of the SPR, the American College of Radiology, the American Society of Radiologic Technologists, and the American Association of Physicists in Medicine. This group has since expanded enormously and has gained support from other organizations throughout the world. The group has developed educational activities including conferences discussing updates and issues, a volume of Pediatric Radiology containing publications from conference presentations[33] and a Web site, www.image-gently.org. This Web site is expansive and includes material for parents, pediatricians, technologists, and radiologists. Educational modules are available for technologists and radiologists to update their training. Anyone desiring more information on methods to decrease radiation exposure from imaging should visit this site.

The approach currently approved by the Image Gently Alliance is

1. Current estimates of radiation risk are predicted based on the linear no threshold model, which assumes that there is a risk of solid cancer incidence at low radiation levels.
2. It is difficult to accurately estimate radiation dosimetry from PET and CT due to varying morphology, site, and tissue kinetics.
3. At present, it is accepted that radiation dose and risk are additive.
4. The goal with current protocols is to decrease effective dose.

REFERENCES

1. NCI. SEER cancer statistics review 1975–2006. Bethesda (MD): National Cancer Institute; 2008.
2. Cowen AR, Davies AG, Kengyelics SM. Advances in computed radiography systems and their physical imaging characteristics. Clin Radiol 2007;62(12):1132–41.
3. Cowen AR, Kengyelics SM, Davies AG. Solid-state, flat-panel, digital radiography detectors and their physical imaging characteristics. Clin Radiol 2008;63(5):487–98.
4. Lee CH, Goo JM, Ye HJ, et al. Radiation dose modulation techniques in the multidetector CT era: from basics to practice. Radiographics 2008;28(5):1451–9.
5. Koch BL. Avoiding sedation in pediatric radiology. Pediatr Radiol 2008;38(Suppl 2):S225–6.
6. Brenner D, Elliston C, Hall E, et al. Estimated risks of radiation-induced fatal cancer from pediatric CT. AJR Am J Roentgenol 2001;176(2):289–96.
7. Fricke BL, Donnelly LF, Frush DP, et al. In-plane bismuth breast shields for pediatric CT: effects on radiation dose and image quality using experimental and clinical data. AJR Am J Roentgenol 2003;180(2):407–11.
8. Fahey FH, Palmer MR, Strauss KJ, et al. Dosimetry and adequacy of CT-based attenuation correction for pediatric PET: phantom study. Radiology 2007;243(1):96–104.
9. Greess H, Nomayr A, Wolf H, et al. Dose reduction in CT examination of children by an attenuation-based on-line modulation of tube current (CARE dose). Eur Radiol 2002;12(6):1571–6.
10. Frush DP, Soden B, Frush KS, et al. Improved pediatric multidetector body CT using a size-based color-coded format. AJR Am J Roentgenol 2002;178(3):721–6.
11. Catuzzo P, Aimonetto S, Fanelli G, et al. Dose reduction in multislice CT by means of bismuth shields: results of in vivo measurements and computed evaluation. Radiol Med 2010;115(1):152–69.
12. Coursey C, Frush DP, Yoshizumi T, et al. Pediatric chest MDCT using tube current modulation: effect on radiation dose with breast shielding. AJR Am J Roentgenol 2008;190(1):W54–61.
13. Gunn ML, Kanal KM, Kolokythas O, et al. Radiation dose to the thyroid gland and breast from multidetector computed tomography of the cervical spine: does bismuth shielding with and without a cervical collar reduce dose? J Comput Assist Tomogr 2009;33(6):987–90.
14. Rigsby CK, Gasber E, Seshadri R, et al. Safety and efficacy of pressure-limited power injection of

iodinated contrast medium through central lines in children. AJR Am J Roentgenol 2007;188(3):726–32.

15. Donnelly LF, Dickerson J, Racadio JM. Is hand injection of central venous catheters for contrast-enhanced CT safe in children? AJR Am J Roentgenol 2007;189(6):1530–2.

16. Zaidi H, Vees H, Wissmeyer M. Molecular PET/CT imaging-guided radiation therapy treatment planning. Acad Radiol 2009;16(9):1108–33.

17. Broome DR, Girguis MS, Baron PW, et al. Gadodiamide-associated nephrogenic systemic fibrosis: why radiologists should be concerned. AJR Am J Roentgenol 2007;188:586–92.

18. Meyer JS, Nadel HR, Marina N, et al. Imaging guidelines for children with Ewing sarcoma and osteosarcoma: a report from the Children's Oncology Group Bone Tumor Committee. Pediatr Blood Cancer 2008; 51(2):163–70.

19. Meyer JS, Nadel HR, Marina N, et al. Response to "Imaging guidelines for children with ewing sarcoma and osteoscaroma": a report form the Children's Oncology Group Bone Tumor Committee. Pediatr Blood Cancer 2008;51(2):163–70.

20. Shaaban A, Rezvani M. Ovarian cancer: detection and radiologic staging. Clin Obstet Gynecol 2009; 52(1):73–93.

21. Kumar J, Seith A, Kumar A, et al. Whole-body MR imaging with the use of parallel imaging for detection of skeletal metastases in pediatric patients with small-cell neoplasms: comparison with skeletal scintigraphy and FDG PET/CT. Pediatr Radiol 2008;38(9):953–62.

22. Koh DM, Collins DJ. Diffusion-weighted MRI in the body: applications and challenges in oncology. AJR Am J Roentgenol 2007;188(6):1622–35.

23. Komori T, Narabayashi I, Matsumura K, et al. 2-[Fluorine-18]-fluoro-2-deoxy-D-glucose positron emission tomography/computed tomography versus whole-body diffusion-weighted MRI for detection of

malignant lesions: initial experience. Ann Nucl Med 2007;21(4):209–15.

24. Russell M, Yoshimi A. Ultrasmall superparamagnetic iron oxide enhanced MR imaging for lymph nodes metastases. Radiography 2007;12(Suppl 1):e73–84.

25. Thrall JH, Ellis BI. Skeletal metastases. Radiol Clin North Am 1987;25(6):1155–70.

26. Shulkin BL, Shapiro B. Current concepts on the diagnostic use of MIBG in children. J Nucl Med 1998; 39(4):679–88.

27. Vik TA, Pfluger T, Kadota R, et al. (123)I-mIBG scintigraphy in patients with known or suspected neuroblastoma: results from a prospective multicenter trial. Pediatr Blood Cancer 2009;52(7):784–90.

28. Rozovsky K, Koplewitz BZ, Krausz Y, et al. Added value of SPECT/CT for correlation of MIBG scintigraphy and diagnostic CT in neuroblastoma and pheochromocytoma. AJR Am J Roentgenol 2008;190(4):1085–90.

29. Hudson MM, Krasin MJ, Kaste SC. PET imaging in pediatric Hodgkin's lymphoma. Pediatr Radiol 2004; 34(3):190–8.

30. Sharp SE, Shulkin BL, Gelfand MJ, et al. 123I-MIBG scintigraphy and 18F-FDG PET in neuroblastoma. J Nucl Med 2009;50(8):1237–43.

31. Garcia C, Bandaru V, Van Nostrand D, et al. Study: controlling temp prior to PET scan reduces brown fat FDG uptake. Mol Imaging Biol 2010;12(6):625–6.

32. Alessio AM, Kinahan PE, Manchanda V, et al. Weight-based, low-dose pediatric whole-body PET/CT protocols. J Nucl Med 2009;50(10):1570–7.

33. Frush DP, Frush KS. The ALARA concept in pediatric imaging. Building bridges between radiology and emergency medicine: consensus conference on imaging safety and quality for children in the emergency setting. Pediatr Radiol 2008;38(Suppl 4):S629–32.

Imaging Tumors of the Pediatric Central Nervous System

Michael J. Paldino, MD[a],*, Eric N. Faerber, MD[b],
Tina Young Poussaint, MD[c]

KEYWORDS

- Magnetic resonance imaging • Perfusion • Diffusion
- Spectroscopy • Pediatric • Brain tumor

Primary tumors of the central nervous system (CNS) are the second most common neoplasms of childhood, exceeded in incidence only by lymphoproliferative disorders.[1] These tumors occur with an annual incidence of 3 per 100,000 and are a leading cause of death in children.[2] Although supratentorial and infratentorial tumors occur with nearly equal incidence when the pediatric population is considered as a whole, the relative frequency by location varies with the age of the patient.[3] Supratentorial tumors are more common in infants and children up to the age of 3 years and after the age of 10 years; from 4 to 10 years of age, infratentorial tumors predominate.[4]

Although there is some overlap with pathologic entities in adults, pediatric brain tumors have a higher degree of pathologic heterogeneity.[5] Furthermore, treatment strategies and outcomes vary widely with the specific tumor pathology and histologic grade. Although a specific pathologic diagnosis is not possible in many cases, thorough noninvasive characterization of pediatric brain tumors is of potential value to optimal patient management.[6] The goal of this article is not to provide an exhaustive description of all pediatric tumors occurring in the CNS. For such purposes, the reader is referred to other outstanding sources.[7] Rather, this review is intended to provide an overview of the typical imaging appearance of the most common childhood tumors and tumorlike conditions, with a focus on suggestive or differential features. Where appropriate, relevant advanced imaging techniques (eg, magnetic resonance spectroscopy [MRS], diffusion-weighted imaging [DWI], and perfusion techniques) are discussed. Despite the superb and diverse tissue contrasts now available with state-of-the-art MR imaging, tumor location remains critical to the generation of an appropriate differential diagnosis. Location forms the organizational basis of this article.

INFRATENTORIAL TUMORS

Cerebellar astrocytoma is one of the most common posterior fossa tumors of childhood, (second only to medulloblastoma), accounting for 40% of all astrocytomas in the pediatric population.[4,7] These tumors occur throughout childhood, with a peak incidence from birth to 9 years of age.[8] Astrocytomas throughout the brain occur with increased frequency in neurofibromatosis type 1 (NF-1), and the posterior fossa is no exception.[4,9,10] Pathology shows juvenile pilocytic astrocytoma (JPA) in most cases.[11–13] These tumors have an excellent prognosis, with a 95% 25-year survival rate.[13] However, diffuse astrocytomas, including glioblastoma multiforme (GBM), do occur, with a tendency toward older patients; survival is of significantly shorter

[a] Division of Neuroradiology, Department of Radiology, Children's Hospital Boston, 300 Longwood Avenue, Boston, MA 02115, USA
[b] Department of Radiology, St Christopher's Hospital for Children, Drexel University School of Medicine, East Erie Avenue & North Front Street, Philadelphia, PA 19134, USA
[c] Department of Radiology, Children's Hospital Boston, Harvard Medical School, 300 Longwood Avenue, Boston, MA 02115, USA
* Corresponding author.
E-mail address: michael.paldino@childrens.harvard.edu

Radiol Clin N Am 49 (2011) 589–616
doi:10.1016/j.rcl.2011.05.011
0033-8389/11/$ – see front matter © 2011 Elsevier Inc. All rights reserved.

duration.[11,14] Although cerebellar astrocytomas frequently originate near the midline, lateral extension tends to result in a mass centered in the cerebellar hemisphere.[10]

Approximately 50% of posterior fossa JPAs show a classic cyst and mural nodule appearance.[15] In these cases, the mural nodule shows intense, diffuse enhancement; the cyst approximates cerebrospinal fluid (CSF) on all imaging sequences (Fig. 1). The remaining tumors tend to have a heterogeneous, cystic, and solid appearance.[15] Less than 10% are completely solid.[16] Solid portions of these tumors tend to show low density on computed tomography (CT) and high signal on T2-weighted

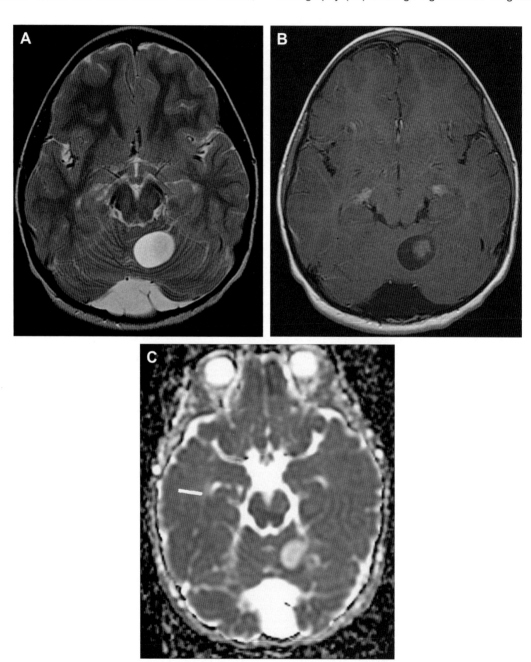

Fig. 1. Cerebellar astrocytoma. Axial T2-weighted (A) and postcontrast T1-weighted (B) images show a cystic and solid mass centered in the left cerebellar hemisphere. As is typical for pilocytic tumors, the solid component of the tumor is hyperintense to brain parenchyma on the T2-weighted images and enhances after the administration of paramagnetic contrast agent. Increased diffusion on the apparent diffusion coefficient (ADC) map (C) is consistent with the low cellularity of these tumors.

images relative to brain parenchyma.[17,18] These characteristics are believed to relate to the relatively low cell density or nuclear/cytoplasm ratio of these tumors. These same histologic features likely account for the increased apparent diffusion coefficient (ADC) in these tumors.[19] Solid components tend to enhance, most frequently in a heterogeneous fashion, after the administration of contrast agent.[17] Mineralization may be seen in up to 20% of cases.[20] The use of advanced imaging modalities in astrocytomas is discussed in the section on hemispheric astrocytoma.

Medulloblastoma

Medulloblastoma is a primitive neuroectodermal tumor (PNET) arising from the fetal granular layer of the cerebellum or the posterior medullary velum.[21–24] Signaling pathways implicated in tumorigenesis include the sonic hedgehog pathway, WNT/WG pathway, receptor kinase family ErbB. It is the most common infratentorial tumor of childhood and accounts for approximately 25% of CNS tumors in the pediatric population.[4,25] The peak age range is 6 to 11 years, although these tumors may also occur in young adults.[26–28] Medulloblastomas occur with increased frequency in patients with basal cell nevus (Gorlin) syndrome, Turcot syndrome, Li-Fraumeni syndrome, ataxia-telangiectasia, xeroderma pigmentosum, and blue rubber bleb syndrome,[5,29] These tumors typically originate in the midline from the roof of the fourth ventricle, with encroachment on and growth into the ventricle. Later in life, origin from the cerebellar hemisphere is more common; tumors in this location tend to be desmoplastic and are associated with a better prognosis.[30]

On CT, medulloblastoma appears as a midline vermian mass, typically hyperdense to cerebellar white matter.[31,32] This hyperdensity is a reliable discriminator from cerebellar astrocytoma, whose solid portions tend to show low attenuation relative to the cerebellar parenchyma. Calcification is rare, but may be detected in up to 10% of cases.[33] The MR imaging appearance of medulloblastoma is variable. T2-weighted images tend to show a heterogeneous appearance. A vermian tumor the solid components of which show hypointensity or isointensity to gray matter on T2-weighted images is suggestive of the diagnosis in the appropriate age group (**Fig. 2**).[5,32,34–37] Relatively short T2 is believed to relate to high cell density or nuclear/cytoplasm ratio; these histologic features also account for relatively restricted diffusion in these tumors.[19,38] In most cases, medulloblastomas show enhancement, which may be heterogeneous or diffuse, after the administration of iodinated (CT)

or paramagnetic (MR imaging) contrast agents.[34] Leptomeningeal dissemination, within the brain or spine, is relatively common and may be found at diagnosis or as a manifestation of tumor recurrence (see **Fig. 2**).[35,36] Distant metastases are uncommon, but have been reported, most commonly to bone or lymph nodes.[39]

Recent work by several groups has shown the usefulness of MR spectroscopy in the differentiation of posterior fossa tumors. Medulloblastoma tends toward a more exaggerated increase of choline level than either ependymoma or astrocytoma, although there is a high degree of overlap between different pathologic entities.[40,41] Medulloblastoma may also show an abnormal taurine peak, a finding which has been reported to allow for accurate differentiation from other infratentorial tumors.[42,43] Other groups have used pattern analyses (quantifying multiple molecular peaks) to provide the most robust prediction of pathologic diagnosis of infratentorial tumors.[6]

Diffusion tensor imaging has been used to assess the effects of radiation therapy in children with medulloblastoma. A reduction in fractional anisotropy (FA) was found in the white matter of medulloblastoma survivors, even in white matter with a normal appearance on T2-weighted images.[44,45] Moreover, the degree of decreased FA correlated with the age at which radiation was administered as well as with deterioration in school performance.[44,45] This work was then corroborated in an animal model, confirming the parallel between tissue anisotropy and the histologic changes of radiation-induced white matter injury.[46] Together, these data support the use of FA as a noninvasive biomarker to monitor the deleterious effects of radiation therapy.

Ependymoma

Ependymoma is a tumor of glial origin accounting for approximately 15% of posterior fossa tumors in the pediatric age group.[47] Although they may occur at any age, peak incidence is from 0 to 5 years of age.[48,49] Ependymoma originates from the ependymal cells lining the ventricular system, most commonly from the floor of the fourth ventricle, with growth into the fourth ventricle.[50] Extension of tumor through the outlet foramina of the fourth ventricle is common and represents an important differential feature. Although medulloblastoma may also protrude into these foramina, thin, fingerlike projections of tumor are highly suggestive of ependymoma.[4,51]

At imaging, ependymoma typically presents as a fourth ventricular mass, the solid components of which tend to show, at least in part,

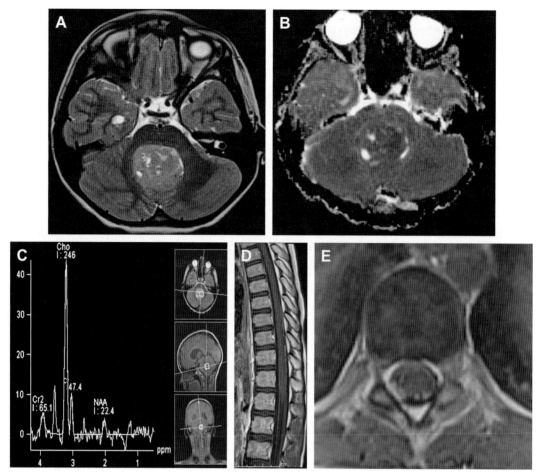

Fig. 2. Medulloblastoma. (A) Axial T2-weighted image shows a mildly heterogeneous mass centered in the fourth ventricle. Signal intensity within the tumor approximates that of gray matter. (B) ADC map shows decreased diffusion within the same regions of tumor, consistent with high cell density. MRS (C) shows decreased N-acetyl-aspartate and a marked increase of choline level. Sagittal (D) and axial (E) postcontrast T1-weighted images through the spine show nodular enhancement along the surface of the cord, consistent with leptomeningeal dissemination of tumor.

isointensity or hypointensity to gray matter on T2-weighted images (Fig. 3).[5,47,52,53] Mineralization, necrosis, and hemorrhage are relatively common, accounting for the characteristic heterogeneity observed on cross-sectional imaging.[29,47,54] These tumors typically enhance in a heterogeneous fashion.[4,47,55] Leptomeningeal dissemination of ependymoma is rare at presentation (in contradistinction to medulloblastoma), but may occur as a manifestation of recurrence. Tumor seeding at the time of diagnosis of an ependymal cell neoplasm suggests anaplastic ependymoma or ependymoblastoma.[4] In most cases, the major differential consideration is medulloblastoma; in addition to the aforementioned suggestive features, ependymoma tends to occur in a younger age group (0–5 years, as noted earlier). The clinical

and imaging presentations of these tumors have significant overlap, and differentiation may not be possible before pathologic evaluation. Increased myoinositol (MI) levels at MRS may have some usefulness in differentiating ependymoma from other posterior fossa tumors, although care must be taken to distinguish MI from glycine, which resonates nearby (3.56 ppm) and may be present in medulloblastoma.[5,6]

Atypical Teratoid Rhabdoid Tumor

Although these tumors have historically been diagnosed as medulloblastoma, newer pathologic techniques have allowed distinction of atypical teratoid rhabdoid tumor (ATRT) from other PNETs[56] These tumors commonly show mutation or deletion

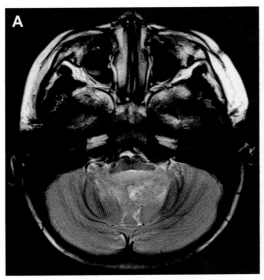
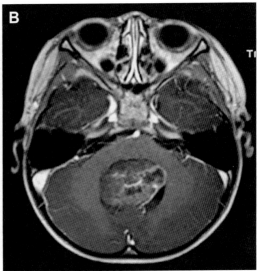

Fig. 3. Ependymoma. (A) Axial T2-weighted image shows a heterogeneous fourth ventricular tumor. Much of the tumor has signal characteristics that approximate that of gray matter. In this case, there is extension of tumor through the foramina of Luschka. (B) Axial postcontrast T1-weighted image shows heterogeneous enhancement of this ependymoma.

of both copies of the hSNF5/INI1 gene that maps to chromosome band 22q11.2, observed in approximately 70% of cerebral ATRT.[57]

The imaging appearance of ATRT is similar to that of medulloblastoma, with solid portions showing attenuation (CT) and signal intensity (MR imaging) similar to that of gray matter (**Fig. 4**).[58,59] This rare tumor should be considered in the differential diagnosis of medulloblastoma and ependymoma; in particular, marked heterogeneity resulting from frequent necrosis and sometimes hemorrhage, cerebellar hemispheric centricity, and young age (median age at diagnosis <2 years) should raise the possibility of an ATRT.[58] MRS may help to differentiate ATRT from medulloblastoma: ATRT is characterized by lower choline levels and the absence of a taurine peak.[60]

Brainstem Tumors

Brainstem glioma is a relatively common tumor of childhood, accounting for approximately 25% of posterior fossa neoplasms.[51] These tumors typically present in the first decade of life, but can occur into adulthood.[15] Brainstem tumors can be further divided based on their site of origin, with pontine tumors being the most common, and whether they are focal or diffuse. In general terms, pontine gliomas tend to be diffuse (ie, involve ≥75% of the cross-sectional area of the pons) and show fibrillary histology. These tumors have an extremely poor prognosis, with median survival of approximately 1 year.[61,62] On CT, diffuse

intrinsic pontine glioma (DIPG) appears as an infiltrative, poorly marginated low-density mass centered in the pons.[4] Mineralization is uncommon and correlates with less aggressive disease.[63] Despite narrowing of the fourth ventricle, hydrocephalus is rare at presentation. MR imaging is the modality of choice, in part because of the absence of beam-hardening artifact, showing an infiltrative mass with long T1 and T2 associated with marked expansion of the pons (**Fig. 5**).[64–66] Anterior growth narrows the pontine cistern and characteristically engulfs the basilar artery. Diffuse tumors rarely enhance significantly after the administration of contrast.[51] Overall, the appearance is characteristic, and therapy is initiated at many institutions without a tissue diagnosis. However, this practice limits therapeutic stratification in these patients. The relative rarity of pathologic samples from these tumors has also contributed to a paucity of knowledge regarding potential molecular targets in this disease. Although at diagnosis DIPG tends to show low choline, high citrate, low cerebral blood volume (CBV), and high ADC (ie, low cellularity), transformation to more biologically aggressive tumors is paralleled by increasing choline, increasing perfusion, and decreasing ADC.[5,60,67]

Medullary and midbrain gliomas are more commonly focal in nature, and may be at least partly exophytic.[68,69] These tumors tend to show pilocytic histology, with a substantially better prognosis than DIPG.[63] Like JPAs elsewhere in the posterior fossa, focal brainstem gliomas

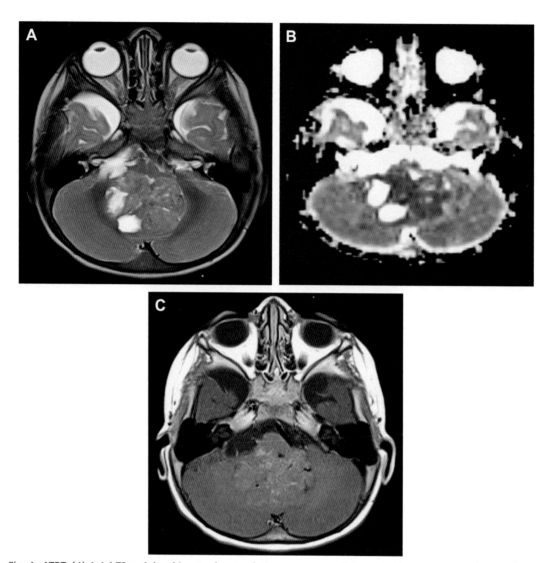

Fig. 4. ATRT. (*A*) Axial T2-weighted image shows a heterogeneous, solid, and cystic mass centered in the fourth ventricle. Solid components of tumor are isointense and hypointense to gray matter. (*B*) ADC map shows decreased diffusion within solid components, consistent with high cell density. Although medulloblastoma often has a similar appearance, the heterogeneity combined with the age of the patient (11 months) suggest that this may be an ATRT. (*C*) Postcontrast images show low-level, heterogeneous enhancement throughout the solid portion of the tumor.

show low attenuation on CT and hyperintensity on T2-weighted images when compared with normal brain parenchyma. Contrast enhancement, typically heterogeneous in nature, is identified in most such tumors.[70]

Tectal or quadrigeminal plate glioma is a specific midbrain tumor that presents with signs and symptoms of increased intracranial pressure resulting from obstruction at the cerebral aqueduct.[71] The imaging appearance is the same as that described for pilocytic astrocytomas in other locations.[72] Differentiation from other brainstem tumors is warranted based on its benign course

and specific therapeutic options (ie, CSF diversion to relieve hydrocephalus and nothing else). There is good evidence to suggest that MR imaging can be used to identify those tectal tumors that are likely to require further treatment. In 1 study, tumor size greater than 2.5 cm in diameter or enhancement on MR imaging were significant radiologic predictors of those patients needing treatment beyond CSF diversion.[73] In another study of 40 children with tectal tumors, tumor volume at presentation was the only factor predictive of tumor enlargement ($P = .002$).[74] Lesions with a volume less than 4 cm^3 were likely to follow

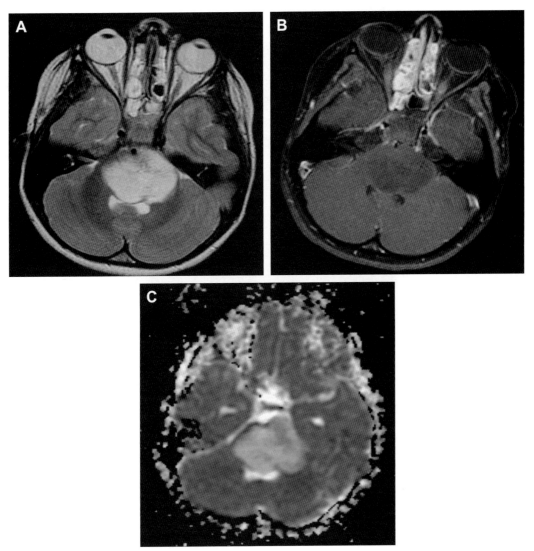

Fig. 5. Diffuse intrinsic brainstem glioma. (A) Axial T2-weighted image shows an infiltrative, hyperintense mass centered in the pons. Marked expansion of the pons narrows the pontine cistern and engulfs the basilar artery. These tumors rarely enhance significantly (B) and tend to show increased diffusion (C) at diagnosis.

a benign course. All large lesions, defined as a volume greater than 10 cm³ at presentation, eventually required treatment.

Choroid Plexus Tumors

Although the fourth ventricle is the most common location of choroid plexus papilloma (CPP) in adults, pediatric tumors occur more commonly in the lateral ventricle. The imaging appearance of choroid plexus lesions is described in detail in the section on supratentorial tumors later in this article.

Hemangioblastoma

Hemangioblastoma is a rare benign tumor of vascular origin accounting for 1% to 2% of all

intracranial neoplasms.[51] Peak incidence occurs in early adulthood, with fewer than 20% of all hemangioblastomas occurring in the pediatric population.[29] These tumors occur with increased frequency in patients with von Hippel-Lindau disease; in such cases, tumors tend to present at an earlier age, and multiple lesions are frequently encountered in the same patient. Hemangioblastomas most commonly originate from the cerebellar hemisphere, typically in a paramedian location. The clinical presentation is often nonspecific, although polycythemia may occur on the basis of erythropoietin secretion.[29,75]

Although many tumors are entirely solid, hemangioblastoma classically appears as a cystic mass with an enhancing mural nodule. Solid components of this tumor are highly vascular and show intense, homogeneous enhancement after the administration of contrast. Flow voids on MR imaging are an important discriminator from cerebellar astrocytoma, a tumor that might otherwise have an identical appearance. Along the same lines, high relative CBV at perfusion MR imaging has been used to accurately distinguish hemangioblastoma from JPA.[76] In rare instances, it may be difficult to differentiate these tumors from an arachnoid cyst; in such cases, the use of contrast medium may be necessary to identify a small mural nodule.[70]

EMBRYONIC TUMORS
Dermoid/epidermoid

Embryonic tumors arise from rests of ectodermal tissue left behind during neural tube closure. Whereas epidermoid cysts are derived from solely from the epidermis (ectoderm), dermoid cysts also contain dermal appendages, which are derived from mesoderm. Within the intracranial compartment, epidermoids are significantly more common.

On CT, a dermoid cyst appears as an extra-axial, fat density mass that has a tendency to occur in the midline.[29] On MR imaging, these tumors show heterogeneous T1 hyperintensity; fat saturation techniques and chemical shift artifact may aid in excluding substances other than fat that produce short T1 signal.[77] Dermoids do not enhance unless they become infected. Like epidermoid cysts (see later discussion), dermoids show diffusion characteristics similar to those of brain parenchyma.[78] Approximately 20% of dermoid cysts are associated with a dermal sinus tract. When in communication with the skin surface, these tracts may be a source of intracranial infection. Close attention should be paid to identifying these tracts in every patient with a dermoid cyst.

Compared with dermoids, epidermoid cysts are less likely to occur in the midline.[4,29] On CT, the appearance is that of a cerebral spinal fluid (CSF) density, extra-axial mass. The presence of mass effect on adjacent structures is typically the only finding to suggest its presence. On MR imaging, the signal characteristics of an epidermoid approximate those of CSF. Fluid attenuated inversion recovery (FLAIR) images often show a heterogeneous internal architecture slightly hyperintense to CSF, a finding that distinguishes an epidermoid cyst from an arachnoid cyst. Definitive differentiation from an arachnoid cyst can be accomplished with DWI: arachnoid cysts show signal approximating CSF on DWI, whereas epidermoids show relatively decreased water motion.[78–80] In some instances, an epidermoid may show hyperintense T1 signal, potentially causing confusion with a dermoid or lipoma; these rare cases can be correctly identified by the absence of chemical shift artifact or by using fat-saturated sequences.[4]

SUPRATENTORIAL TUMORS
Tumors Occurring Within the Cerebral Hemispheres

Hemispheric astrocytoma
Astrocytomas are the most common childhood tumors of the CNS, constituting approximately one-third of all pediatric supratentorial tumors.[1,81] These tumors occur throughout childhood, with peaks in incidence from 2 to 4 years of age and in early adolescence.[15] In addition to the cerebral hemispheres, astrocytomas also commonly originate from the thalamus, hypothalamus, and basal ganglia.[1] Hemispheric astrocytoma occurs with increased frequency in patients with NF-1.[51] As in the cerebellum, most of these tumors are low grade. However, high-grade neoplasms including GBM do occur; in such cases, the imaging appearance is identical to that of adult high-grade primary brain tumors.[82]

On imaging, low-grade hemispheric astrocytomas tend to have a heterogeneous, cystic, and solid appearance. Solid portions of these tumors show low density on CT and high signal on T2-weighted images relative to brain parenchyma as well as heterogeneous enhancement.[5,62,70,83] Like low-grade astrocytomas that develop elsewhere, low cell density or nuclear/cytoplasm ratio accounts for relatively high diffusivity within these tumors.[84] The cyst and mural nodule appearance classically described in the posterior fossa is less common in this location.[85,86]

Gliomatosis cerebri is a rare tumor characterized by diffuse overgrowth of glial elements, typically of astrocytic origin, which occurs predominantly in children and young adults.[49] This tumor may be difficult to appreciate on CT, and signs of mild mass effect may be the only indication of its presence. MR imaging shows mild, diffuse T2 (and sometimes T1) prolongation.[49,87,88] Mass effect is generally mild, and enhancement is typically absent.[49,87–89]

Pleomorphic xanthoastrocytoma (PXA) is a rare astrocytic neoplasm that tends to involve the leptomeninges.[51] These tumors show a peripheral hemispheric predominance, most commonly originating in the temporal lobe.[90] At imaging, PXA classically appears as a cystic and solid peripheral hemispheric mass, although completely solid tumors are not uncommon (**Fig. 6**).[90,91] Solid

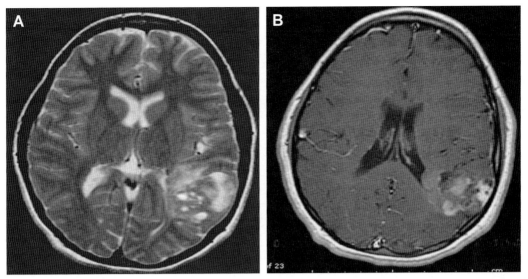

Fig. 6. PXA. (A) Axial T2-weighted images show a heterogeneous, cystic, and solid mass centered in the left parietal lobe. Solid components show T2 signal approximating that of gray matter, which would be atypical in other hemispheric cystic masses. (B) Axial postcontrast T1-weighted images (at a different level) show heterogeneous enhancement.

components tend to show signal intensity approximating that of normal gray matter, a finding that may help to distinguish these tumors from hemispheric astrocytoma and ganglioglioma. PXA typically shows heterogeneous enhancement after the administration of intravenous contrast agent.[92]

In general terms, astrocytic tumors show increased choline, decreased N-acetyl-aspartate, and occasionally a lactate peak on MRS.[93] Increased choline concentration and the presence of lactate tend to be associated with more aggressive tumors.[94] Spectra from pilocytic tumors (World Health Organization [WHO] grade I tumors) are paradoxic in this regard, with metabolite profiles approximating those of high-grade tumors.[95] JPA also tends to show high relative cerebral blood volume (rCBV), a finding that otherwise has been shown to correlate with tumor grade.[96,97] In a recent study in adult patients with primary brain tumors, rCBV was found to be a better predictor of tumor behavior than pathologic evaluation.[98] However, studies in childhood brain tumors have been less consistent in their findings, possibly relating to the frequency of pilocytic tumors.[60,96,97] DWI seems to have some prognostic value in these patients: for example, when WHO grades 2 to 4 are considered, a negative correlation between the ADC and tumor grade has been reported.[84] Increased citrate at diagnosis (similar to that seen in DIPG) has been reported in low-grade astrocytomas that show rapid disease progression.[5,60] This finding raises the possibility that citrate may be a marker of

low-grade tumors with a propensity toward unexpectedly aggressive behavior.[5,60]

Ependymal cell tumors

Supratentorial ependymoma arises from ependymal cell rests within white matter or from ventricular ependyma.[29] Although this tumor may occur at any age, the peak incidence is from 0 to 5 years of age.[48,49] However, unlike tumors occurring in the posterior fossa, supratentorial ependymoma are rarely intraventricular in location. Rather, they tend to occur in a periventricular location.

On imaging, supratentorial ependymoma typically appears as a heterogeneously enhancing, intra-axial mass, the solid components of which tend to show, at least in part, isodensity or hyperdensity to gray matter on CT and isointensity or hypointensity to gray matter on T2-weighted images.[4,47,55] Mineralization, necrosis, and hemorrhage are common, accounting for the characteristic heterogeneity seen in these tumors. Isointensity to gray matter should distinguish ependymoma from hemispheric astrocytoma, whereas a periventricular location and marked heterogeneity help to differentiate it from PXA. In most cases, the major differential considerations are supratentorial PNET and ATRT. Although MRS may be helpful in some cases (see earlier discussion), definitive differentiation from these tumors often requires pathologic evaluation.

Oligodendroglioma

Oligodendroglioma is a glial neoplasm that occurs most frequently in adults (peak incidence fourth and fifth decades of life).[99] These tumors account for approximately 1% of CNS tumors in the pediatric population[99,100] and can occur as either well-differentiated oligodendrogliomas (WHO grade II) or as less common anaplastic oligodendroglioma (WHO grade III). Oligodendroglioma is a slow-growing tumor that tends to have a peripheral location. Osseous remodeling of the inner table of the skull is a common finding.

MR imaging shows a predominantly solid mass centered peripherally in the cerebral hemispheres. Solid components tend to show homogeneous T1 and T2 prolongation.[101] Prominent cortical thickening may help to distinguish these tumors from astrocytic neoplasms.[51] Mineralization is a frequent finding, particularly on CT. The presence of dense, nodular calcification suggests the diagnosis of oligodendroglioma, although it occurs less commonly in children than in adults.[101] Enhancement is variable. Noncalcified lesions are impossible to differentiate from glioneuronal and astrocytic tumors without pathologic evaluation.

PNETs

PNET refers to a rare group of malignant tumors, distinguished from other neoplasms by an extremely high proportion of undifferentiated cells.[102,103] Supratentorial PNETs occur mainly in the first decade of life, with peak incidence from birth to 5 years of age.[1] PNETs account for approximately 5% of all supratentorial tumors in the pediatric population.

On imaging, supratentorial PNET tends to present as a large, heterogeneous mass centered in the deep white matter of the brain.[104] Necrosis, cystic degeneration, and hemorrhage are common, contributing to the heterogeneous appearance of this tumor.[104,105] With respect to gray matter, solid portions of the tumor tend to show isodensity on CT and isointensity on T2-weighted MR images (**Fig. 7**).[105,106] These solid regions also tend toward increased CBV and decreased ADC.[5,60,84] Enhancement after contrast administration is the rule, and is typically heterogeneous in appearance.[105,107] Calcification and osseous erosion are best shown at CT, whereas MR imaging is the study of choice to identify leptomeningeal dissemination. High-grade glioma, supratentorial ATRT, and ependymoma should be considered in the differential diagnosis of a mass with these imaging characteristics.

Recent evidence suggests MRS may aid in the differentiation of PNET from other supratentorial tumors. Like medulloblastoma (posterior fossa PNET), supratentorial PNET tends to show markedly increased choline levels in addition to an abnormal taurine peak.[60] The prospective performance of these imaging features has yet to be fully characterized.

NEOPLASMS WITH NEURONAL ELEMENTS
Ganglioglioma and Gangliocytoma

Ganglioglioma and gangliocytoma are tumors that consist, at least in part, of neuronal elements.[108] Ganglioglioma is characterized by the coexistence of neoplastic glial cells, whereas gangliocytoma consists solely of neuronal elements.[109] Together, these tumors account for 3% of brain tumors and 6% of supratentorial tumors in children.[110] Peak incidence is in adolescents and in young adults, although they can present at any age.[29] These tumors tend to involve the cerebral cortex, most commonly in the temporal lobes[111,112]; the common association with complex partial seizures is not unexpected.

The imaging appearances of ganglioglioma and gangliocytoma are identical. These tumors present as a peripherally located, intra-axial mass that may be wholly solid or partly cystic in appearance.[113–116] Mineralization is a common finding on CT.[113] On MR imaging, solid components of these tumors show T1 and T2 prolongation relative to gray matter.[114–116] Enhancement after intravenous contrast administration is a variable finding. Differential considerations in these cases include primarily low-grade neoplasms such as dysembryoplastic neuroepithelial tumor (DNET), astrocytoma, and oligodendroglioma. Mineralization and the absence of enhancement may suggest the diagnosis, especially given the relative rarity of oligodendroglioma in the pediatric population, but ultimately these findings are nonspecific. On the other hand, high CBV on MR perfusion may aid in distinguishing ganglioglioma from low-grade glial neoplasms.[117]

DNET

DNETs are low-grade neoplasms that may share a common origin with malformations of cortical development.[118] Most DNETs occur in the temporal lobes and are always centered in the cerebral cortex, with most of the remainder occurring in the frontal lobes.[109,118] Patients typically present with partial complex seizures without other neurologic findings.

On CT, DNET appears as a peripherally located, low-density mass.[119] The MR imaging appearance is classic (ie, a circumscribed mass centered within the cerebral cortex that shows prolonged T1 and T2 (**Fig. 8**)).[115,119] Involvement of the subcortical white matter is not uncommon and, when present, tends to show a centripetal tapering; this finding may reflect its origin in

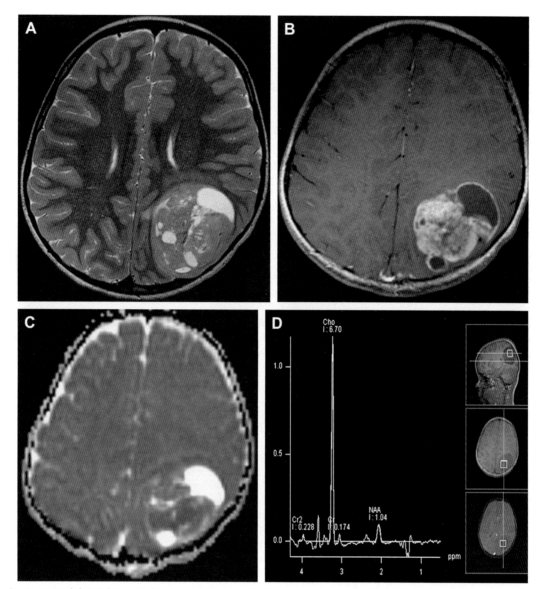

Fig. 7. PNET. (*A*) Axial T2-weighted image shows a heterogeneous mass centered in the left parietal lobe. Solid portions of tumor show signal characteristics similar to those of gray matter as well as heterogeneous enhancement (*B*) and decreased diffusion relative to brain parenchyma (*C*). (*D*) MRS (echo time = 144) shows decreased *N*-acetyl-aspartate, markedly increased choline level, and an inverted lactate peak.

cortical development, analogous to the white matter tail associated with many focal cortical dysplasias. Cystic components are common and may impart a soap bubble appearance.[115,119] A complete or incomplete hyperintense rim on FLAIR images, which may correspond to the presence of peripheral loose neuroglial elements, is an additional finding that has been reported in patients with DNETs. This ring sign may have some potential to differentiate these tumors from low-grade gliomas and gangliogliomas.[120] Contrast enhancement, which is identified in the minority of

tumors, tends to be nodular. Although the differential includes other low-grade neoplasms such as ganglioglioma, astrocytoma, and oligodendroglioma, in our experience the diagnosis is suggested by the imaging characteristics described earlier.

On MRS, DNETs tend to show a normal metabolic spectra.[121] DWI may also lend support to the diagnosis, because DNET tends to show higher ADC than do glial and other glioneuronal tumors.[84] This same study reported 100% accuracy in differentiating DNET from all other tumors on the basis of diffusion characteristics.

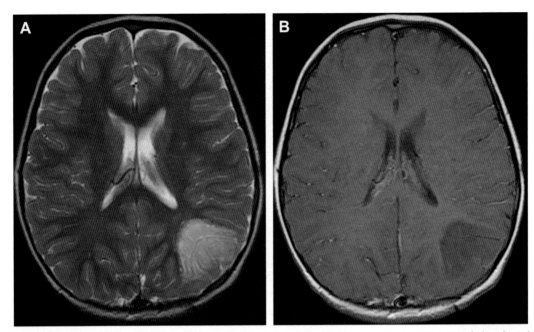

Fig. 8. DNET. (*A*) Axial T2-weighted image shows a peripheral, hyperintense mass that prominently involves the cortex. Centripetal tapering toward the left lateral ventricle is typical and may reflect an origin in cortical development. These tumors rarely show significant enhancement (*B*).

Desmoplastic Infantile Ganglioglioma

Desmoplastic infantile ganglioglioma (DIG) is a rare neoplasm characterized by glial and neuronal elements within a prominent desmoplastic stroma.[122] Peak incidence is in the first year of life; occurrence after 3 years of age is uncommon.[123,124] Imaging typically shows a large, predominantly cystic, intra-axial mass associated with peripheral, solid elements that frequently present in the frontal and parietal lobes (**Fig. 9**).[125] Solid components of tumor, which tend to involve the meninges, show signal intensity approximating that of gray matter as well as intense, homogeneous enhancement.[126,127]

SELLAR AND PARASELLAR TUMORS
Optic Pathway and Hypothalamic Astrocytoma

Optic pathway/hypothalamic astrocytomas are tumors of early childhood, with peak incidence between the ages of 2 and 6 years.[7] Optic pathway astrocytoma accounts for approximately 15% of all supratentorial tumors in the pediatric population.[7] Most astrocytomas in this location show pilocytic histology.[128] These tumors occur with increased frequency in patients with NF-1.[129] Identification of bilateral optic gliomas is highly suggestive of this diagnosis.

On imaging, these tumors typically present as heterogeneous, cystic, and solid suprasellar masses.[4,128,130] Heterogeneous enhancement of solid components is identified in most tumors. Homogeneous, fusiform expansion of the optic nerves is an additional common appearance, although contrast enhancement is less consistent in these cases.[4,128,130] Although CT affords excellent inherent contrast between the optic nerves and intraorbital fat and may help to characterize the intracanalicular and orbital involvement, MR imaging is clearly the modality of choice for evaluating the intracranial extent of these tumors.[15] Regardless of the morphology of the tumor, solid components typically show hypodensity on CT and hyperintensity on MR with T2-weighted images, respectively.[83,131] This finding may help discriminate astrocytoma from other suprasellar masses discussed later. T2 signal abnormality frequently extends along the optic radiations, although rarely beyond the lateral geniculate bodies; it is difficult in these cases to differentiate edema from nonenhancing tumor.[4,15]

Craniopharyngioma

Craniopharyngiomas arise from squamous cell rests, possibly occurring as remnants of the Rathke craniopharyngeal pouch.[132] Most pediatric craniopharyngiomas show adamantinomatous histology. Peak incidence is in the second decade of life, although they may be seen at any age.[132]

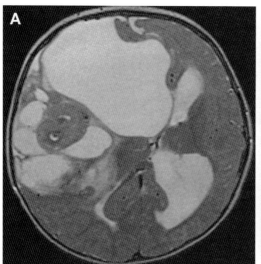
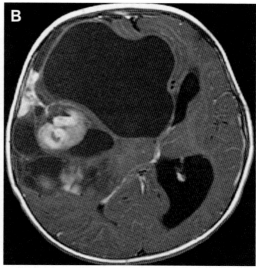

Fig. 9. DIG. (*A*) Axial T2-weighted image shows a large, predominantly cystic, intra-axial mass associated with peripheral, solid elements involving the right frontal and parietal lobes. Solid components of tumor tend to show signal intensity approximating that of gray matter as well as intense, homogeneous enhancement (*B*).

There is a second peak of craniopharyngioma in the fourth to sixth decades of life; however, these tumors differ in both histology (papillary) and imaging appearance. Craniopharyngioma tends to originate within the sella or suprasellar region, with most of the remainder occurring in the third ventricle.[133,134] Extension into the anterior, middle, or posterior cranial fossa is common.[135]

The CT appearance is characteristic, with most tumors showing cystic, solid enhancing, and mineralized components.[136] MR imaging shows a multilobulated, cystic, and solid sellar/suprasellar mass.[137,138] Solid components enhance (as do the cyst walls) after the administration of paramagnetic contrast, typically in heterogeneous fashion.[137,138] Although cystic components are highly variable in appearance, T1 hyperintensity may be identified on the basis of either high cholesterol or protein content.[137–139] This finding helps to differentiate these tumors from astrocytoma, the cystic components of which rarely show high T1 signal. However, the absence of short T1 does not exclude craniopharyngioma. In such cases, evidence of mineralization on CT is a helpful differential feature.

Germ Cell Tumors

Germinoma constitutes most suprasellar germ cell tumors. These tumors originate in the hypothalamus and typically extend into the infundibulum.[140,141] In most instances, patients present with central diabetes insipidus (DI), believed to develop because of interrupted transport of the vasopressin neurosecretory granules along the hypothalamic-neurohypophyseal pathway.[140–142] Unlike those occurring in the pineal region, suprasellar germinomas occur with equal frequency in males and females.[51]

Early in the course of disease, MR imaging may show mild thickening and homogeneous enhancement of the infundibulum (**Fig. 10**).[141,143,144] This appearance is indistinguishable from that of lymphocytic hypophysitis and Langerhans cell histiocytosis (LCH). Clinical presentation can be helpful in these cases because DI is significantly more common at diagnosis in patients with germinoma. Later in the course of the disease, imaging shows a solid or predominantly solid, suprasellar mass with signal characteristics approximating that of gray matter.[143] The bright spot normally evident in the posterior pituitary is generally absent. Solid components of these tumors typically show diffuse enhancement. Isointensity to gray matter combined with absence of prominent cystic components further distinguish this tumor from other common suprasellar masses such as astrocytoma and craniopharyngioma. On imaging, it may be difficult to differentiate LCH from other granulomatous infectious and inflammatory diseases. Serum markers, including human chorionic gonadotropin, α-fetoprotein, and placental alkaline phosphatase, can be a helpful adjunctive measure in these cases. Because central DI and the absence of the normal posterior pituitary bright spot may precede other clinical and imaging features of hypothalamic tumor by months or years, follow-up MR imaging with gadolinium is recommended in all such patients.[145]

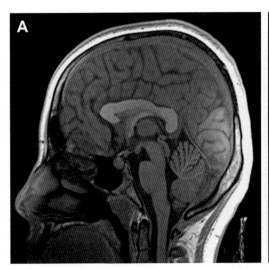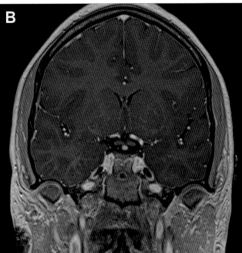

Fig. 10. Suprasellar germinoma. (*A*) Sagittal T1-weighted image shows absence of the posterior pituitary bright spot. There is also the suggestion of nodular thickening of the proximal infundibulum, which is confirmed on the coronal postcontrast images (*B*).

LCH

LCH is a reticuloendothelial disorder characterized by proliferation of a specific subset of histiocytes. The imaging appearance is identical to that of germinoma. The identification of characteristic calvarial (and other skeletal) lytic lesions should suggest the diagnosis.[146,147]

Tumors of Pituitary Origin

The incidence of pituitary adenomas, once considered to be extremely rare in childhood, has increased with improved detection, primarily related to advances in MR imaging. Adenomas now comprise approximately 3% of all supratentorial tumors in childhood.[148] The clinical presentation depends on tumor size, hormonal activity, and extrasellar extent. Pituitary adenomas are divided into hormonally active and inactive types. Most are hormonally active, most commonly prolactin secreting. Most of these lesions measure less than 1 cm in diameter (microadenomas) and present with neuroendocrine symptoms. Macroadenomas (>1 cm in diameter) may be prolactin secreting or hormonally inactive, presenting with neuroendocrine symptoms, visual field deficits, or headache. Macroadenomas in adolescence have a significant male predominance.[149]

The appearance of pituitary adenomas is nearly identical to that in adults, although macroadenomas are more common in the pediatric population.[150] Tumors may be isointense or hypointense (compared with the normal pituitary gland) on T1-weighted images and isointense to hyperintense on T2-weighted images.[150,151] Detection of microadenoma is primarily based on relative hypoenhancement compared with normal surrounding pituitary glandular tissue after the administration of paramagnetic contrast agent.[150–152] Macroadenomas are heterogeneous masses that tend to involve both the sella and suprasellar regions, often with a waist at the sellar diaphragm; a significant fraction of macroadenomas in this age group are hemorrhagic.[149]

Hypothalamic Hamartoma

Hypothalamic hamartoma (HH; hamartoma of the tuber cinereum) is a rare congenital lesion composed of nonneoplastic neuronal tissue.[153] Patients most commonly present early in life with precocious puberty.[154,155] Epilepsy, including gelastic type seizures, is another common presentation.[156] These lesions occur in association with multiple congenital abnormalities, including hypoplasia of the olfactory bulbs; absence of the pituitary gland; cardiac and renal anomalies; imperforate anus; craniofacial anomalies; syndactyly and a short metacarpal: clinical features that characterize the autosomal-dominant Pallister-Hall syndrome.[157,158]

On CT, HH appears as a gray matter density, suprasellar mass. MR imaging shows a round or ovoid mass centered at or pedunculated from the tuber cinereum.[154] These lesions show isointensity and isointensity or slight hyperintensity to gray matter on T1-weighted and T2-weighted images, respectively (**Fig. 11**).[159,160] Contrast

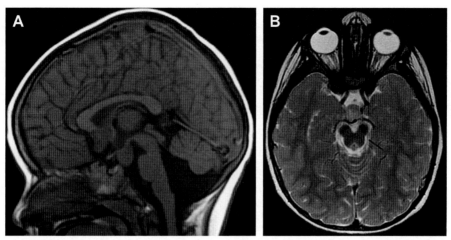

Fig. 11. HH. (A) Sagittal T1-weighted image shows an ovoid mass immediately posterior to the infundibulum, which is isointense to gray matter. (B) Axial T2-weighted image shows signal intensity slightly hyperintense to that of gray matter. Postcontrast images (not shown) showed no abnormal enhancement in this lesion, which has an imaging appearance characteristic for HH.

enhancement should suggest an alternative diagnosis such as LCH or germinoma.

PINEAL REGION TUMORS

The diverse tumors occurring in the pineal region can be classified into several groups: (1) germ cell tumors, (2) tumors of pineal cell origin, (3) glial tumors, and (4) other extra-axial tumors, including meningioma, melanoma, and nonneoplastic cysts.[15]

Germ Cell Tumors

Germinoma
Germinoma is the most common intracranial germ cell tumor and the most common tumor of the pineal region.[161,162] Patients with pineal region germinoma show a marked male predominance.[51] These tumors can occur throughout the first 3 decades of life, with peak incidence in adolescence.[4] Pineal region germinoma has an identical imaging appearance to those occurring in a suprasellar location (see earlier discussion). Differentiation from pineoblastoma may be difficult, as described later in the section on tumors of pineal cell origin. In the appropriate clinical setting, the coexistence of a suprasellar mass should suggest the diagnosis of germinoma (Fig. 12). Serum markers may also be helpful as discussed earlier in the section on germ cell tumors.

Teratoma
Teratoma is a neoplasm derived from all 3 germ layers. It is the second most common germ cell tumor of the pineal region and the single

most common intracranial tumor occurring in the neonatal period.[163]

Benign teratoma has a characteristic imaging appearance, showing marked heterogeneity resulting from the coexistence of cystic, solid enhancing, fatty, and mineralized components. Even in the absence of all 4 findings in the same tumor, fat density is still highly suggestive of the diagnosis. The presence of an associated solid, enhancing component should discriminate this tumor from a dermoid cyst and lipoma (Fig. 13). Malignant teratoma has a less specific imaging appearance. In such cases, MR imaging typically shows a predominantly solid, enhancing mass, without associated fat or mineralization.[164]

Tumors of pineal cell origin
Parenchymal tumors of the pineal gland, pineoblastoma and pineocytoma, account for up to 40% of all tumors occurring in the pineal region.[1] Pineoblastoma is a small round cell tumor, the histology of which is similar to that of PNET.[165,166] Peak incidence is in the first decade of life.[29] Pineocytoma may occur in childhood, but is more common in adults.[29]

At imaging, pineocytoma typically appears as a partially cystic mass, commonly associated with mineralization. Associated hydrocephalus is uncommon.[167] These tumors tend to show heterogeneous enhancement after the administration of contrast.[168] Pineoblastoma tends to be larger and more heterogeneous than pineocytoma (as a result of frequent necrosis and hemorrhage); it is also associated with hydrocephalus in most cases.[4,169] Like other high-grade tumors, solid

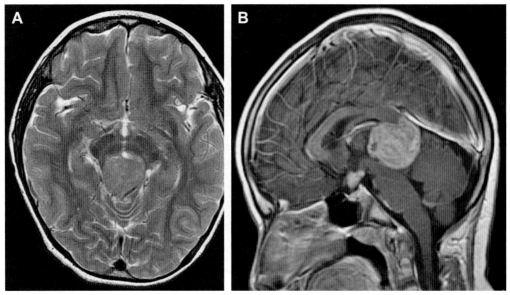

Fig. 12. Pineal germinoma. (*A*) Axial T2-weighted image from an adolescent male shows a pineal region mass that is homogeneously isointense to gray matter. (*B*) Sagittal postcontrast T1-weighted image shows homogeneous enhancement of this mass as well as an additional enhancing mass in the suprasellar cistern. These imaging characteristics are typical for germinoma and should suggest the diagnosis in the appropriate patient population.

components of pineoblastoma tend to show either hyperdensity and isointensity or hypointensity to gray matter on CT and T2-weighted images, respectively.[72,168,169] Postcontrast sequences show enhancement of its solid components.[170–172]

Poorly defined margins with adjacent parenchymal structures are typical, consistent with its invasive nature.[171] Leptomeningeal dissemination may occur at diagnosis or as a manifestation of recurrence.[107] The primary differential consideration in most cases

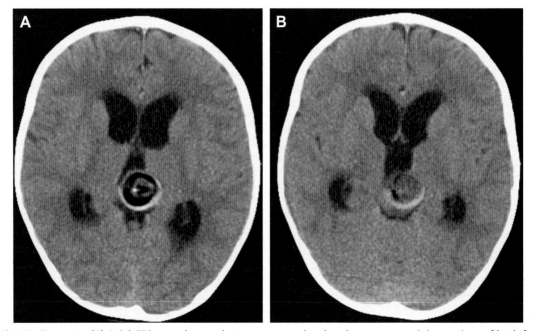

Fig. 13. Teratoma. (*A*) Axial CT image shows a heterogeneous pineal region mass containing regions of both fat and calcium. (*B*) Additional axial CT image (inferior to the plane in *A*) shows a prominent soft tissue component that enhanced after the administration of iodinated contrast agent (*not shown*). Both images also show enlargement of the ventricular system in this patient with obstructive hydrocephalus.

is germinoma. Although definitive differentiation is often not possible, germinoma commonly contains intrinsic tumoral calcification, whereas pineal parenchymal tumors typically displace preexisting normal pineal calcifications peripherally.[173] In these cases, mineralization may adopt an exploded appearance. Furthermore, pineal germinoma tends to occur in older patients (peak in adolescence) and rarely in female patients.

Tectal glioma

Tectal glioma is a specific intrinsic midbrain tumor that tends to present with raised intracranial pressure as a result of aqueductal stenosis.[15] These tumors are discussed in detail in the section on brainstem tumors.

INTRAVENTRICULAR TUMORS
Choroid Plexus Tumors

CPP and choroid plexus carcinoma (CPC) both arise from the epithelium of the choroid plexus.[174] These neoplasms comprise 10% to 20% of CNS tumors in the first year of life, and 3% to 5% of all intracranial tumors of childhood.[175] Peak incidence is from birth to 5 years of age, with CPP tending to present earlier than carcinoma.[176,177] In children, choroid plexus tumors occur most frequently within the lateral ventricle, particularly the trigone.[178] Hydrocephalus is associated with most of these tumors at presentation, which may result from CSF overproduction, obstruction of CSF by the tumor, or impaired CSF absorption secondary to repeated hemorrhage.

Cross-sectional imaging shows a markedly lobulated, often frondlike, solid mass centered within the ventricle (**Fig. 14**).[179] These tumors enhance after the administration of intravenous contrast, typically in homogeneous fashion.[51] Mineralization may be identified in up to 20% of cases.[180] Aggressive lesions may show invasion through the ependyma into the hemispheric parenchyma. Although differentiation cannot be reliably made at imaging, CPC tends to have a more heterogeneous appearance and is more frequently associated with parenchymal invasion and CSF dissemination.[181,182] A CPC may be difficult to distinguish from an intraventricular PNET.

CPP has a characteristic metabolic profile at MRS, with a marked increase of MI level.[40] This finding should distinguish CPP from most other intraventricular tumors, including CPC. The rare intraventricular ependymoma may show a similar MRS profile, as discussed in the section on ependymoma. On the other hand, MRS in CPC typically shows a marked increase of choline level, a finding that has not been reported in CPP.[183]

Subependymal Giant Cell Astrocytoma

Subependymal giant cell astrocytoma (SEGA) is a low-grade astrocytic neoplasm that occurs almost exclusively in patients with tuberous sclerosis (TS).[184] Peak incidence is in the first decade of life, although they may occur at any age. These tumors are characteristically located within the lateral ventricle, centered in the region of the foramen of Monro.[185]

Cross-sectional imaging shows a circumscribed, homogeneously enhancing mass in this characteristic location.[183–187] These findings are effectively diagnostic of SEGA when in association with other CNS stigmata of TS. Distinction from enhancing subependymal nodules in patients with TS can be reliably made on the basis of interval growth. In rare instances, these tumors may occur without additional intracranial manifestations of TS.

Ependymoma

Supratentorial ependymoma occurs more commonly in the cerebral hemispheres. When located within the ventricular system, the appearance is identical to that of infratentorial ependymoma, as discussed earlier in the section on intraventricular tumors.

MISCELLANEOUS EXTRA-AXIAL TUMORS
Schwannoma

Schwannoma is a benign neoplasm arising from the cells that form axonal myelin sheaths.[29] These tumors are rare in children and should raise the possibility of neurofibromatosis type 2.[4,50] The most frequent location is the internal auditory canal (IAC)/cerebellopontine angle cistern; such tumors originate from the vestibular division of the eighth cranial nerve.[188] The trigeminal nerve is the next most common site of origin.[188]

On imaging, the appearance of schwannoma is that of an enhancing, extra-axial mass.[189–191] In most of these tumors, hyperintensity to gray matter is observed on T2-weighted imaging.[4] In some cases, a target appearance, which results from relatively low T2 signal fibrous components centrally, may be identified.[191] Vestibular tumors originate from the peripheral portion of the eighth cranial nerve, and therefore commonly remodel and expand the acoustic meatus. In the authors' experience, this finding can help to differentiate vestibular schwannoma from other cerebellopontine angle tumors, which extend into the IAC secondarily. Trigeminal and other schwannomas tend to grow along the course of the nerve of origin, resulting in a characteristic fusiform shape.[4]

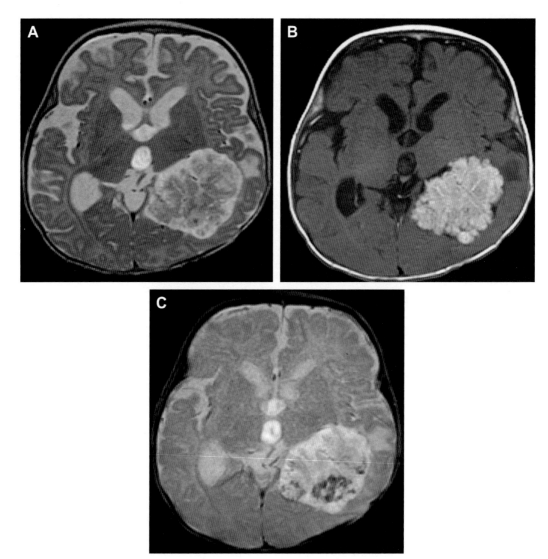

Fig. 14. CPP. (*A*) Axial T2-weighted image shows a lobulated mass centered within the atrium of the left lateral ventricle. (*B*) Axial postcontrast T1-weighted image shows homogeneous enhancement of the mass and highlights the typical frondlike appearance of these tumors. (C) Although better shown by CT, a gradient echo image shows susceptibility-related signal loss in the tumor related to mineralization.

Diffuse enhancement is typical in solid portions of tumor.[188–190]

Meningeal Tumors

Meningioma is a rare tumor of childhood and adolescence.[192] Like schwannoma, identification of a meningioma in a child should raise the possibility of neurofibromatosis type 2.[193] Although the appearance is identical to those occurring in the adult population, pediatric meningioma occurs most commonly in the lateral ventricle, typically within the trigone.[194] Radiation-induced meningiomas have been reported as a late effect of treatment of a variety of childhood neoplasms, notably lymphoblastic leukemia.[195,196]

In the absence of mineralization, meningioma in any location tends to show CT density and MR signal intensity similar to that of gray matter.[197,198] Intense, homogeneous enhancement is the rule.[192,199] Hyperostosis of adjacent osseous structures, best appreciated on CT, is a highly suggestive finding.[200,201] Mineralization or, more rarely, cystic or lipomatous components may be observed.[202–205] Other intrinsic meningeal tumors, including myofibroma, plasma cell granuloma, and meningeal sarcoma, may have an identical imaging appearance.

Embryonic Tumors

Supratentorial dermoid and epidermoid cysts have an identical appearance to those occurring in the posterior fossa, such as was described earlier in this review.

Metastatic Disease

Metastatic involvement of the CNS may result from hematogenous dissemination, leptomeningeal seeding, or direct extension. Although leptomeningeal seeding most commonly results from a wide spectrum of primary brain tumors, notably medulloblastoma, it may also occur in the setting of non-CNS primary tumors and systemic malignancies.[206,207] In these cases, the imaging appearance is identical to that of leptomeningeal dissemination occurring secondary to a primary CNS tumor.[20,206]

Hematogenous metastases to the cranium or dura most commonly result from neuroblastoma, leukemia, and lymphoma. These lesions appear as aggressive lytic calvarial lesions or as nonspecific, enhancing dural masses (**Fig. 15**).[107,208] Hematogenously disseminated metastases to the brain parenchyma are uncommon in the pediatric population. In those rare instances when they do occur, they generally arise from sarcomas, particularly rhabdomyosarcoma and Ewing sarcoma.[209] Rhabdoid tumors of the kidney are also found in association with parenchymal brain masses, although it remains unclear whether these represent metastatic lesions or synchronous intracranial tumors.[210] Parenchymal metastatic lesions tend to be multiple, located at the gray-white junction, and associated with prominent vasogenic edema.[211,212] Enhancement is the rule because nonbrain primaries are devoid of the blood-brain barrier.[213]

Lymphoproliferative Disorders

The CNS may be involved by lymphoproliferative disorders in 3 main forms: (1) solid intra-axial masses; (2) diffuse leptomeningeal infiltration; and (3) focal/multifocal extra-axial masses involving the dura or regional osseous structures.[29] The CNS is the most frequent site of relapsed acute lymphocytic leukemia of childhood.[15,214]

Primary CNS lymphoma (PCNSL) is rare in children, accounting for less than 1% of all intracranial tumors.[215] Most are non-Hodgkin lymphomas (NHLs) of B cell origin, frequently occurring in the setting of immunosuppression.[216–218] PCNSL tends to involve the brain parenchyma, may be single or multifocal, and most commonly originates within deep gray and white matter structures.[219] These tumors tend to show homogeneous hyperdensity on CT and isointensity to gray matter on T2-weighted imaging.[219,220] Diffuse enhancement is common, although tumors occurring in immunosuppressed patients have a greater tendency toward ring enhancement.[221] In such cases, patients are typically treated empirically for toxoplasmosis; the diagnosis of PCNSL can then be made by the absence of appropriate response. Imaging with fluorodeoxyglucose positron emission tomography, which shows increased uptake in lymphoma, may help to differentiate these

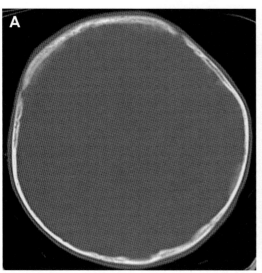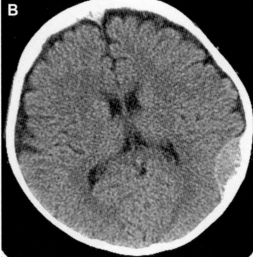

Fig. 15. Metastatic neuroblastoma. (*A*) Axial CT image on bone windows shows extensive regions of permeative lucency and periosteal reaction involving the calvarium. (*B*) The same CT image on soft tissue windows shows an epidural soft tissue mass along the inner table of the left parietal bone.

entities prospectively.[222] DWI tends to show decreased diffusivity compared with brain parenchyma, believed to result from high cell density or nuclear/cytoplasm ratio.[19] Similar to other CNS malignancies, an inverse correlation between ADC and prognosis has been shown.[223] Secondary involvement of the brain parenchyma in patients with systemic NHL, although less common, may be indistinguishable from PCNSL.

Extra-axial manifestations of systemic lymphoma and leukemia have already been discussed, in the section on miscellaneous extra-axial tumors. Although most frequently occurring in the setting of systemic disease, lymphomatous involvement of the leptomeninges, dura, and calvarium can occur as a manifestation of PCNSL.[224] Granulocytic sarcoma (chloroma) is an extra-axial manifestation of leukemia, typically associated with a specific subtype of myelogenous malignancy.[225] Like PCNSL, these tumors tend to show high attenuation on CT, low T2 signal, restricted diffusion, and diffuse enhancement after contrast administration (**Fig. 16**).[226]

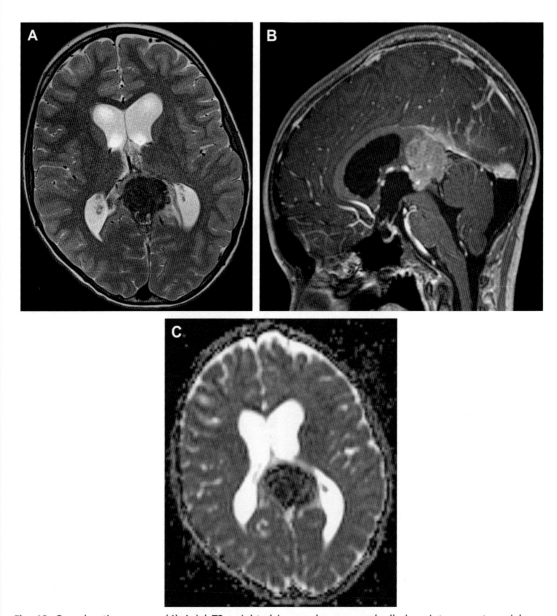

Fig. 16. Granulocytic sarcoma. (*A*) Axial T2-weighted image shows a markedly hypointense, extra-axial mass centered in the pineal region. (*B*) Sagittal postcontrast T1-weighted image shows relatively homogeneous enhancement. (*C*) ADC map shows markedly decreased diffusion relative to brain parenchyma, consistent with the high cell density seen pathologically in these tumors.

SUMMARY

The challenges inherent to imaging tumors of the pediatric CNS are myriad and complex. Specific considerations in this patient population (eg, developmental age, cognitive level, psychosocial status, and concomitant conditions) can make the process of medical decision making difficult at best. Further complicating management of these patients are the diverse pathologic diagnoses that must be considered when evaluating an intracranial mass. Rare neoplasms and atypical presentations of common neoplasms abound, and even optimal interpretation of state-of-the-art imaging frequently fails to accurately predict the pathologic diagnosis.

However, in the past decade we have witnessed a revolution in the development of advanced MR imaging technologies such as DWI, perfusion, and MR spectroscopy that have improved our ability to detect, diagnose, and treat CNS tumors of childhood. Yet without a comprehensive understanding of how each of these tumors appears on anatomic imaging, the potential of these techniques to enhance our diagnostic capabilities is significantly limited. The overarching objective of this review, therefore, is to offer a primer on the typical imaging features of tumors of the pediatric CNS. It is hoped that this body of information (with its focus on suggestive or differential features), when leveraged by these powerful imaging technologies, will produce more rapid, accurate diagnoses, leading, in turn, to disease management tailored to the unique needs of each child.

REFERENCES

1. Heideman RL, Packer RJ, Albright LA, et al. Tumors of the central nervous system. In: Pizzo PA, Poplack DG, editors. Principles and practice of pediatric oncology. Philadelphia: JB Lippincott; 1989. p. 505–53.
2. Altekruse S, Kosary C, Krapcho M, et al. SEER Cancer Statistics Review, 1975–2007. Bethesda (MD): National Cancer Institute; 2010. Available at: http://seer.cancer.gov/csr/1975_2007/. based on November 2009 SEER data submission, posted to the SEER web site, 2010. Accessed April, 2010.
3. Edwards-Brann SK. Supratentorial brain tumors. Neuroimaging Clin N Am 1994;4:437–55.
4. Maroldo TV, Barkovich AJ. Pediatric brain tumors. Semin Ultrasound CT MR 1992;13:412–48.
5. Panigrahy A, Bluml S. Neuroimaging of pediatric brain tumors: from basic to advanced magnetic resonance imaging (MRI). J Child Neurol 2009;24:1343–65.
6. Davies NP, Wilson M, Harris LM, et al. Identification and characterisation of childhood cerebellar tumours by in vivo proton MRS. NMR Biomed 2008;21:908–18.
7. Burkhard C, Di Patre PL, Schuler D, et al. A population-based study of the incidence and survival rates in patients with pilocytic astrocytoma. J Neurosurg 2003;98:1170–4.
8. Gjerris F, Klinken L. Long-term prognosis in children with benign cerebellar astrocytoma. J Neurosurg 1978;49:179–84.
9. Kibirige MS, Birch JM, Campbell RH, et al. A review of astrocytoma in childhood. Pediatr Hematol Oncol 1989;6:319–29.
10. Ringertz N, Nordenstam H. Cerebellar astrocytoma. J Neuropathol Exp Neurol 1951;10:343–67.
11. Bonner K, Siegel KR. Pathology, treatment and management of posterior fossa brain tumors in childhood. J Neurosci Nurs 1988;20:84–93.
12. Koeller KK, Henry JM. From the archives of the AFIP: superficial gliomas: radiologic-pathologic correlation. Armed Forces Institute of Pathology. Radiographics 2001;21:1533–56.
13. Zee CS. Infratentorial tumors in children. Neuroimaging Clin N Am 1993;3:705–13.
14. DeAngelis LM. Brain tumors. N Engl J Med 2001; 344:114–23.
15. Faerber EN, Roman NV. Central nervous system tumors of childhood. Radiol Clin North Am 1997; 35:1301–28.
16. Vassilyadi M, Shamji MF, Tataryn Z, et al. Postoperative surveillance magnetic resonance imaging for cerebellar astrocytoma. Can J Neurol Sci 2009;36: 707–12.
17. Higano S, Takahashi S, Kurihara N, et al. Supratentorial primary intra-axial tumors in children. MR and CT evaluation. Acta Radiol 1997;38:945–52.
18. Kingsley DP, Kendall BE. The CT scanner in posterior fossa tumours of childhood. Br J Radiol 1979; 52:769–76.
19. Guo AC, Cummings TJ, Dash RC, et al. Lymphomas and high-grade astrocytomas: comparison of water diffusibility and histologic characteristics. Radiology 2002;224:177–83.
20. Gusnard DA. Cerebellar neoplasms in children. Semin Roentgenol 1990;25:263–78.
21. Pfister S, Hartmann C, Korshunov A. Histology and molecular pathology of pediatric brain tumors. J Child Neurol 2009;24:1375–86.
22. Provias JP, Becker LE. Cellular and molecular pathology of medulloblastoma. J Neurooncol 1996; 29:35–43.
23. Radner H, Blumcke I, Reifenberger G, et al. The new WHO classification of tumors of the nervous system 2000. Pathology and genetics. Pathologe 2002;23:260–83 [in German].
24. Rossi A, Caracciolo V, Russo G, et al. Medulloblastoma: from molecular pathology to therapy. Clin Cancer Res 2008;14:971–6.

25. Pollack IF. Brain tumors in children. N Engl J Med 1994;331:1500–7.

26. Alston RD, Newton R, Kelsey A, et al. Childhood medulloblastoma in northwest England 1954 to 1997: incidence and survival. Dev Med Child Neurol 2003;45:308–14.

27. Deorah S, Lynch CF, Sibenaller ZA, et al. Trends in brain cancer incidence and survival in the United States: surveillance, epidemiology, and end results program, 1973 to 2001. Neurosurg Focus 2006; 20:E1.

28. McNeil DE, Cote TR, Clegg L, et al. Incidence and trends in pediatric malignancies medulloblastoma/ primitive neuroectodermal tumor: a SEER update. Surveillance epidemiology and end results. Med Pediatr Oncol 2002;39:190–4.

29. Russell DS, Rubenstein LJ. Pathology of tumors of the nervous system. 5th edition. Baltimore (MD): Williams & Wilkins; 1989. p. 251–79.

30. Zimmerman RA, Bilaniuk LT, Pahlajani H. Spectrum of medulloblastomas demonstrated by computed tomography. Radiology 1978;126:137–41.

31. Bourgouin PM, Tampieri D, Grahovac SZ, et al. CT and MR imaging findings in adults with cerebellar medulloblastoma: comparison with findings in children. AJR Am J Roentgenol 1992;159:609–12.

32. Tortori-Donati P, Fondelli MP, Rossi A, et al. Medulloblastoma in children: CT and MRI findings. Neuroradiology 1996;38:352–9.

33. Fitz CR, Rao KC. Primary tumors in children. In: Lee H, Rao KC, editors. Cranial tomography. New York: McGraw-Hill; 1983. p. 295–343.

34. Chawla A, Emmanuel JV, Seow WT, et al. Paediatric PNET: pre-surgical MRI features. Clin Radiol 2007; 62:43–52.

35. Malheiros SM, Carrete H Jr, Stavale JN, et al. MRI of medulloblastoma in adults. Neuroradiology 2003;45:463–7.

36. Buhring U, Strayle-Batra M, Freudenstein D, et al. MRI features of primary, secondary and metastatic medulloblastoma. Eur Radiol 2002;12:1342–8.

37. Mueller DP, Moore SA, Sato Y, et al. MRI spectrum of medulloblastoma. Clin Imaging 1992;16:250–5.

38. Rumboldt Z, Camacho DL, Lake D, et al. Apparent diffusion coefficients for differentiation of cerebellar tumors in children. AJNR Am J Neuroradiol 2006; 27:1362–9.

39. Brutschin P, Culver GJ. Extracranial metastases from medulloblastomas. Radiology 1973;107:359–62.

40. Panigrahy A, Krieger MD, Gonzalez-Gomez I, et al. Quantitative short echo time 1H-MR spectroscopy of untreated pediatric brain tumors: preoperative diagnosis and characterization. AJNR Am J Neuroradiol 2006;27:560–72.

41. Wang Z, Sutton LN, Cnaan A, et al. Proton MR spectroscopy of pediatric cerebellar tumors. AJNR Am J Neuroradiol 1995;16:1821–33.

42. Kovanlikaya A, Panigrahy A, Krieger MD, et al. Untreated pediatric primitive neuroectodermal tumor in vivo: quantitation of taurine with MR spectroscopy. Radiology 2005;236:1020–5.

43. Moreno-Torres A, Martinez-Perez I, Baquero M, et al. Taurine detection by proton magnetic resonance spectroscopy in medulloblastoma: contribution to noninvasive differential diagnosis with cerebellar astrocytoma. Neurosurgery 2004;55: 824–9 [discussion: 829].

44. Khong PL, Kwong DL, Chan GC, et al. Diffusion-tensor imaging for the detection and quantification of treatment-induced white matter injury in children with medulloblastoma: a pilot study. AJNR Am J Neuroradiol 2003;24:734–40.

45. Khong PL, Leung LH, Chan GC, et al. White matter anisotropy in childhood medulloblastoma survivors: association with neurotoxicity risk factors. Radiology 2005;236:647–52.

46. Wang S, Wu EX, Qiu D, et al. Longitudinal diffusion tensor magnetic resonance imaging study of radiation-induced white matter damage in a rat model. Cancer Res 2009;69:1190–8.

47. Yuh EL, Barkovich AJ, Gupta N. Imaging of ependymomas: MRI and CT. Childs Nerv Syst 2009; 25:1203–13.

48. Kun LE, Kovnar EH, Sanford RA. Ependymomas in children. Pediatr Neurosci 1988;14:57–63.

49. Yanaka K, Kamezaki T, Kobayashi E, et al. MR imaging of diffuse glioma. AJNR Am J Neuroradiol 1992;13:349–51.

50. Amador LV. Brain tumors in the young. Springfield (IL): Charles C Thomas; 1983. p. 1–453.

51. Barkovich AJ. Intracranial, orbital, and neck masses of childhood. In: Barkovich AJ, editor. Pediatric neuroimaging. 4th edition. New York: Lippincott, Williams & Wilkins; 2005. p. 506–658.

52. Lefton DR, Pinto RS, Martin SW. MRI features of intracranial and spinal ependymomas. Pediatr Neurosurg 1998;28:97–105.

53. Tortori-Donati P, Fondelli MP, Cama A, et al. Ependymomas of the posterior cranial fossa: CT and MRI findings. Neuroradiology 1995;37:238–43.

54. Spoto GP, Press GA, Hesselink JR, et al. Intracranial ependymoma and subependymoma: MR manifestations. AJNR Am J Neuroradiol 1990;11: 83–91.

55. Asa SL, Bilbao JM, Kovacs K, et al. Hypothalamic neuronal hamartoma associated with pituitary growth hormone cell adenoma and acromegaly. Acta Neuropathol 1980;52:231–4.

56. Gessi M, Giangaspero F, Pietsch T. Atypical teratoid/rhabdoid tumors and choroid plexus tumors: when genetics "surprise" pathology. Brain Pathol 2003;13:409–14.

57. Biegel JA. Molecular genetics of atypical teratoid/ rhabdoid tumor. Neurosurg Focus 2006;20:E11.

58. Biswas A, Goyal S, Puri T, et al. Atypical teratoid rhabdoid tumor of the brain: case series and review of literature. Childs Nerv Syst 2009;25:1495–500.

59. Warmuth-Metz M, Bison B, Dannemann-Stern E, et al. CT and MR imaging in atypical teratoid/rhabdoid tumors of the central nervous system. Neuroradiology 2008;50:447–52.

60. Panigrahy A, Nelson MD Jr, Bluml S. Magnetic resonance spectroscopy in pediatric neuroradiology: clinical and research applications. Pediatr Radiol 2010;40:3–30.

61. Frappaz D, Schell M, Thiesse P, et al. Preradiation chemotherapy may improve survival in pediatric diffuse intrinsic brainstem gliomas: final results of BSG 98 prospective trial. Neuro Oncol 2008;10: 599–607.

62. Tibbetts KM, Emnett RJ, Gao F, et al. Histopathologic predictors of pilocytic astrocytoma event-free survival. Acta Neuropathol 2009;117:657–65.

63. Duffner PK, Klein DM, Cohen ME. Calcification in brainstem gliomas. Neurology 1978;28:832–4.

64. Kwon JW, Kim IO, Cheon JE, et al. Paediatric brainstem gliomas: MRI, FDG-PET and histological grading correlation. Pediatr Radiol 2006;36:959–64.

65. Sun B, Wang CC, Wang J. MRI characteristics of midbrain tumours. Neuroradiology 1999;41:158–62.

66. Bruggers CS, Friedman HS, Fuller GN, et al. Comparison of serial PET and MRI scans in a pediatric patient with a brainstem glioma. Med Pediatr Oncol 1993;21:301–6.

67. Thakur SB, Karimi S, Dunkel IJ, et al. Longitudinal MR spectroscopic imaging of pediatric diffuse pontine tumors to assess tumor aggression and progression. AJNR Am J Neuroradiol 2006;27: 806–9.

68. Yousry I, Muacevic A, Olteanu-Nerbe V, et al. Exophytic pilocytic astrocytoma of the brain stem in an adult with encasement of the caudal cranial nerve complex (IX-XII): presurgical anatomical neuroimaging using MRI. Eur Radiol 2004;14:1169–73.

69. Ozawa Y, Katsumata Y, Maehara T. Exophytic pontine glioma mimicking acoustic neurinoma: CT and MRI appearance. Radiat Med 1993;11:217–9.

70. Barkovich AJ. Neuroimaging of pediatric brain tumors. Neurosurg Clin N Am 1992;3:739–69.

71. May PL, Blaser SI, Hoffman HJ, et al. Benign intrinsic tectal "tumors" in children. J Neurosurg 1991;74:867–71.

72. Satoh H, Uozumi T, Kiya K, et al. MRI of pineal region tumours: relationship between tumours and adjacent structures. Neuroradiology 1995;37: 624–30.

73. Poussaint TY, Kowal JR, Barnes PD, et al. Tectal tumors of childhood: clinical and imaging follow-up. AJNR Am J Neuroradiol 1998;19:977–83.

74. Ternier J, Wray A, Puget S, et al. Tectal plate lesions in children. J Neurosurg 2006;104:369–76.

75. Cramer F, Kimsey W. The cerebellar hemangioblastomas. Review of 53 cases, with special reference to cerebellar cysts and the association of polycythemia. AMA Arch Neurol Psychiatry 1952;67: 237–52.

76. Bing F, Kremer S, Lamalle L, et al. Value of perfusion MRI in the study of pilocytic astrocytoma and hemangioblastoma: preliminary findings. J Neuroradiol 2009;36:82–7 [in French].

77. Simon J, Szumowski J, Totterman S, et al. Fat-suppression MR imaging of the orbit. AJNR Am J Neuroradiol 1988;9:961–8.

78. Maeda M, Kawamura Y, Tamagawa Y, et al. Intravoxel incoherent motion (IVIM) MRI in intracranial, extraaxial tumors and cysts. J Comput Assist Tomogr 1992;16:514–8.

79. Tsuruda JS, Chew WM, Moseley ME, et al. Diffusion-weighted MR imaging of the brain: value of differentiating between extraaxial cysts and epidermoid tumors. AJR Am J Roentgenol 1990;155: 1059–65 [discussion: 1066–8].

80. Tsuruda JS, Chew WM, Moseley ME, et al. Diffusion-weighted MR imaging of the brain: value of differentiating between extraaxial cysts and epidermoid tumors. AJNR Am J Neuroradiol 1990;11: 925–31 [discussion: 932–4].

81. Rorke LB, Gilles FH, Davis RL, et al. Revision of the World Health Organization classification of brain tumors for childhood brain tumors. Cancer 1985; 56:1869–86.

82. Dohrmann GJ, Farwell JR, Flannery JT. Glioblastoma multiforme in children. J Neurosurg 1976;44: 442–8.

83. Cummings TJ, Provenzale JM, Hunter SB, et al. Gliomas of the optic nerve: histological, immunohistochemical (MIB-1 and p53), and MRI analysis. Acta Neuropathol 2000;99:563–70.

84. Yamasaki F, Kurisu K, Satoh K, et al. Apparent diffusion coefficient of human brain tumors at MR imaging. Radiology 2005;235:985–91.

85. Drayer B, Johnson B, Bird C. Magnetic resonance imaging and glioma. BNI Q 1987;3:44–55.

86. Vezina LG. Imaging of central nervous system tumors in children: advances and limitations. J Child Neurol 2008;23:1128–35.

87. Jayawant S, Neale J, Stoodley N, et al. Gliomatosis cerebri in a 10-year-old girl masquerading as diffuse encephalomyelitis and spinal cord tumour. Dev Med Child Neurol 2001;43:124–6.

88. Porta-Etessam J, Berbel A, Martinez-Salio A, et al. Gliomatosis cerebri. MRI, SPECT and the study of pathology. Rev Neurol 1999;29:287–8 [in Spanish].

89. Faerber EN. Intracranial tumors. In: Faerber EN, editor. CNS magnetic resonance imaging in infants and children. London: Mackeith Press; 1995. p. 164–97.

90. Fouladi M, Jenkins J, Burger P, et al. Pleomorphic xanthoastrocytoma: favorable outcome after

complete surgical resection. Neuro Oncol 2001;3: 184–92.

91. Frank S, Cordier D, Tolnay M, et al. A 28-year-old man with headache, visual and aphasic speech disturbances. Brain Pathol 2009;19:163–6.

92. Sugita Y, Irie K, Ohshima K, et al. Pleomorphic xanthoastrocytoma as a component of a temporal lobe cystic ganglioglioma: a case report. Brain Tumor Pathol 2009;26:31–6.

93. Byrd SE, Tomita T, Palka PS, et al. Magnetic resonance spectroscopy (MRS) in the evaluation of pediatric brain tumors, Part II: clinical analysis. J Natl Med Assoc 1996;88:717–23.

94. Fayed N, Modrego PJ. The contribution of magnetic resonance spectroscopy and echoplanar perfusion-weighted MRI in the initial assessment of brain tumours. J Neurooncol 2005;72:261–5.

95. Cecil KM, Jones BV. Magnetic resonance spectroscopy of the pediatric brain. Top Magn Reson Imaging 2001;12:435–52.

96. Ball WS Jr, Holland SK. Perfusion imaging in the pediatric patient. Magn Reson Imaging Clin N Am 2001;9:207–30, ix.

97. Tzika AA, Vajapeyam S, Barnes PD. Multivoxel proton MR spectroscopy and hemodynamic MR imaging of childhood brain tumors: preliminary observations. AJNR Am J Neuroradiol 1997;18:203–18.

98. Law M, Young RJ, Babb JS, et al. Gliomas: predicting time to progression or survival with cerebral blood volume measurements at dynamic susceptibility-weighted contrast-enhanced perfusion MR imaging. Radiology 2008;247:490–8.

99. Mork SJ, Lindegaard KF, Halvorsen TB, et al. Oligodendroglioma: incidence and biological behavior in a defined population. J Neurosurg 1985;63: 881–9.

100. Favier J, Pizzolato GP, Berney J. Oligodendroglial tumors in childhood. Childs Nerv Syst 1985;1:33–8.

101. Koeller KK, Rushing EJ. From the archives of the AFIP: oligodendroglioma and its variants: radiologic-pathologic correlation. Radiographics 2005;25:1669–88.

102. De Tommasi A, De Tommasi C, Occhiogrosso G, et al. Primary intramedullary primitive neuroectodermal tumor (PNET)–case report and review of the literature. Eur J Neurol 2006;13:240–3.

103. Hart MN, Earle KM. Primitive neuroectodermal tumors of the brain in children. Cancer 1973;32: 890–7.

104. Figeroa RE, el Gammal T, Brooks BS, et al. MR findings on primitive neuroectodermal tumors. J Comput Assist Tomogr 1989;13:773–8.

105. Robles HA, Smirniotopoulos JG, Figueroa RE. Understanding the radiology of intracranial primitive neuroectodermal tumors from a pathological perspective: a review. Semin Ultrasound CT MR 1992;13:170–81.

106. Rorke LB. The cerebellar medulloblastoma and its relationship to primitive neuroectodermal tumors. J Neuropathol Exp Neurol 1983;42:1–15.

107. Davis PC. Tumors of the brain. In: Cohen MD, Edwards MK, editors. Magnetic resonance imaging of children. Philadelphia: BC Decker; 1990. p. 155–220.

108. Courville CB. Ganglioma: tumor of the central nervous system. Review of literature and report of two cases. Arch Neurol Psychiatry 1930;24: 439–91.

109. Pasquier B, Peoc HM, Fabre-Bocquentin B, et al. Surgical pathology of drug-resistant partial epilepsy. A 10-year-experience with a series of 327 consecutive resections. Epileptic Disord 2002;4:99–119.

110. Sutton LN, Packer RJ, Rorke LB, et al. Cerebral gangliogliomas during childhood. Neurosurgery 1983;13:124–8.

111. Demierre B, Stichnoth FA, Hori A, et al. Intracerebral ganglioglioma. J Neurosurg 1986;65:177–82.

112. Garrido E, Becker LF, Hoffman HJ, et al. Gangliogliomas in children. A clinicopathological study. Childs Brain 1978;4:339–46.

113. Benitez WI, Glasier CM, Husain M, et al. MR findings in childhood gangliogliomas. J Comput Assist Tomogr 1990;14:712–6.

114. Chan A, McAbee G, Queenan J, et al. Ganglioneurocytoma mimicking a malignant tumor: case report with a literature review of the MRI appearance of neurocytomas and gangliogliomas. J Neuroimaging 2001;11:47–50.

115. Urbach H. MRI of long-term epilepsy-associated tumors. Semin Ultrasound CT MR 2008;29:40–6.

116. Zhang D, Henning TD, Zou LG, et al. Intracranial ganglioglioma: clinicopathological and MRI findings in 16 patients. Clin Radiol 2008;63:80–91.

117. Law M, Meltzer DE, Wetzel SG, et al. Conventional MR imaging with simultaneous measurements of cerebral blood volume and vascular permeability in ganglioglioma. Magn Reson Imaging 2004;22: 599–606.

118. Bilginer B, Yalnizoglu D, Soylemezoglu F, et al. Surgery for epilepsy in children with dysembryoplastic neuroepithelial tumor: clinical spectrum, seizure outcome, neuroradiology, and pathology. Childs Nerv Syst 2009;25:485–91.

119. Ostertun B, Wolf HK, Campos MG, et al. Dysembryoplastic neuroepithelial tumors: MR and CT evaluation. AJNR Am J Neuroradiol 1996;17: 419–30.

120. Parmar HA, Hawkins C, Ozelame R, et al. Fluid-attenuated inversion recovery ring sign as a marker of dysembryoplastic neuroepithelial tumors. J Comput Assist Tomogr 2007;31:348–53.

121. Bulakbasi N, Kocaoglu M, Ors F, et al. Combination of single-voxel proton MR spectroscopy and apparent diffusion coefficient calculation in the

evaluation of common brain tumors. AJNR Am J Neuroradiol 2003;24:225–33.

122. Bhardwaj M, Sharma A, Pal HK. Desmoplastic infantile ganglioglioma with calcification. Neuropathology 2006;26:318–22.

123. Onguru O, Celasun B, Gunhan O. Desmoplastic non-infantile ganglioglioma. Neuropathology 2005; 25:150–2.

124. Tamburrini G, Colosimo C Jr, Giangaspero F, et al. Desmoplastic infantile ganglioglioma. Childs Nerv Syst 2003;19:292–7.

125. Balaji R, Ramachandran K. Imaging of desmoplastic infantile ganglioglioma: a spectroscopic viewpoint. Childs Nerv Syst 2009;25:497–501.

126. Nikas I, Anagnostara A, Theophanopoulou M, et al. Desmoplastic infantile ganglioglioma: MRI and histological findings case report. Neuroradiology 2004;46:1039–43.

127. Trehan G, Bruge H, Vinchon M, et al. MR imaging in the diagnosis of desmoplastic infantile tumor: retrospective study of six cases. AJNR Am J Neuroradiol 2004;25:1028–33.

128. Muller-Forell W. Intracranial pathology of the visual pathway. Eur J Radiol 2004;49:143–78.

129. von Deimling A, Krone W, Menon AG. Neurofibromatosis type 1: pathology, clinical features and molecular genetics. Brain Pathol 1995;5:153–62.

130. Wiegand W. The optic nerve pathology in magnetic resonance imaging. Metab Pediatr Syst Ophthalmol 1990;13:60–6.

131. Buffa A, Vannelli S, Peretta P. NF1 and gliomas: the importance of the MRI. Minerva Pediatr 2008;60: 259–60 [in Italian].

132. Miller DC. Pathology of craniopharyngiomas: clinical import of pathological findings. Pediatr Neurosurg 1994;21(Suppl 1):11–7.

133. Hammock MK, Milhorat TH. Cranial computed tomography in infancy and childhood. Baltimore (MD): Williams & Wilkins; 1981.

134. Majd M, Farkas J, LoPresti JM, et al. A large calcified craniopharyngioma in the newborn. Radiology 1971;99:399–400.

135. Harwood-Nash DC, Fitz CR. Neuroradiology in infants and children. St Louis (MO): CV Mosby; 1976. p. 754–61.

136. Hamamoto Y, Niino K, Adachi M, et al. MR and CT findings of craniopharyngioma during and after radiation therapy. Neuroradiology 2002;44:118–22.

137. Choi SH, Kwon BJ, Na DG, et al. Pituitary adenoma, craniopharyngioma, and Rathke cleft cyst involving both intrasellar and suprasellar regions: differentiation using MRI. Clin Radiol 2007; 62:453–62.

138. Warakaulle DR, Anslow P. Differential diagnosis of intracranial lesions with high signal on T1 or low signal on T2-weighted MRI. Clin Radiol 2003;58: 922–33.

139. Cakirer S, Karaarslan E, Arslan A. Spontaneously T1-hyperintense lesions of the brain on MRI: a pictorial review. Curr Probl Diagn Radiol 2003; 32:194–217.

140. Edouard T, Stafford DE, Oliver I, et al. Isolated lymphocytic infiltration of pituitary stalk preceding the diagnosis of germinoma in 2 prepubertal children treated with growth hormone. Horm Res 2009;72:57–62.

141. Antoine V, Moret C, Schmitt E, et al. MRI imaging of the neural pituitary. Ann Endocrinol (Paris) 2008;69: 181–92 [in French].

142. Ghirardello S, Garre ML, Rossi A, et al. The diagnosis of children with central diabetes insipidus. J Pediatr Endocrinol Metab 2007;20:359–75.

143. Liang L, Korogi Y, Sugahara T, et al. MRI of intracranial germ-cell tumours. Neuroradiology 2002; 44:382–8.

144. Kanagaki M, Miki Y, Takahashi JA, et al. MRI and CT findings of neurohypophyseal germinoma. Eur J Radiol 2004;49:204–11.

145. Appignani B, Landy H, Barnes P. MR in idiopathic central diabetes insipidus of childhood. AJNR Am J Neuroradiol 1993;14:1407–10.

146. Makras P, Papadogias D, Samara C, et al. Langerhans' cell histiocytosis in an adult patient manifested as recurrent skull lesions and Diabetes Insipidus. Hormones (Athens) 2004;3:59–64.

147. Gibson SE, Prayson RA. Primary skull lesions in the pediatric population: a 25-year experience. Arch Pathol Lab Med 2007;131:761–6.

148. Kane LA, Leinung MC, Scheithauer BW, et al. Pituitary adenomas in childhood and adolescence. J Clin Endocrinol Metab 1994;79:1135–40.

149. Poussaint TY, Barnes PD, Anthony DC, et al. Hemorrhagic pituitary adenomas of adolescence. AJNR Am J Neuroradiol 1996;17:1907–12.

150. Rutka JT, Hoffman HJ, Drake JM, et al. Suprasellar and sellar tumors in childhood and adolescence. Neurosurg Clin N Am 1992;3:803–20.

151. Kulkarni MV, Lee KF, McArdle CB, et al. 1.5-T MR imaging of pituitary microadenomas: technical considerations and CT correlation. AJNR Am J Neuroradiol 1988;9:5–11.

152. Pojunas KW, Daniels DL, Williams AL, et al. MR imaging of prolactin-secreting microadenomas. AJNR Am J Neuroradiol 1986;7:209–13.

153. Chong BW, Newton TH. Hypothalamic and pituitary pathology. Radiol Clin North Am 1993;31: 1147–53.

154. Ng SM, Kumar Y, Cody D, et al. Cranial MRI scans are indicated in all girls with central precocious puberty. Arch Dis Child 2003;88:414–8 [discussion: 414–8].

155. Zuniga OF, Tanner SM, Wild WO, et al. Hamartoma of CNS associated with precocious puberty. Am J Dis Child 1983;137:127–33.

156. Breningstall GN. Gelastic seizures, precocious puberty, and hypothalamic hamartoma. Neurology 1985;35:1180–3.

157. Hall JG, Pallister PD, Clarren SK, et al. Congenital hypothalamic hamartoblastoma, hypopituitarism, imperforate anus and postaxial polydactyly–a new syndrome? Part I: clinical, causal, and pathogenetic considerations. Am J Med Genet 1980;7:47–74.

158. Celedin S, Kau T, Gasser J, et al. Fetal MRI of a hypothalamic hamartoma in Pallister-Hall syndrome. Pediatr Neurol 2010;42:59–60.

159. Lona Soto A, Takahashi M, Yamashita Y, et al. MRI findings of hypothalamic hamartoma: report of five cases and review of the literature. Comput Med Imaging Graph 1991;15:415–21.

160. Barral V, Brunelle F, Brauner R, et al. MRI of hypothalamic hamartomas in children. Pediatr Radiol 1988;18:449–52.

161. Fernandes VS, Bisi H, Camargo RY, et al. Retrospective analysis of the incidence of midline supratentorial neoplasms in children and young patients: craniopharyngiomas, hypophyseal and pineal neoplasms. Rev Paul Med 1990;108:71–7 [in Portuguese].

162. Goodwin TL, Sainani K, Fisher PG. Incidence patterns of central nervous system germ cell tumors: a SEER Study. J Pediatr Hematol Oncol 2009;31:541–4.

163. Buetow PC, Smirniotopoulos JG, Done S. Congenital brain tumors: a review of 45 cases. AJNR Am J Neuroradiol 1990;11:793–9.

164. Fujimaki T, Matsutani M, Funada N, et al. CT and MRI features of intracranial germ cell tumors. J Neurooncol 1994;19:217–26.

165. Sato K, Kubota T. Pathology of pineal parenchymal tumors. Prog Neurol Surg 2009;23:12–25.

166. Hirato J, Nakazato Y. Pathology of pineal region tumors. J Neurooncol 2001;54:239–49.

167. Weisberg LA. Clinical and computed tomographic correlations of pineal neoplasms. Comput Radiol 1984;8:285–92.

168. Korogi Y, Takahashi M, Ushio Y. MRI of pineal region tumors. J Neurooncol 2001;54:251–61.

169. Lagrange C, Froment JC, Leclercq R, et al. Tumors of the pineal region: MRI aspects. Apropos of 20 cases. Ann Radiol (Paris) 1989;32:251–8 [in French].

170. Reis F, Faria AV, Zanardi VA, et al. Neuroimaging in pineal tumors. J Neuroimaging 2006;16:52–8.

171. Nakamura M, Saeki N, Iwadate Y, et al. Neuroradiological characteristics of pineocytoma and pineoblastoma. Neuroradiology 2000;42:509–14.

172. Chiechi MV, Smirniotopoulos JG, Mena H. Pineal parenchymal tumors: CT and MR features. J Comput Assist Tomogr 1995;19:509–17.

173. Gouliamos AD, Kalovidouris AE, Kotoulas GK, et al. CT and MR of pineal region tumors. Magn Reson Imaging 1994;12:17–24.

174. Gaudio RM, Tacconi L, Rossi ML. Pathology of choroid plexus papillomas: a review. Clin Neurol Neurosurg 1998;100:165–86.

175. Zimmerman RA, Bilaniuk LT. Computed tomography of choroid plexus lesions. J Comput Tomogr 1979;3:93–103.

176. Ambrosino MM, Hernanz-Schulman M, Genieser NB, et al. Brain tumors in infants less than a year of age. Pediatr Radiol 1988;19:6–8.

177. Radkowski MA, Naidich TP, Tomita T, et al. Neonatal brain tumors: CT and MR findings. J Comput Assist Tomogr 1988;12:10–20.

178. Hopper KD, Foley LC, Nieves NL, et al. The interventricular extension of choroid plexus papillomas. AJNR Am J Neuroradiol 1987;8:469–72.

179. Guermazi A, De Kerviler E, Zagdanski AM, et al. Diagnostic imaging of choroid plexus disease. Clin Radiol 2000;55:503–16.

180. Rovit RL, Schecter MM, Chodroff P. Choroid plexus papillomas: observations on radiographic diagnosis. Am J Roentgenol Radium Ther Nucl Med 1970;110:608–17.

181. Connor SE, Chandler C, Bodi I, et al. Preoperative and early postoperative magnetic resonance imaging in two cases of childhood choroid plexus carcinoma. Eur Radiol 2002;12:883–8.

182. Taylor MB, Jackson RW, Hughes DG, et al. Magnetic resonance imaging in the diagnosis and management of choroid plexus carcinoma in children. Pediatr Radiol 2001;31:624–30.

183. Krieger MD, Panigrahy A, McComb JG, et al. Differentiation of choroid plexus tumors by advanced magnetic resonance spectroscopy. Neurosurg Focus 2005;18:E4.

184. Ech-Cherif El Kettani N, Salaheddine T, El Quessar A, et al. Neuro-imaging of tuberous sclerosis. J Radiol 2006;87:109–13 [in French].

185. Clarke MJ, Foy AB, Wetjen N, et al. Imaging characteristics and growth of subependymal giant cell astrocytomas. Neurosurg Focus 2006;20:E5.

186. Braffman BH, Bilaniuk LT, Naidich TP, et al. MR imaging of tuberous sclerosis: pathogenesis of this phakomatosis, use of gadopentetate dimeglumine, and literature review. Radiology 1992;183:227–38.

187. Martin N, Debussche C, De Broucker T, et al. Gadolinium-DTPA enhanced MR imaging in tuberous sclerosis. Neuroradiology 1990;31:492–7.

188. Pinto RS, Kricheff II. Neuroradiology of intracranial neuromas. Semin Roentgenol 1984;19:44–52.

189. VandeVyver V, Lemmerling M, Van Hecke W, et al. MRI findings of the normal and diseased trigeminal nerve ganglion and branches: a pictorial review. JBR-BTR 2007;90:272–7.

190. Imhof H, Henk CB, Dirisamer A, et al. CT and MRI characteristics of tumours of the temporal bone and the cerebello-pontine angle. Radiologe 2003;43:219–26 [in German].

191. Kovacsovics B, Davidsson L, Harder H, et al. MRI screening of the cerebellopontine angle and inner ear with fast spin-echo T2 technique. Arch Ital Biol 2000;138:87–92.

192. Arivazhagan A, Devi BI, Kolluri SV, et al. Pediatric intracranial meningiomas–do they differ from their counterparts in adults? Pediatr Neurosurg 2008; 44:43–8.

193. Nunes F, MacCollin M. Neurofibromatosis 2 in the pediatric population. J Child Neurol 2003;18: 718–24.

194. Merten DF, Gooding CA, Newton TH, et al. Meningiomas of childhood and adolescence. J Pediatr 1974;84:696–700.

195. Banerjee J, Paakko E, Harila M, et al. Radiation-induced meningiomas: a shadow in the success story of childhood leukemia. Neuro Oncol 2009;11: 543–9.

196. Maniar TN, Braunstein I, Keefe S, et al. Childhood ALL and second neoplasms. Cancer Biol Ther 2007;6:1525–31.

197. Darling CF, Byrd SE, Reyes-Mugica M, et al. MR of pediatric intracranial meningiomas. AJNR Am J Neuroradiol 1994;15:435–44.

198. Shah MV, Haines SJ. Pediatric skull, skull base, and meningeal tumors. Neurosurg Clin N Am 1992;3:893–924.

199. Wilson PE, Oleszek JL, Clayton GH. Pediatric spinal cord tumors and masses. J Spinal Cord Med 2007;30(Suppl 1):S15–20.

200. Kizana E, Lee R, Young N, et al. A review of the radiological features of intracranial meningiomas. Australas Radiol 1996;40:454–62.

201. Terstegge K, Schorner W, Henkes H, et al. Hyperostosis in meningiomas: MR findings in patients with recurrent meningioma of the sphenoid wings. AJNR Am J Neuroradiol 1994;15:555–60.

202. Buschmann U, Gers B, Hildebrandt G. Uncommon case of a cystic papillary meningioma in an adolescent. Childs Nerv Syst 2005;21:322–6.

203. Harmouch T, Colombat M, El Amri A, et al. Lipomatous meningioma: two case reports. Ann Pathol 2005;25:389–92 [in French].

204. Lake P, Heiden JS, Minckler J. Cystic meningioma. Case report. J Neurosurg 1973;38:638–41.

205. Matyja E, Naganska E, Zabek M, et al. Meningioma with the unique coexistence of secretory and lipomatous components: a case report with immunohistochemical and ultrastructural study. Clin Neuropathol 2005;24:257–61.

206. Yousem DM, Patrone PM, Grossman RI. Leptomeningeal metastases: MR evaluation. J Comput Assist Tomogr 1990;14:255–61.

207. Kobayashi Z, Tsuchiya K, Machida A, et al. Metastatic CNS lymphoma presenting with periventricular dissemination–MRI and neuropathological findings in an autopsy case. J Neurol Sci 2009;277:109–13.

208. Russell EJ, Geremia GK, Johnson CE, et al. Multiple cerebral metastases: detectability with Gd-DTPA-enhanced MR imaging. Radiology 1987; 165:609–17.

209. Bouffet E, Doumi N, Thiesse P, et al. Brain metastases in children with solid tumors. Cancer 1997; 79:403–10.

210. Alavi S, Rashidi A, Khatami AR, et al. Rhabdoid tumor of the kidney presenting with hemiplegia: report of a case. Pediatr Hematol Oncol 2007;24: 123–8.

211. Bisese JH. MRI of cranial metastasis. Semin Ultrasound CT MR 1992;13:473–83.

212. Kim SY, Kim JS, Park HS, et al. Screening of brain metastasis with limited magnetic resonance imaging (MRI): clinical implications of using limited brain MRI during initial staging for non-small cell lung cancer patients. J Korean Med Sci 2005;20:121–6.

213. Pedersen H, McConnell J, Harwood-Nash DC, et al. Computed tomography in intracranial, supratentorial metastases in children. Neuroradiology 1989;31:19–23.

214. Aur RJ, Simone JV, Hustu HO, et al. A comparative study of central nervous system irradiation and intensive chemotherapy early in remission of childhood acute lymphocytic leukemia. Cancer 1972; 29:381–91.

215. Jellinger K, Radaskiewicz TH, Slowik F. Primary malignant lymphomas of the central nervous system in man. Acta Neuropathol 1975;(Suppl 6): 95–102.

216. Hochberg FH, Miller G, Schooley RT, et al. Central-nervous-system lymphoma related to Epstein-Barr virus. N Engl J Med 1983;309:745–8.

217. Lehrich JR, Richardson EP Jr. Malignant lymphoma histiocytic type with Sjogren's syndrome. N Engl J Med 1978;299:1349–59.

218. Lipsmeyer EA. Development of malignant cerebral lymphoma in a patient with systemic lupus erythematosus treated with immunosuppression. Arthritis Rheum 1972;15:183–6.

219. Jack CR Jr, O'Neill BP, Banks PM, et al. Central nervous system lymphoma: histologic types and CT appearance. Radiology 1988;167:211–5.

220. Henry JM, Heffner RR Jr, Dillard SH, et al. Primary malignant lymphomas of the central nervous system. Cancer 1974;34:1293–302.

221. Snanoudj R, Durrbach A, Leblond V, et al. Primary brain lymphomas after kidney transplantation: presentation and outcome. Transplantation 2003; 76:930–7.

222. Hoffman JM, Waskin HA, Schifter T, et al. FDG-PET in differentiating lymphoma from nonmalignant central nervous system lesions in patients with AIDS. J Nucl Med 1993;34:567–75.

223. Barajas RF Jr, Rubenstein JL, Chang JS, et al. Diffusion-weighted MR imaging derived apparent

diffusion coefficient is predictive of clinical outcome in primary central nervous system lymphoma. AJNR Am J Neuroradiol 2010;31:60–6.

224. Sugie M, Ishihara K, Kato H, et al. Primary central nervous system lymphoma initially mimicking lymphomatosis cerebri: an autopsy case report. Neuropathology 2009;29(6):704–7.

225. Noh BW, Park SW, Chun JE, et al. Granulocytic sarcoma in the head and neck: CT and MR imaging findings. Clin Exp Otorhinolaryngol 2009;2:66–71.

226. Caner BE, Mezaki Y, Suto Y, et al. Scintigraphic and MRI studies in a patient with granulocytic sarcoma accompanied with CML and myelofibrosis. Radiat Med 1989;7:165–8.

Imaging of Pediatric Neck Masses

Elliott R. Friedman, MD, Susan D. John, MD*

KEYWORDS
• Mass • Neck • Children • Ultrasound • MRI

Palpable neck masses are a common indication for pediatric imaging. Such lesions may be caused by infectious, inflammatory, tumoral, traumatic, lymphovascular, immunologic, or congenital etiologies. Many are asymptomatic and noticed incidentally by patients or on physical examination, whereas others are brought to clinical attention because of the mass effect on, or compromise of, the aerodigestive tract; fever or symptoms related to acute infection; inflammatory disease; pain; or cosmetic deformity.

As compared with adults, where contrast-enhanced computed tomography (CT) is the mainstay of initial assessment for palpable or symptomatic lesions in the neck, radiological assessment of neck masses in young children should be tailored based on patient presentation and physical examination, as well as clinical suspicion. The goal of imaging should be to help arrive at a diagnosis or limited differential in an efficient manner while minimizing radiation exposure. Plain film radiography, particularly the lateral soft-tissue neck view, is the most appropriate initial assessment of the toxic-appearing child or the child with potential airway compromise. Although radiographs provide little direct information about the composition of a neck mass in many cases, the lateral neck radiograph allows quick and reliable information about the presence of a retropharyngeal mass or other causes of airway obstruction, and guides further imaging workup. Proper technique is crucial because poor inspiratory effort or lack of neck extension can produce buckling of the retropharyngeal soft tissues, which can mimic pathology.

Ultrasound (US) should serve as the primary initial imaging modality in children for palpable masses and assessment of superficial glandular structures, such as the thyroid and salivary glands. Because of the smaller neck size and less subcutaneous fat, sonographic penetration and resolution is generally improved as compared with adults. Additional advantages include ready availability and quick interpretation, lower cost as compared with cross-sectional imaging, and lack of radiation exposure. US easily determines the solid or cystic composition of a lesion, and color Doppler can assess vascularity of solid masses. Lymph nodes are the most common palpable neck masses in children and have a characteristic appearance. Sonography often allows accurate diagnosis of neck lesions without additional imaging workup (**Fig. 1**).

Both magnetic resonance (MR) imaging and CT are used for additional evaluation of neck masses in children, when necessary. MR imaging is advantageous because it imparts no ionizing radiation exposure, and evaluation of tissue signal intensity and enhancement characteristics allows confidant assessment of many lesions. However, MR imaging requires sedation in infants and young children, which can be problematic. CT is usually more readily available, particularly in the emergent setting, and quicker scan times lessen the potential for motion degradation of scan quality or need for sedation. CT findings often complement MR imaging, particularly in the assessment of osseous involvement.

INFECTIOUS/INFLAMMATORY LESIONS

Lymphoid hyperplasia within Waldeyer's ring is a common finding in the pediatric population and a frequent cause of upper airway obstruction.[1]

The authors have nothing to disclose.
Department of Diagnostic & Interventional Imaging, University of Texas Health Science Center at Houston, 6431 Fannin-MSB2.130B, Houston, TX 77030, USA
* Corresponding author.
E-mail address: Susan.D.John@uth.tmc.edu

Radiol Clin N Am 49 (2011) 617–632
doi:10.1016/j.rcl.2011.05.005

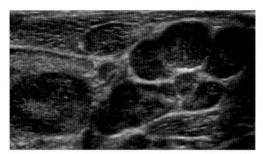

Fig. 1. Cervical lymphadenopathy. Multiple hypoechoic nodules representing enlarged lymph nodes in a child with Bartonella infection.

Lateral radiographs should be obtained with the neck extended, during nasal inspiration with the mouth closed. Adenoidal size is age dependent, enlarging rapidly after birth, reaching a maximum size between 7 and 10 years old, and then progressively decreasing (**Fig. 2**).[2] The presence of small nasopharyngeal cysts is common and should not be confused with a tumor. Palatine tonsillar hypertrophy appears as smooth, rounded, or oval soft-tissue masses on either side of the oropharynx. Hypertrophic palatine tonsils are generally hyperintense to muscle on T2-weighted images and isointense and isoattenuating to muscle on T1-weighted images and CT, respectively (**Fig. 3**). Hypertrophic lingual tonsils are

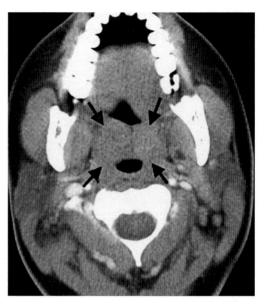

Fig. 3. Hypertrophied tonsils. Axial CT shows bilateral palatine tonsillar hypertrophy (*arrows*) with apposition in the midline.

similar in appearance to palatine tonsils, but they occur at the tongue base, often filling the vallecula.

Anecdotally, lymph nodes account for the most common palpable neck mass in a child. The most common cause of cervical adenitis is viral infection, typically presenting with small bilateral lymph nodes most commonly involving the submandibular and upper internal jugular chains. Acute unilateral lymph node enlargement is most often caused by a bacterial infection originating in the oropharynx or elsewhere along the drainage pathway.[3] Retropharyngeal lymph nodes are a common location for cervical adenitis in children aged 1 to 5 years, because these nodes serve as a drainage pathway for infections of the nasopharynx and tonsil. Infected retropharyngeal nodes may suppurate and perforate into the retropharyngeal or parapharyngeal spaces. Lateral soft tissue neck radiographs are often the initial radiological evaluation ordered. Typical findings include thickening of the retropharyngeal soft tissues, with smooth, curved anterior displacement of the cervical airway, and loss of the normal step off of the posterior hypopharyngeal wall and posterior wall of the trachea.[4]

US reliably distinguishes simple lymphadenopathy from suppurative lymph nodes and developing abscess. Simple adenopathy appears as discrete round-to-oval lesions or confluent masses. Color Doppler imaging demonstrates increased blood flow to inflamed lymph nodes. With suppuration, the central portion of the node becomes hypoechoic.

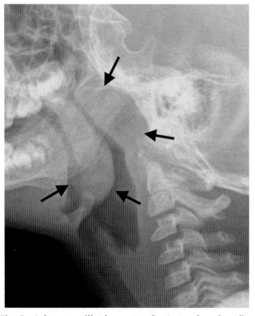

Fig. 2. Adenotonsillar hypertrophy. Lateral neck radiograph demonstrating adenoidal and palatine tonsillar enlargement (*arrows*) with associated narrowing of the nasopharyngeal and oropharyngeal airway.

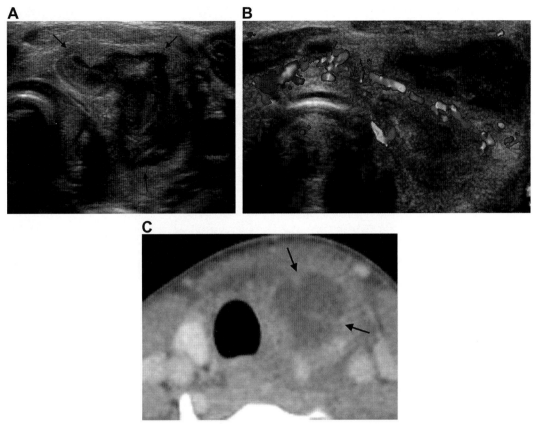

Fig. 4. Neck abscess secondary to infected fourth branchial cleft cyst. (A) US of an anterior neck abscess shows a central hypoechoic fluid collection with internal debris, surrounded by a thick rim of solid tissue (arrows). The abscess involves the left lobe of the thyroid gland. (B) Color Doppler imaging reveals increased blood flow around the fluid collection and within the internal septations. (C) Contrast enhanced CT demonstrates the peripherally enhancing abscess (arrows) but with less soft-tissue detail.

Abscesses appear as hypoechoic to anechoic masses with a variably thick rim of solid tissue (Fig. 4). Contrast-enhanced CT is considered the investigation of choice for assessing deep cervical space neck infections. Cellulitis generally appears as low attenuation soft tissue and muscular edema, which obliterates normal fat planes, typically without rim enhancement. The most characteristic appearance of a deep neck abscess is low attenuation and complete rim enhancement; however, this appearance usually overlaps with phlegmon or cellulitis (Fig. 5).[5] Multiple studies have demonstrated that CT is highly sensitive but not specific for the diagnosis of a deep neck space abscess, because phlegmonous changes and frank pus often have a similar imaging appearance. Individual imaging findings have variable predictive value. Lucency is highly sensitive but has low specificity, whereas complete rim enhancement is more specific but less sensitive in identifying a drainable abscess.[6] In general,

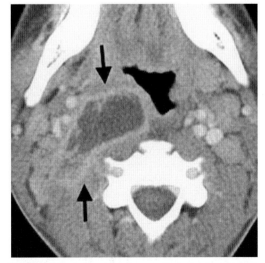

Fig. 5. Retropharyngeal abscess. Note the peripherally enhancing, centrally low attenuation abscess in the lateral retropharyngeal space (arrows), with a retropharyngeal edema.

US is more specific but less sensitive than contrast enhanced CT for abscess detection. Recently, methicillin-resistant *Staphylococcus aureus* (MRSA) abscess has become more prevalent (**Fig. 6**).

Nontuberculous mycobacteria (NTM) are responsible for most granulomatous lesions of the head and neck in immunocompetent children in the United States. Characteristic clinical manifestations include slowly enlarging solitary or clustered unilateral submandibular or preauricular nodal masses. Nodes progress to liquefaction and suppuration in approximately 50% of patients, with sinus tract formation in approximately 10%. Nodal calcifications are more suggestive of tuberculous adenitis.[7] Tuberculosis (TB) of the neck, most frequently found in children with HIV, usually produces bilateral adenopathy that is more diffuse than NTM, most commonly involving the posterior cervical, high internal jugular chain, and submandibular nodes. In the early granulomatous stage, the involved nodes demonstrate homogenous enhancement with or without a minimal amount of necrosis. The enhancing regions of granulation tissue are hyperintense on T2-weighted images. Tuberculous adenitis progresses to central necrosis, the most common imaging manifestation. At this stage, a conglomerate nodal mass may demonstrate low density on CT or increased signal intensity on T2-weighted MR imaging, with a thick rim of peripheral enhancement and minimally effaced fascial planes (**Fig. 7**). With advanced disease, the nodal capsule may rupture, resulting in multiple adherent nodes and loss of adjacent soft-tissue planes, forming a *cold abscess*, a frank abscess that may drain through

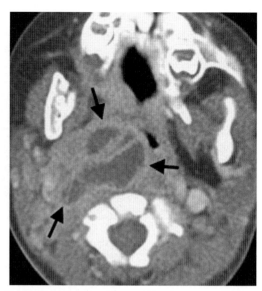

Fig. 7. Tuberculous abscess. This abscess manifests as conglomerate adenopathy progressing to central necrosis, involving the retropharyngeal, high internal jugular, and posterior cervical regions (*arrows*).

a sinus tract to the skin.[8] Treated TB typically appears as fibrocalcified nodes.[9]

VASCULAR MALFORMATIONS AND HEMANGIOMAS

According to the classification initially proposed by Mulliken and Glowacki,[10] vascular malformations are distinguished from hemangiomas, which represent vasoformative tumors. Hemangiomas are proliferative endothelial cell lesions and, therefore, demonstrate increased mitotic activity. Vascular malformations are caused by errors in vascular morphogenesis, have normal endothelial cell mitotic activity, and are classified according to vessel type and hemodynamics.[10] Vascular malformations are present at birth, grow slowly, commensurate with patients, and do not spontaneously regress. There is no associated gender or racial predilection. Clinically, vascular malformations tend to be compressible. Infantile hemangiomas are rarely present at birth; however, 90% become clinically apparent during the first month of life. Hemangiomas are more common in preterm infants, girls, and Caucasians. Hemangiomas are characterized by a rapid proliferative phase during the first year of life, followed by a period of gradual spontaneous involution, which may continue for several years.[11,12] Hemangiomas may arise in or around critical structures, such as the airway, and rapid growth can result in progressive stridor and airway compromise. Clinically,

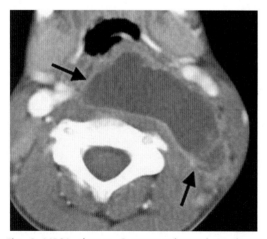

Fig. 6. MRSA abscess. Contrast-enhanced CT shows a multilocular low-attenuation retropharyngeal collection extending to the carotid space (*arrows*).

hemangiomas are often firm or rubbery and less commonly involve bone than vascular malformations. Additional vascular tumors include congenital hemangioma, hemangioendothelioma, and angiosarcoma. Congenital hemangiomas differ from the infantile type in that they are typically fully formed at birth, do not demonstrate accelerated or disproportionate postnatal growth, and do not express the GLUT1 transporter. Based on their natural history, congenital hemangiomas are divided into rapidly involuting and noninvoluting subtypes.[13–15]

Lymphatic malformations (LMs) are cystic masses composed of dysplastic endothelium-lined lymphatic channels filled with protein-rich fluid. LMs may be detected antenatally, but usually present at birth or within the first few years of life, grow proportionately with the child, and do not spontaneously regress. LMs may suddenly enlarge as a consequence of hemorrhage or infection. Skeletal distortion and overgrowth may occur with extensive lesions. The majority of LMs are sporadic, but they may occur as part of a syndrome, such as Turner syndrome; Noonan syndrome; or trisomy 21, 13, or 18.[11,12] On clinical examination, LMs may present as a localized cystic, solid, or spongy mass or cause diffuse infiltration and enlargement of the affected region. The most common locations in the suprahyoid neck are the masticator and submandibular spaces, whereas the posterior cervical space is the most common location in the infrahyoid neck. LMs tend to be trans-spatial, often insinuating between normal structures without significant mass effect on them. Fluid-fluid levels may be present. LMs are usually cystic lesions with multiple thin, irregular septations.[12] Macrocystic LMs are most common and are easily identified by US as a multi-loculated cystic mass. Color Doppler imaging reveals blood flow only within the walls and septations of these lesions. Microcystic LMs appear hyperechoic because of numerous interfaces (Fig. 8). Uncomplicated LMs usually appear hypodense on CT, and low signal intensity on T1-weighted and markedly hyperintense on T2-weighted MR images. However, the density on CT and signal intensity on MR imaging vary, depending on the protein content and the presence of blood products (Fig. 9). Vascular flow voids and flow-related enhancements are not characteristic of LMs, and suggest the presence of a high-flow vascular malformation. Following the administration of contrast, the cyst walls and septations enhance, but the fluid contained within the cystic space does not enhance. In the absence of prior treatment, areas of enhancement within the lesion may represent venous rests within a mixed lymphaticovenous malformation (Fig. 10).[12] The main differential diagnosis for multi-septated macrocystic lesions in the fetus or newborn is teratoma and venous malformation. The presence of fluid-fluid levels, lack of enhancement, and absence of phleboliths differentiate LM from venous malformation. The absence of fat or calcification within the lesion differentiates LM from teratoma. Microcystic LMs may be more confusing because tiny cystic spaces may simulate a diffusely enhancing lesion. Macrocystic LMs are treated with surgical excision or sclerotherapy. Microcystic LMs are usually treated with staged resections.[11,12]

Venous malformations (VMs) are low-flow vascular malformations that consist of dysplastic endothelium-lined venous channels. Clinical examination typically reveals blue or purplish discoloration of the skin and a soft or spongy, compressible mass that expands with the Valsalva

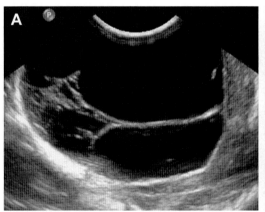
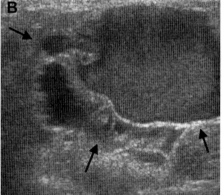

Fig. 8. Cervical lymphangioma (cystic hygroma). (A) US demonstrates the cystic nature of this lesion with numerous, thin internal septations. (B) US in a different patient shows echogenic debris suspended in the fluid in one of the locules of this multi-septated lymphangioma (arrows), caused by internal hemorrhage.

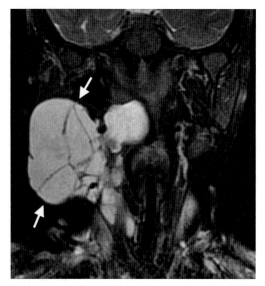

Fig. 9. Lymphatic malformation. Fat-suppressed T2-weighted coronal MR imaging demonstrates multilocular, trans-spatial cystic mass with hyperintense signal intensity (*arrows*).

maneuver or with dependent positioning. VMs grow proportionately with the child, but may enlarge during puberty or following trauma or attempted surgical resection.[13] VMs are most commonly located in the buccal region, masticator space, sublingual space, orbit, tongue, and dorsal neck. VMs can be trans-spatial, and mixed lymphaticovenous malformations are common. Lesions may involve superficial or deep tissues and be localized or diffuse. The characteristic imaging finding of VMs is the presence of phleboliths, easily demonstrated as rounded, calcific densities on CT or depicted as signal voids on MR imaging. VMs are typically isodense to muscle

on nonenhanced CT, variably hypointense to isointense as compared with muscle on T1-weighted MR imaging and hyperintense on T2-weighted imaging with more intense signal in malformations with larger vascular channels (**Fig. 11**). VMs with smaller vascular channels may have a more solid appearance. VMs may also contain venous lakes, which appear as discrete areas of homogenous high T2 signal intensity.[12,16] Enhancement within VMs is variable. Adjacent fat hypertrophy may be present. Magnetic resonance angiography (MRA) is normal, but magnetic resonance venography (MRV) may demonstrate enlarged or anomalous veins in the vicinity of the VM.[12] US demonstrates a compressible collection of variably sized vascular channels without evidence of high flow. Doppler evaluation shows monophasic, low-velocity venous flow. Phleboliths appear as circumscribed signal voids with acoustic shadowing. Treatment options include sclerotherapy and surgical resection.[12,13]

Infantile hemangiomas are the most common tumor of the head and neck in infancy. US accurately identifies most hemangiomas and arteriovenous malformations (AVMs). In most cases, hemangiomas appear heterogeneously echogenic or hypoechoic. There may be small hypoechoic areas that demonstrate flow with color Doppler. Prominent intralesional vessels are more likely to be seen with vascular malformations on grayscale images. Hemangiomas tend to be comprised of more solid tissue, whereas AVMs consist predominantly of vascular structures. Color Doppler shows multiple internal vessels, usually with a high vessel density (**Fig. 12**). Mean peak venous velocity tends to be higher in AVMs than hemangiomas because of greater arteriovenous. On CT, proliferating hemangiomas appear as

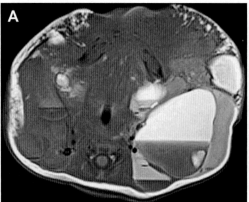
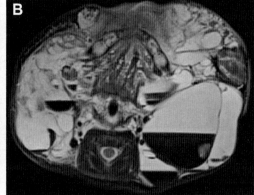

Fig. 10. Lymphaticovenous malformation. T1-weighted (*A*) and T2-weighted with fat saturation (*B*) axial images demonstrating large multilocular and trans-spatial, insinuating lesion with hemorrhage-fluid levels.

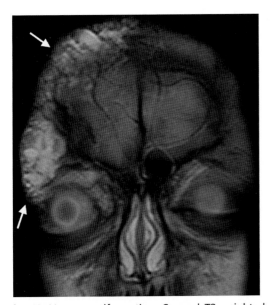

Fig. 11. Venous malformation. Coronal T2-weighted image demonstrating diffuse, infiltrating hyperintense lesion in the scalp (*arrows*) that extends into the right orbit.

lobulated solid tumors that are isodense with muscle, and they enhance rapidly and intensely following the administration of contrast and demonstrate rapid washout of contrast. Phleboliths and calcifications are not characteristic of infantile hemangiomas and should suggest a different diagnosis.[12] Calcifications are found in a minority of congenital hemangiomas.[17] Involuting hemangiomas may contain foci of fat. During the proliferative phase, hemangiomas appear as a lobulated mass isointense to muscle on T1-weighted MR imaging and moderately hyperintense with flow voids on T2-weighted MR imaging. Hemangiomas demonstrate robust enhancement (**Fig. 13**).[12] Small soft-tissue satellite lesions may be present adjacent to or distant from the dominant mass. Involuting hemangiomas are characterized by the accumulation of fibrofatty tissue with increased heterogeneity on both T1- and T2-weighted imaging, fewer signs of fast-flow vascularity, and variable enhancement.[16]

Hemangiomas are rarely found in the airway, most commonly localized to the subglottic larynx (SGH), where they can be associated with airway

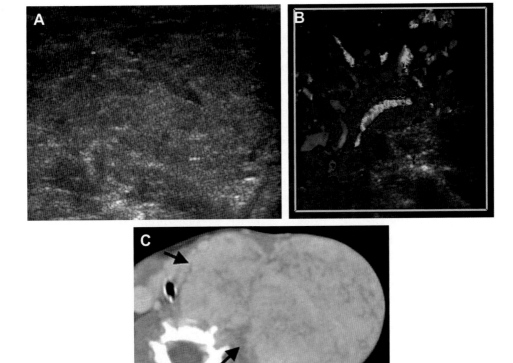

Fig. 12. Hemangioma. (*A*) US appearance of hemangioma with heterogeneous echotexture and a few tubular hypoechoic structures representing blood vessels. (*B*) Color Doppler imaging demonstrates numerous vessels coursing through the mass. (*C*) With contrast-enhanced CT, the mass enhances strongly. CT better outlines the extent of this large lesion (*arrows*).

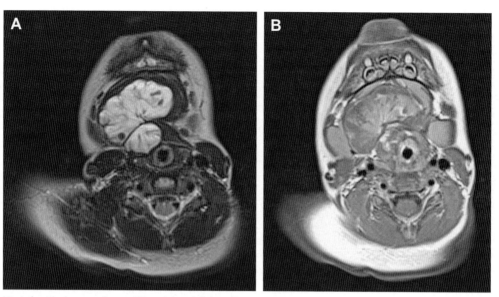

Fig. 13. Infantile hemangioma. T2-weighted (*A*) and postcontrast T1-weighted (*B*) axial images demonstrate well-defined, T2 hyperintense, enhancing, solid sublingual mass with central flow voids.

obstruction, and most commonly present with biphasic stridor.[18,19] Diagnosis is confirmed by endoscopy, and imaging may not be necessary in children with isolated SGH.[19] Radiographic evaluation is helpful, especially when endoscopic findings are inconclusive, or to evaluate the soft tissue extent of deep lesions that compromise the airway or potentially involve vital structures. Anteroposterior (AP) radiographs in SGH classically show asymmetric subglottic narrowing, unlike the concentric symmetric narrowing of congenital subglottic stenosis. However, 50% of the time, the subglottic narrowing may be symmetric, as occurs in patients with circumferential lesions or hemangiomas located centrally within the airway on the AP projection.[20] The lateral film may reveal a subglottic mass. Approximately half of all children with SGH also have cutaneous hemangiomas, most commonly in a beard distribution (preauricular, chin, lower lip, neck). The PHACES association, manifested by posterior fossa malformations, segmental hemangiomas, arterial anomalies, cardiovascular defects, eye abnormalities, and sternal or ventral defects has been reported to be present in up to 2% of children with facial hemangiomas and 20% of children with segmental facial hemangiomas.[18] In such cases, further evaluation with intracranial MRA and brain MR imaging is recommended. Infantile hemangiomas that do not interfere with vital functions can usually be managed expectantly, anticipating involution.

CONGENITAL LESIONS

Thyroglossal duct cyst (TDC) is the most common congenital neck mass. TDCs can be located anywhere along the course of the thyroglossal duct from the base of the tongue to the thyroid gland, most commonly at the level of the hyoid bone.[21] Suprahyoid and hyoid level TDCs are usually located in the midline, whereas infrahyoid TDCs can be paramedian and are embedded in the strap muscles. Most TDC present as a painless, enlarging neck mass or infection.[22] On US, TDCs appear as hypoechoic or anechoic lesions with a thin outer wall and increased through transmission. Cysts may demonstrate increased heterogeneity secondary to proteinaceous content (**Fig. 14**). Importantly, the sonographic appearance does not correlate with the presence of infection or inflammation. It is necessary to confirm the presence of a normal thyroid gland. CT or MR imaging is performed to characterize the mass, define the extent of the lesion, and exclude other lesions. Simple TDCs are low density, usually unilocular but occasionally septated, well-circumscribed lesions on CT with well-defined walls (**Fig. 15**).[22] On MR imaging, TDCs are usually homogenously hyperintense on T2-weighted imaging. On T1-weighted imaging, signal intensity is variable because of differing protein content. Rim enhancement may be seen following intravenous contrast administration. The treatment of TDCs is surgical excision using the Sistrunk procedure in which the entire

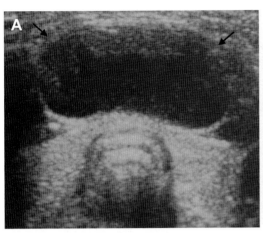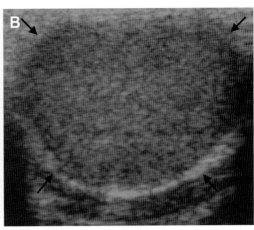

Fig. 14. Thyroglossal duct cyst. (A) US shows a midline, thin-walled, anechoic cyst anterior to the thyroid isthmus (arrow). (B) US in a different child shows a cyst filled with echogenic colloid (arrows).

cyst, tract, and central body of the hyoid bone are resected en bloc. Sistrunk's operative approach has been advocated to reduce the incidence of postoperative recurrence.[21]

A solid mass in association with a presumed TDC may represent ectopic thyroid tissue or, rarely, carcinoma. If ectopic thyroid tissue coexists within a TDC and if this tissue is the patients' only functioning thyroid tissue, resection of the ectopic thyroid with the cyst will render patients permanently hypothyroid. Malignancy is present in less than 1% of TDCs, and the overwhelming majority is papillary thyroid carcinoma.[23] Most patients with TDCs and associated malignancy are adults,

but there are reports of carcinomas occurring in children as young as 6 years of age. Thyroid carcinoma arising in a TDC may be clinically indistinguishable from a benign TDC. Carcinoma should be considered in TDCs that have a mural nodule, calcification, or both.[24]

As opposed to the median/paramedian location of TDCs, cystic anomalies of the branchial apparatus are typically located more laterally in the neck. Second branchial cleft cysts (BCCs) are by far the most common, most often found posterior to the submandibular gland, lateral to the carotid

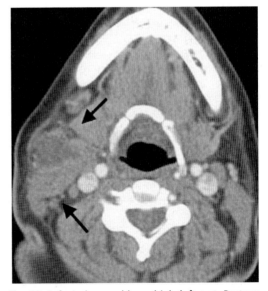

Fig. 16. Infected second branchial cleft cyst. Postcontrast axial CT demonstrates a peripherally enhancing cystic lesion located posterolateral to the submandibular gland just below the angle of the mandible (arrows). Stranding of adjacent soft tissues and loss of fat planes indicates inflammation.

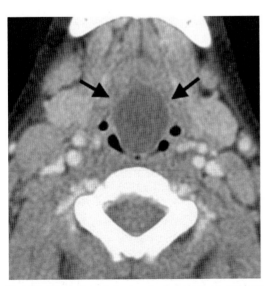

Fig. 15. Thyroglossal duct cyst. Postcontrast axial CT image demonstrating well-defined midline cystic lesion (arrows) exerting mass effect on the airway at the level of the floor of mouth.

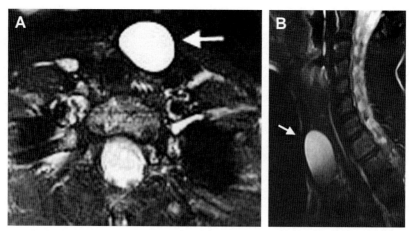

Fig. 17. Third branchial cleft cyst. Axial (*A*) and sagittal (*B*) T2-weighted fat-suppressed images show well-defined T2 hyperintense cystic lesion in the anterior left neck at the level of the thyroid gland (*arrow*), a pathologically proven branchial cleft cyst.

space, and anteromedial to the sternocleidomastoid muscle. Second BCCs may occur anywhere along the tract of the second branchial cleft tract from the palatine tonsil to the supraclavicular region. On imaging, BCCs demonstrate typical cystic appearance, usually without significant wall enhancement, unless infected (**Fig. 16**). The notch sign, a focal projection of the cyst between the internal and external carotid artery bifurcation, is considered pathognomonic for a second BCC.[25]

Third and fourth branchial pouch sinuses arise from the base and apex of the piriform sinus respectively. Anomalies of the third and fourth branchial remnants typically present as recurrent neck infections or abscesses, usually on the left side (**Fig. 17**). Suppurative thyroiditis or recurrent thyroid abscess in children (see **Fig. 4**) have previously been attributed to the fourth branchial pouch sinus tracts; however, they may actually be caused by pyriform sinus fistulas arising from persistence of a patent thymopharyngeal duct.[26] Third BCCs, although rare, are the second most common cystic lesion of the posterior cervical space after lymphatic malformations, located deep or posterior to the sternocleidomastoid muscle and posterior to the common or internal carotid arteries.[27]

Defective pathways of embryologic descent of thymic primordium can present with solid or cystic masses anywhere along the pathway of thymic descent from the angle of the mandible to the superior mediastinum. Ectopic cervical thymus is common at autopsy but usually asymptomatic. US is preferred for initial assessment and may demonstrate characteristic linear echogenic septa and scattered echogenic foci. On MR imaging, thymic tissue has a slightly higher T1 signal than muscle, and a slightly less T2 signal than fat. Cervical thymic cysts are rare lesions derived from the thymopharyngeal duct and are usually intimately associated with the carotid space. Imaging factors that may help distinguish a thymic cyst from a cystic branchial remnant include cigar shape and extension into the superior mediastinum.[28]

An ectopic thyroid can occur anywhere along the initial path of descent of the thyroid, most commonly occurring as lingual thyroid, posterior to the foramen cecum at the base of the tongue. I-123 scintigraphy will demonstrate uptake in the ectopic location and can also identify normally located thyroid tissue. US readily characterizes a mass at the base of the tongue and provides assessment for orthotopic thyroid tissue (**Fig. 18**). Approximately 70% of patients with lingual thyroid have no other functioning thyroid tissue, so

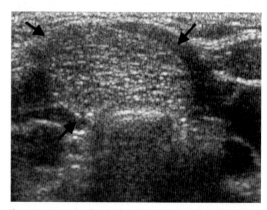

Fig. 18. Ectopic thyroid. US shows a homogeneously echogenic mass (*arrows*) that represents thyroid tissue high in the anterior neck above the thyroid cartilage.

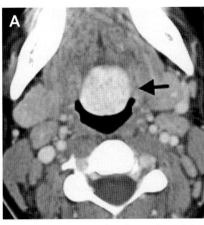
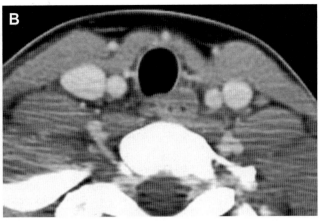

Fig. 19. Lingual thyroid. Enhanced axial CT scans demonstrate high-attenuation, well-defined mass (*arrow*) in the midline base of tongue (*A*) and absence of normal thyroid tissue in the lower neck (*B*).

imaging should include evaluation of the thyroid bed.[29] CT demonstrates typical high attenuation of thyroidal tissue (**Fig. 19**).

Fibromatosis colli is a benign fusiform mass arising within the sternocleidomastoid muscle of a neonate. US is the imaging modality of choice, and characteristic imaging findings in conjunction with clinical features of congenital torticollis usually obviate the need for additional imaging. Most masses are either hyperechoic or mixed echogenicity with a surrounding hypoechoic rim, and move synchronously with the muscle. Involvement is more common on the right side and in the lower third of the muscle (**Fig. 20**).[30]

Laryngoceles are air- or fluid-filled outpouchings of the laryngeal saccule that communicate with the laryngeal ventricle and are a rare cause of airway obstruction in infants. An internal laryngocele remains confined to the supraglottic paraglottic space, lying medial to the thyrohyoid membrane. An external or mixed laryngocele, the more common type, penetrates through the thyrohyoid membrane and may fluctuate in size with alterations in intralaryngeal pressure. The CT density or the MR signal intensity of the laryngocele is variable, depending on whether the cyst is filled with air, fluid, or proteinaceous debris. An infected laryngocele, filled with pus, is a laryngopyocele, demonstrating higher attenuation fluid contents, possible air-fluid level, and a thickened, enhancing rim on CT.[31]

Dermoid cysts are lined by ectodermally derived squamous epithelium, and contain skin appendages within the cyst wall. Approximately 7% of dermoid cysts occur in the head and neck, typically in a midline, suprahyoid location. The floor of the mouth is the most common cervical location. The presence of lipid attenuation or signal intensity material in a unilocular lesion, when present, is helpful in diagnosing dermoid cysts. Small globules of fat within the cyst lumen create a sack-of-marbles appearance, which is essentially pathognomonic for a dermoid cyst (**Fig. 21**). Lipid-fluid levels may be present. The cyst wall may calcify or enhance.[25]

BENIGN AND MALIGNANT TUMORS

Lipomas are benign tumors of fat, most commonly located in the posterior triangle of the neck. These tumors are usually an incidental finding on imaging and fairly uncommon in the first 2 decades of life. Lipomas typically appear as well-defined homogenous fatty masses, echogenic on US, low attenuation on CT, and increased signal intensity on standard spin echo MR imaging sequences.

Multiple localized neurofibromas or larger plexiform neurofibromas are common in children with neurofibromatosis type 1. Localized neurofibromas may involve the skin and subcutaneous tissues or

Fig. 20. Fibromatosis colli. US shows the body of the sternocleidomastoid muscle expanded by a solid, echogenic mass of fibrous tissue. Note the hypoechoic muscle tissue tapering at the margins of the mass (*arrows*).

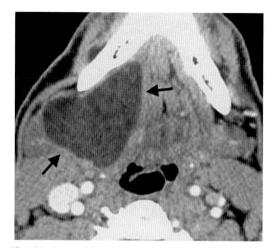

Fig. 21. Dermoid cyst. Postcontrast axial CT at the level of the floor of mouth shows a well-defined, low-attenuation sublingual lesion with sack-of-marbles appearance (*arrows*).

Plexiform neurofibromas are manifested by multiple masses or fusiform enlargement of peripheral nerves, usually involving a long segment of a major nerve trunk and multiple branches, producing a bag-of-worms appearance.[32]

Teratomas are histologically heterogeneous neoplasms usually composed of elements from all 3 germ cell layers, which may have predominantly solid, cystic, or mixed morphology with variable degrees of structural differentiation. Most teratomas in the neck in children are of the mature type and are histologically benign. Teratomas are typically large, heterogeneous masses commonly located in the anterior or lateral neck, often presenting in the newborn period with respiratory distress or feeding difficulties. Teratomas are classically multilocular masses with areas of calcification and macroscopic fat, not infrequently containing foci of thyroid tissue (**Fig. 23**).[33]

Malignancies of the nasopharynx, such as lymphoma, rhabdomyosarcoma, and nasopharyngeal carcinoma, can overlap considerably with respect to their imaging appearance. Although MR imaging appearance may suggest a particular diagnosis, its most important utility is to delineate the extent of disease.

Lymphoma is the most common malignant tumor of the head and neck in children. Hodgkin's lymphoma has a predilection for internal jugular chain lymph nodes, often with involvement of contiguous nodal groups in the mediastinum. Non-Hodgkin lymphoma (NHL) frequently manifests as noncontiguous adenopathy and more commonly demonstrates extranodal disease,

deeper tissues of the neck, or present as multiple bilateral paraspinal masses. Neurofibromas are generally slightly hypoattenuating with respect to muscle on CT. Lesions are hypointense on T1-weighted imaging and hyperintense on T2-weighted imaging with contrast enhancement. A characteristic imaging appearance is the target sign, manifested by a central hypointense region and peripheral hyperintensity on T2-weighted imaging (**Fig. 22**). US may simulate a cyst, with a well-defined hypoechoic mass with distal acoustic enhancement or may show a target sign.

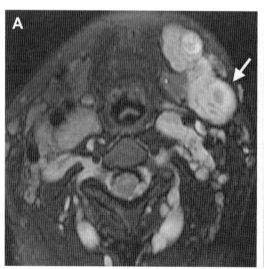
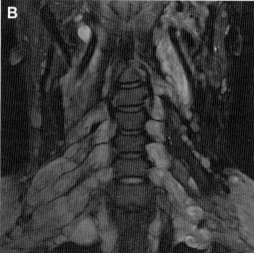

Fig. 22. Neurofibromatosis. Axial (*A*) and coronal (*B*) T2-weighted fat suppressed images demonstrate numerous paraspinal, carotid space, and submandibular region neurofibromas in this child with neurofibromatosis type 1. A target sign is present in the submandibular mass (*arrow*).

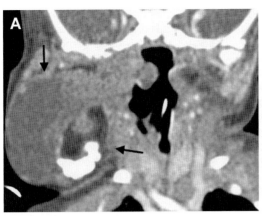

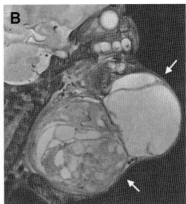

Fig. 23. Teratoma. Coronal CT (*A*) demonstrating heterogeneous mass with areas of soft-tissue, coarse calcification and fat density (*arrows*). Sagittal T2-weighted MR imaging (*B*) shows large multilocular cystic and solid mass (*arrows*).

frequently involving Waldeyer's ring. Retropharyngeal, occipital, parotid, posterior triangle, and submandibular lymphadenopathy should suggest NHL as a possible diagnosis.[34] Enlarged lymph nodes in lymphoma are generally homogenous, and calcifications are rare in the absence of prior therapy, particularly radiation. Enlarged nodes are usually isointense and hyperintense to muscle on T1-weighted and T2-weighted imaging, respectively, and demonstrate variable, usually mild, homogenous enhancement (**Fig. 24**). No reliable size criteria exist for distinguishing benign, reactive from lymphomatous adenopathy. Nodal biopsy is required for diagnosis. Fluorodeoxyglucose (FDG) positron emission tomography typically demonstrates high FDG avidity for nodal and non-nodal disease.

Rhabdomyosarcoma is the most common childhood soft-tissue sarcoma in children younger than 15 years old. Head and neck disease is classified by location into orbital, parameningeal, and nonparameningeal disease. Paramanengeal sites

of involvement include the nasal cavity and paranasal sinuses, pterygoid fossa, nasopharynx, and middle ear cavity.[35] CT usually demonstrates a soft-tissue mass that is isodense to muscle on unenhanced scans, and frequently associated with bone erosion (**Fig. 25**). The skull base should be carefully evaluated for erosion or foraminal widening. On MR imaging, tumors are generally isointense to minimally hyperintense with respect to muscle on T1-weighted images, hyperintense to muscle on T2-weighted images, with avid enhancement. Intratumoral hemorrhage or necrosis may result in an inhomogeneous appearance. Fat-suppressed coronal T1-weighted postcontrast

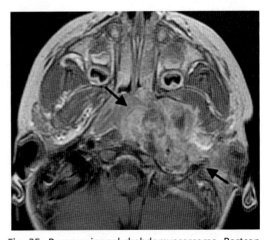

Fig. 25. Parameningeal rhabdomyosarcoma. Postcontrast axial T1-weighted image demonstrates poorly defined, trans-spatial heterogeneously enhancing mass (*arrows*) involving the nasopharyngeal mucosal, parapharyngeal, masticator, and prevertebral spaces with osseous invasion of the clivus and temporal bone. The mass encases and stenoses the internal carotid artery and internal jugular vein.

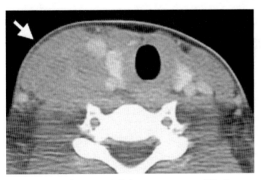

Fig. 24. Lymphoma. Axial postcontrast CT demonstrates bulky right internal jugular chain lymphadenopathy (*arrow*) in this patient with Hodgkin lymphoma.

imaging is helpful to assess for intracranial extension and perineural spread. Metastatic cervical lymphadenopathy has been reported in 12% to 50% of cases.[36] Parameningeal tumors have the poorest prognosis because they are commonly locally invasive with intracranial extension. Adjuvant chemotherapy and radiation are performed after surgical debulking. Postoperative restaging MR imaging should not be performed before 6 weeks postoperatively to minimize confusion between postsurgical changes and residual disease.[35]

Nasopharyngeal carcinoma (NPC) is endemic to Southern China, Southeast Asia, and the Mediterranean Basin. NPC is rare in North America, most commonly affecting patients aged 10 to 20 years. NPC is more common in males and African Americans. The childhood form of NPC is closely linked to Epstein-Barr virus infection, commonly has an undifferentiated histology, and is often associated with locoregionally advanced disease at presentation.[37] Most children have metastatic cervical adenopathy at presentation.[38] The most common clinical presentation is a painless upper neck mass with or without nasal symptoms, such as obstruction, bleeding, or discharge.[37] NPC is characteristically an asymmetric mass arising in the Fossa of Rosenmuller. In children, NPC tends to be slightly hyperintense and moderately hyperintense as compared with muscle on T1- and T2-weighted images, respectively, with homogenous enhancement (**Fig. 26**).[38] Local spread of the tumor into the masticator and parapharyngeal spaces is common. The pharyngobasilar fascia initially acts as a barrier to local spread, directing progression toward the clivus and central skull base. Osseous infiltration is most sensitively detected as a low signal on T1-weighted images. Widening of the petroclival fissure may be seen on CT.[39] Common routes of intracranial spread include extension through foramen lacerum and into the cavernous sinus, direct erosion through the skull base, or perineural spread through foramen ovale.[40] Cervical lymph node involvement is present in 80% to 90% of patients at presentation, 50% of which are bilateral. As opposed to NPC in adults, necrosis within metastatic lymph nodes is uncommon in children.[38] The primary routes of lymphatic drainage from the nasopharynx are the lateral retropharyngeal, high level II, and high level V nodes.[39] Undifferentiated NPC is radiosensitive.[37]

Neuroblastoma may occur anywhere along the sympathetic chain, with up to 5% of primary cases occurring in the neck, primarily in infants. Cervical

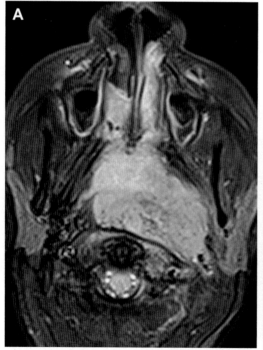
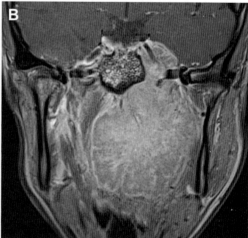

Fig. 26. Nasopharyngeal carcinoma. Axial (*A*) and coronal (*B*) T1-weighted postcontrast images demonstrate a diffusely enhancing trans-spatial, locally invasive nasopharyngeal mass with intracranial extension through a widened foramen lacerum into the cavernous sinus and middle cranial fossa.

neuroblastoma may present as an asymptomatic mass or may cause symptoms by compression of the airway or cranial nerves 9 to 12, Horner syndrome, or heterochromia iridis.[41] On CT, tumors may demonstrate calcification. Internal areas of hemorrhage or necrosis may be present, particularly in larger lesions. Neuroblastomas are mildly hyperintense on T2-weighted imaging with intense enhancement. MR imaging is particularly useful for demonstrating the relationship of the mass to the carotid space. Tumors may invade the skull base with epidural extension. Metaiodobenzylguanidine scintigraphy can be used to detect primary and metastatic neuroblastoma.[42]

REFERENCES

1. Mahboubi S, Marsh RR, Potsic WP, et al. The lateral neck radiograph in adenotonsillar hyperplasia. Int J Pediatr Otorhinolaryngol 1985;10:67–73.

2. Vogler RC, Wippold FJ, Pilgram TK. Age-specific size of the adenoidal fat pad on magnetic resonance imaging. Clin Otolaryngol 2000;25:392–5.

3. Beiler HA, Eckstein TM, Roth H, et al. Specific and nonspecific lymphadenitis in childhood: etiology, diagnosis, and therapy. Pediatr Surg Int 1997;12:108–12.

4. John SD, Swischuk LE. Stridor and upper airway obstruction in infants and children. Radiographics 1992;12:625–43.

5. Malloy KM, Christenson T, Meyer JS, et al. Lack of association of CT findings and surgical drainage in pediatric neck abscesses. Int J Pediatr Otorhinolaryngol 2008;72:235–9.

6. Daya H, Lo S, Papsin BC, et al. Retropharyngeal and parapharyngeal infections in children: the Toronto experience. Int J Pediatr Otorhinolaryngol 2005;69: 81–6.

7. Robson CD, Hazra R, Barnes PD, et al. Nontuberculous mycobacterial infection of the head and neck in immunocompetent children: CT and MR findings. AJNR Am J Neuroradiol 1999;20:1829–35.

8. Hudgins PA. Nodal and nonnodal inflammatory processes of the pediatric neck. Neuroimaging Clin N Am 2000;10:181–92.

9. Robson CD. Imaging of granulomatous lesions of the neck in children. Radiol Clin North Am 2000; 38:969–77.

10. Mulliken JB, Glowacki J. Hemangiomas and vascular malformations in infants and children: a classification based on endothelial characteristics. Plast Reconstr Surg 1982;69:412–22.

11. Sie KC, Tampakopoulou DA. Hemangiomas and vascular malformations of the airway. Otolaryngol Clin North Am 2000;33:209–20.

12. Robertson RL, Robson CD, Barnes PD, et al. Head and neck vascular anomalies of childhood. Neuroimaging Clin N Am 1999;9:115–32.

13. Mulliken JB, Fishman SJ, Burrows PE. Vascular anomalies. Curr Probl Surg 2000;37:517–84.

14. Boon LM, Enjolras O, Mulliken JB. Congenital hemangioma: evidence of accelerated involution. J Pediatr 1996;128:329–35.

15. Krol A, MacArthur CJ. Congenital hemangiomas: rapidly involuting and noninvoluting congenital hemangiomas. Arch Facial Plast Surg 2005;7: 307–11.

16. Baker LL, Dillon WP, Hieshima GB, et al. Hemangiomas and vascular malformations of the head and neck: MR characterization. AJNR Am J Neuroradiol 1993;14:307–14.

17. Gorincour G, Kokta V, Rypens F, et al. Imaging characteristics of two subtypes of congenital hemangiomas: rapidly involuting congenital hemangiomas and non-involuting congenital hemangiomas. Pediatr Radiol 2005;35:1178–85.

18. O-Lee TJ, Messner A. Subglottic hemangioma. Otolaryngol Clin North Am 2008;41:903–11.

19. Zoplewitz BZ, Springer C, Slasky BS, et al. CT of hemangiomas of the upper airway in children. AJR Am J Roentgenol 2005;184:663–70.

20. Cooper M, Slovis TL, Madgy DN, et al. Congenital subglottic hemangioma: frequency of symmetric subglottic narrowing on frontal radiographs of the neck. AJR Am J Roentgenol 1992;159:1269–71.

21. Rosa PA, Hirsch DL, Dierks EL. Congenital neck masses. Oral Maxillofac Surg Clin North Am 2008; 20:339–52.

22. Reede DL, Bergeron RT, Som PM. CT of thyroglossal duct cysts. Radiology 1985;157:121–5.

23. Solomon JR, Rangecroft L. Thyroglossal-duct lesions in childhood. J Pediatr Surg 1984;19:555–61.

24. Branstetter BF, Weissman JL, Kennedy TL, et al. The CT appearance of thyroglossal duct carcinoma. AJNR Am J Neuroradiol 2000;21:1547–50.

25. Koeller KK, Alamo L, Adair CF, et al. Congenital cystic masses of the neck: radiologic-pathologic correlation. Radiographics 1999;19:121–46.

26. Thomas B, Shroff M, Forte V, et al. Revisiting imaging features and the embryologic basis of third and fourth branchial anomalies. AJNR Am J Neuroradiol 2010;31:755–60.

27. Joshi MJ, Provenzano MJ, Sato Y, et al. The rare third branchial cleft cyst. AJNR Am J Neuroradiol 2009;30:1804–6.

28. Burton EM, Mercado-Deane MG, Howell CG, et al. Cervical thymic cysts: CT appearance of two cases including a persistent thymopharyngeal duct cyst. Pediatr Radiol 1995;25:363–5.

29. Rahbar R, Yoon MJ, Connolly LP, et al. Lingual thyroid in children: a rare clinical entity. Laryngoscope 2008;118:1174–9.

30. Chan YL, Cheng JC, Metreweli C. Ultrasonography of congenital muscular torticollis. Pediatr Radiol 1992;22:356–60.

31. Alvi A, Weissman J, Myssiorek D, et al. Computed tomography and magnetic resonance imaging characteristics of laryngocele and its variants. Am J Otolaryngol 1998;19:251–6.

32. Lin J, Martel W. Cross-sectional imaging of peripheral nerve sheath tumors: characteristic signs on CT, MR imaging, and sonography. AJR Am J Roentgenol 2001;176:75–82.

33. Smirniotopoulos JG, Chiechi MV. From the archives of the AFIP. Teratomas, dermoids, and epidermoids of the head and neck. Radiographics 1995;15:1437–55.

34. Aiken AH, Glastonbury C. Imaging Hodgkin and non-Hodgkin lymphoma in the head and neck. Radiol Clin North Am 2008;46:363–78.

35. Lloyd C, McHugh K. The role of radiology in head and neck tumours in children. Cancer Imaging 2010;10:49–61.

36. Yousem DM, Lexa FJ, Bilaniuk LT, et al. Rhabdomyosarcoma in the head and neck: MR imaging evaluation. Radiology 1990;177:683–6.

37. Ayan I, Kaytan E, Ayan N. Childhood nasopharyngeal carcinoma: from biology to treatment. Lancet Oncol 2003;4:13–21.

38. Yabuuchi H, Fukuya T, Murayama S, et al. CT and MR features of nasopharyngeal carcinoma in children and young adults. Clin Radiol 2002;57:205–10.

39. Stambuk HE, Patel SG, Mosier KM, et al. Nasopharyngeal carcinoma: recognizing the radiographic features in children. AJNR Am J Neuroradiol 2005;26:1575–9.

40. Chong VF, Fan YF, Khoo JB. Nasopharyngeal carcinoma with intracranial spread: CT and MR characteristics. J Comput Assist Tomogr 1996;20:563–9.

41. Abramson SJ, Berdon WE, Ruzal-Shapiro C, et al. Cervical neuroblastoma in eleven infants-a tumor with favorable prognosis. Pediatr Radiol 1993;23:253–7.

42. Weber AL, Montandon C, Robson CD. Neurogenic tumors of the neck. Radiol Clin North Am 2000;38:1077–90.

Thoracic Neoplasms in Children

Beverley Newman, MB, BCh

KEYWORDS

• Chest • Pediatric • Neoplasm • Imaging

This article provides an overview of neoplasms that occur in the thorax in childhood, including those of the mediastinum, lung, airway, heart, and chest wall. Different imaging methods and their role in evaluating these lesions are reviewed. Because of the broad topic, the intent is not to cover specific lesions in detail but to emphasize helpful distinguishing features. Non-neoplastic lesions are included only to serve as examples of where they are confused with tumors and should be included as differential diagnostic considerations. The long-term effects of childhood cancer with reference to the thorax are briefly discussed.

IMAGING MODALITIES
Chest Radiographs

Chest radiographs are still usually the first imaging examination obtained in a child with a palpable mass or clinical symptoms referable to the chest.[1] Frontal and lateral views are often helpful in evaluating the location, size, number, and most likely differential diagnostic possibilities when abnormality is visible. The radiographs should be carefully scrutinized for extent of involvement, multiple lesions, and specific features, such as cavitation and calcification as well as pleural, soft tissue, and bone abnormalities. Chest radiographs serve as a triage platform for recommending whether or not and which additional imaging studies are likely to be most useful (**Figs. 1** and **2**). When a neoplasm is suspected or considered, additional cross-sectional imaging, ultrasound (US), CT, or MR imaging is frequently required to better characterize the nature and extent of the mass and its relationship to vital structures (see **Figs. 1** and **2**; **Fig. 3**).

Decubitus views may be obtained to evaluate a suspected pneumothorax, free or loculated pleural fluid, or other fluid-containing lesion. Decubitus views are usually not helpful when there is complete whiteout of a hemithorax. Even if free fluid is present, it cannot be appreciated without any adjacent air or aerated lung.

Fluoroscopic evaluation of the chest still has occasional value, including assessment of an airway foreign body or other airway obstruction, laryngotracheobronchomalacia, or a pulsatile vascular mass. Since the advent of high-quality cross-sectional chest imaging, an esophagram is rarely part of the imaging assessment of a vascular ring or mediastinal mass.

Ultrasound Imaging

There are several questions that can be readily answered, at least partially, on sonographic imaging.[2,3] The thymus is the most common cause of an unusual upper mediastinal contour (see **Fig. 3**). Ectopic thymic tissue in the neck or behind the superior vena cava is a frequent cause of concern for a mediastinal mass. In addition, many anterior mediastinal neoplastic lesions, both benign and malignant, commonly infiltrate or involve the thymus (see **Fig. 1**). The thymus has a characteristic appearance on US and normal thymic tissue or lesions in or adjacent to the thymus are often readily visualized because there is no intervening air-filled lung between the transducer and anterior mediastinum (see **Fig. 3**).[2] Other masses in the anterior mediastinum as well as lesions of the chest wall and pleura often are seen on sonography, allowing characterization of free fluid versus cystic or solid lesions as well as information on vascular flow with spectral and

Financial disclosure: the author has nothing to disclose.

Lucile Packard Children's Hospital at Stanford University School of Medicine, Department of Radiology, 725 Welch Road, Room 1677, Stanford, CA 94305-5913, USA

E-mail address: Bev.newman@stanford.edu

Radiol Clin N Am 49 (2011) 633–664

doi:10.1016/j.rcl.2011.05.010

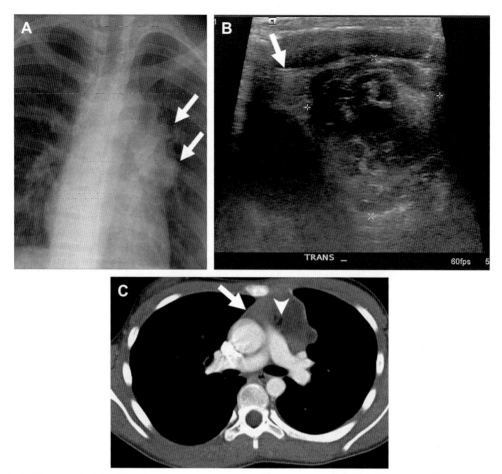

Fig. 1. A 12-year-old girl with a benign anterior mediastinal teratoma. (*A*) Outside chest radiograph contains a large amount of linear artifact. A prominent lobulated left superior mediastinal mass (*arrows*) is, however, appreciated. The lack of silhouetting of the aortic arch and descending aorta suggests an anterior mediastinal location. (*B*) Transverse US and (*C*) axial CT (mediastinal window) of the upper mediastinum shows that the anterior mediastinal mass is probably originating within the thymus. Note the adjacent normal thymic tissue to the right (*arrow*). Multiple hypoechoic cystic and echogenic solid components are evident on US (*B*). On the CT (*C*), solid, fluid, and fatty (*arrowhead*) components are identified.

color Doppler imaging.[1–4] Fat and calcification may also be identified or suspected on US imaging (see **Fig. 1**).

With the advent of routine prenatal US, many chest masses are first imaged in utero. The majority of these lesions are bronchopulmonary malformations but also occasional chest and cardiac neoplasms.

CT

CT is an excellent modality for imaging the chest.[5] Evaluation of a potential thoracic neoplasm typically entails contiguous axial slices between 1 and 5 mm depending on the size of the child and anatomic detail required. Dynamic intravenous contrast injection (2–3 mL/kg) is desirable in

almost all cases, especially in small children who have little natural tissue contrast or fat to separate adjacent structures. A timed or fluoroscopically triggered CT angiogram may be obtained when specific vascular detail is needed. Multiplanar 2-D as well as maximum intensity projection, minimum intensity projection, and 3-D reconstructions are readily obtained with CT and MR images, so that the location, extent, and characteristics of a lesion can be optimally displayed and measured. This helps with therapeutic decisions, surgical planning, and follow-up.

CT imaging has the advantage of being fast, especially with newer multislice or dual-head scanners, so that sedation or anesthesia is only required in small children or those who cannot cooperate with keeping still or holding their breath.

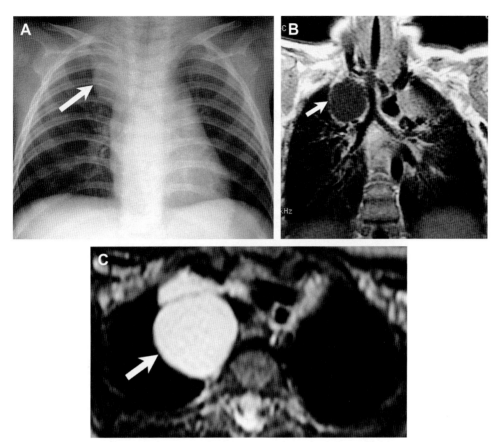

Fig. 2. A 4-year-old boy with a cough—bronchogenic cyst. (*A*) The frontal chest radiograph demonstrates a smooth bulging mass in the right superior mediastinum (*arrow*). (*B*) Coronal T1-weighted image (postcontrast) and (*C*) axial T2-weighted image demonstrate a typical well-defined fluid filled cyst, dark on T1 with rim enhancement and bright on T2-weighted images, located close to the airway (*arrows*).

CT provides excellent spatial resolution with details of pulmonary parenchyma optimally visualized on CT as opposed to MR imaging. Calcification is usually better appreciated on CT than MR imaging whereas fat is typically well characterized on both CT (see **Fig. 1**) and MR imaging and fluid may be more reliably appreciated on MR imaging (T2 bright) (see **Fig. 2**).[6] Proteinaceous fluids, such as blood or lymph, may have soft tissue attenuation on CT and bright signal on T1-weighted MR images, creating difficulty in separating a cystic from a solid lesion; US may be helpful in these circumstances.

The disadvantage of CT imaging is exposure to ionizing radiation at levels considerably higher than plain radiographs.[6] This is especially important in young children who are much more sensitive to ionizing radiation than adults. Careful attention must be paid to having clear clinical indications for obtaining CT and tailoring the study to the needs of the patient. Parameters, such as milliampere second, kilovolt (peak), pitch, collimation,

and slice thickness should be chosen to obtain diagnostic quality imaging with the lowest possible dose. The thyroid should be kept out of the imaging field whenever possible and breast shields can be added in female patients to further decrease breast dose. Multiple series, such as noncontrast followed by contrast scans or late delayed scans, should be avoided unless needed. Electrocardiographically gated CT is associated with a much higher radiation dose and should be reserved for specific indications, such as detailed intracardiac and coronary evaluation. Where appropriate, US or MR imaging should be considered as a substitute for CT.

Iodinated contrast should be used with caution in patients with renal dysfunction, especially with a creatinine level greater than 2 mg/dL. Prehydration with fluids and use of bicarbonate and *N*-acetylcysteine before CT have been advocated to mitigate the nephrotoxic effects of contrast. Patients on dialysis can have their contrast CT scheduled to coordinate with subsequent dialysis.

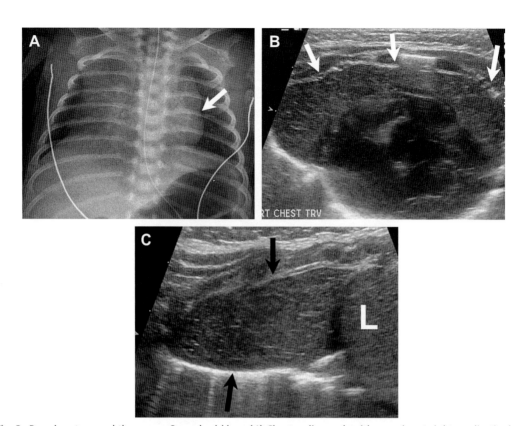

Fig. 3. Prominent normal thymus—a 3-week-old boy. (*A*) Chest radiograph with prominent right mediastinal soft tissue extending to the diaphragm, thought to probably represent normal asymmetric prominence of the thymus. A normal thymic wave sign (indentation of the margin of the thymus by the adjacent ribs) is seen on the left (*arrow*). (*B*) Transverse US and (*C*) right sagittal US images demonstrate the normal sonographic appearance of the anterior thymus (*arrows*) (hypoechoic with small punctate and linear areas of echogenicity) with asymmetric prominence of the right lobe (*B*) extending down to the right hemidiaphragm (*C*). L, liver.

Although contrast-related allergic reactions are uncommon in children, vigilant monitoring by trained staff with quick access to support equipment and drugs is essential. Nonionic contrast agents tend to be used because of fewer allergic and other contrast reactions, such as vomiting. If contrast is needed in children who had a prior contrast reaction, they can be pretreated with oral steroids beginning 24 hours before the imaging study. If intravenous contrast cannot be used for CT, there should be careful reconsideration of the value of the study and whether other alternatives, such as US and MR imaging, might substitute.

MR Imaging

MR imaging provides a great deal of anatomic information as well as tissue characterization with regard to lesions of the chest. MR imaging is superior to CT for evaluating most lesions of the chest wall but suboptimal for assessing lung parenchyma.[4] MR imaging is often equivalent to CT for mediastinal lesions and superior when spine evaluation is required (eg, neuroblastoma).[6] MR imaging is more often used than CT for evaluating cardiac anatomy with the exception of coronary evaluation. MR imaging is superior to CT for cardiac functional assessment, including ventricular volumes and mass, ejection fraction, and cardiac output as well as quantifying volume and direction of vascular flow, valvular regurgitation, and shunts.

The major disadvantage of MR imaging is the length of the examination and, therefore, increased need for sedation or anesthesia as compared with CT. The need for well-trained staff, who are skilled in monitoring and managing children, and constant vigilance regarding the safety of a child imaged by either CT or MR imaging cannot be overemphasized.

New faster sequences are allowing for more rapid MR imaging scanning with improved spatial resolution. New contrast agents allow for improved and prolonged vascular opacification.

Both MR imaging and CT should be used with caution in patients with renal dysfunction. MR imaging contrast is generally contraindicated with an estimated glomerular filtration rate of less than 30 mL/min because of the potential risk of nephrogenic systemic sclerosis, although few cases have been reported in children. Allergic reactions to MR imaging contrast agents are rare.

MR imaging safety is paramount: metallic and personal electronic objects must be removed and all equipment must be MR imaging compatible. Patients, parents, and personnel need to be carefully screened before entering the scanner. Major contraindications to MR imaging include presence of a pacemaker, intracranial vascular clips. and orbital metal.

Prenatal MR imaging is commonly used to further evaluate and follow the nature and extent of thoracic masses picked up on antenatal US examinations. MR imaging is contraindicated in the first trimester of pregnancy and MR imaging contrast agent use is discouraged throughout pregnancy.

Nuclear Imaging

Chest nuclear imaging in children currently has a limited role. Ventilation and perfusion imaging may be used to evaluate airway and vascular pathology and assess for pulmonary emboli or differential lung flow. Bone scan, gallium scan, white blood cell scan, or iodine scan or *m*-iodobenzylguanidine (MIBG) might be used in specific instances to evaluate for bone lesions, infection, thyroid tissue, or neuroblastoma, respectively.

Fluorodeoxyglucose positron emission tomography (FDG PET) detects metabolically active processes, including tumors and inflammation. FDG PET and FDG PET-CT, where the PET metabolic activity and CT anatomic images can be superimposed, are increasingly used to evaluate and follow malignant tumors, especially lymphoma (**Figs. 4** and **5**).[7] One disadvantage of FDG PET and PET-CT is the high dose of ionizing radiation.

MEDIASTINAL MASSES

- Mediastinal masses are more common than intrapulmonary masses in children and have a greater likelihood of being malignant (**Box 1**).
- Compartmentalization of the mediastinum is useful in generating likely differential diagnoses.
- Several lesions, especially adenopathy, lymphoma, and vascular/lymphatic lesions, can occur in multiple different compartments.
- Large lesions often span more than one compartment.

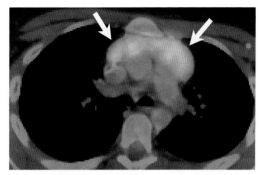

Fig. 4. A 10 year old with thymic rebound. Prior history of large cell lymphoma with increasing soft tissue fullness in the anterior mediastinum. Axial cut from a PET-CT demonstrates homogeneous diffuse uptake of the agent in the normal prominent thymus (*arrows*).

The mediastinum is conveniently divided into 3 spaces that span from superior to inferior. The anterior mediastinum or prevascular space is located in front of the heart and great vessels; the middle mediastinum or vascular space encompasses the heart and most of the major great vessels; and the posterior mediastinum or postvascular space extends from behind the heart to the spine. Special consideration should be given to the inferior mediastinum where masses may be due to diaphragmatic lesions especially diaphragmatic or hiatal hernias.

When necessary, CT or MR imaging can be obtained to define the nature, origin, and extent of a mediastinal lesion.[6] Frequently, a specific diagnosis can be suggested (see **Figs. 1** and **5**). Malignant lymphoma, benign thymic enlargement, teratomas, foregut cysts, and neurogenic tumors account for 80% of mediastinal masses in children.[5]

Anterior Mediastinum

The common masses in the anterior mediastinum or prevascular compartment are remembered most easily by the letter, T, and include thymus, teratoma, thyroid, and T-cell lymphoma.

Normal variations of the thymus include bilateral or unilateral prominence (most often right), thymic hyperplasia, or rebound (see **Figs. 3** and **4**) and ectopic thymic tissue (most often retrocaval or extending into the neck). These variations are a common reason for suspecting a mediastinal mass on a chest radiograph in a child. The concern can frequently be put to rest and additional studies avoided when chest radiographs are reviewed by an experienced pediatric radiologist. When concern persists as to whether the findings represent

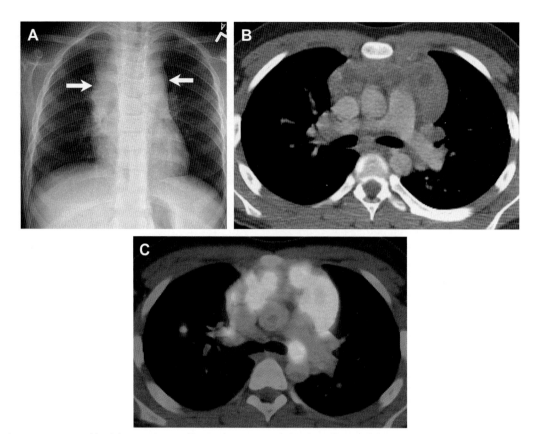

Fig. 5. A 7 year old with anterior mediastinal mass—Hodgkin lymphoma. (*A*) Chest radiograph demonstrates widening of the mediastinum with irregular contours (*arrows*). Note the heterogeneous lumpy appearance of the infiltrated thymus on both CT (*B*) and corresponding PET-CT (*C*) images. There are small abnormal nodes in the hila bilaterally as well as several small pulmonary nodules that take up the FDG, suspicious for intrapulmonary involvement with lymphoma. (*Reprinted from* Rudolph C, Rudolph A, Lister G, et al. Imaging the chest. In: Rudolph's textbook of pediatrics. 22nd edition. United States: McGraw-Hill; 2011 [Fig. 9]; with permission.)

a variation of normal thymus, directed US imaging by an experienced pediatric imager is often helpful in identifying normal hypoechoic thymic tissue versus thymic infiltration or other mass (see **Figs. 1** and **3**).

Normal thymic tissue is characterized by its uniform homogeneous appearance as well as lack of mass effect on adjacent structures. In young infants it tends to be quadrilateral in shape and more triangular in older adolescents with progressive fatty infiltration. Ectopic or atypical thymus is similar in appearance and enhancement and usually directly contiguous with the intrathoracic thymus.[3] Thymic cysts are common, especially in ectopic thymus in the neck. The thymus itself is frequently the site of origin or directly infiltrated by anterior mediastinal neoplastic lesions, including lymphangioma, histiocytosis, teratoma/germ cell tumors (see **Fig. 1**), lymphoma (see **Fig. 5**), thymolipoma, and thymic carcinoma (**Fig. 6**).[6,8]

Lymphoma is the most common cause of a mediastinal tumor in childhood.[9] Both Hodgkin and non-Hodgkin lymphoma (especially T-cell lymphoblastic leukemia/lymphoma type) commonly affect the mediastinum.[7] In Hodgkin lymphoma, a large anterior heterogeneous lobulated mediastinal mass involving the thymus and adjacent nodes with contiguous neck adenopathy is typical (see **Fig. 5**). There are frequently areas of necrosis within the mass. Encasement of adjacent mediastinal vessels and displacement and compression of the airway in children is common in lymphoma.[7,9] CT or MR imaging with sedation or anesthesia must be undertaken with great care in patients with a potentially compromised airway.

Non-Hodgkin lymphoma is more common in younger children and is similar in appearance on imaging to Hodgkin lymphoma, with more frequent involvement of hilar, subcarinal, posterior mediastinal, and paracardiac nodes as well as noncontiguous tumor in the abdomen occurring more fat and calcification (see **Fig. 1**). Malignant germ cell tumors have a male predilection and may be difficult to definitively distinguish from benign teratoma. Suggestive features are a larger, less well-defined mass with extensive central necrosis. There is a propensity for local invasion and pleural and pericardial effusions as well as distant spread. Nonseminomatous germ cell tumors are associated with hematologic malignancies and Klinefelter syndrome.[10]

Thymoma and thymic carcinoma are uncommon in children. Thymomas are slow growing, potentially malignant neoplasms capable of invasive behavior and metastases.[8,11] They are associated with myasthenia gravis (30%–50%), red cell aplasia, or hypogammaglobulinemia.[8,10] A thymoma is usually a unilateral solid/cystic soft tissue mass in the anterior mediastinum. Diffuse implants on pleural, mediastinal, and pericardial surfaces are seen with invasive thymoma; however, pleural effusion is uncommon.[10] Thymomas may occasionally arise in locations other than the anterior mediastinum, including neck, elsewhere in the mediastinum, heart, or in the lung.[8,12] Thymic carcinoma is a rare aggressive thymic neoplasm. This entity is difficult to differentiate by imaging from invasive thymoma, although pleural and pericardial effusions are more common in association with local spread of thymic carcinoma (see **Fig. 6**). Distant metastases are common, including lymph nodes, lung, bone, brain, and liver.[8,10]

Ectopic thyroid and parathyroid tissue may rarely occur in the anterior mediastinum in children. Thyroid and parathyroid neoplasms, both benign and malignant, are likewise uncommon. An anterior mediastinal neoplasm may also be simulated by paramediastinal upper lobe atelectasis, upper lobe airless bronchial atresia, or lung consolidation.

commonly.[7] Lymphoma is optimally staged and followed using FDG PET-CT (see **Fig. 5**).

A mature benign mediastinal teratoma is typically a well-defined soft tissue mass containing

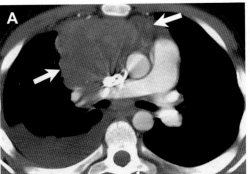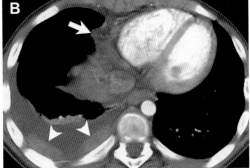

Fig. 6. A 10-year-old—thymic carcinoma. Two axial CT slices (*A, B*) viewed on mediastinal windows illustrate a large inhomogeneous lobulated predominantly anterior medistinal mass (*arrows*). There is contiguous infiiltration of the pleura with multiple areas of pleural enhancing tumor (*arrowheads*) and effusion.

Middle Mediastinum

The middle mediastinum encompasses the vascular space. Adenopathy, bronchopulmonary foregut lesions (bronchogenic cyst predominantly) (see **Fig. 2**), and vascular masses (aneurysm, vascular ring, and vascular/lymphatic malformation) predominate in this compartment. Cardiac and pericardial lesions overlap with middle mediastinal masses. They are discussed later.

Prominent reactive adenopathy often accompanies bacterial infection in children, is less common in most viral infections (adenovirus is an exception), and is particularly prominent with granulomatous inflammation, including tuberculosis, histoplasmosis, and sarcoidosis. Granulomatous adenopathy, especially tuberculosis, as well as atypical mycobacteria is characterized by low attenuation or cavitating nodes. Fibrosing mediastinitis, also known as fibroinflammatory lesion of the mediastinum,[13] may be related to histoplasmosis infection or idiopathic. It is uncommon in children. The ensuing infiltrative fibrous soft tissue that encases and obliterates vessels and airways may be difficult to differentiate from infiltrating mediastinal neoplasms.

Another benign entity that can produce prominent mediastinal adenopathy is Castleman disease (**Fig. 7**).[7] This is a poorly understood rare lymphoproliferative disorder that occurs in both nodal and extranodal sites. The hyaline vascular type is more common and less aggressive than the plasma cell form. A characteristic feature is adenopathy that has increased signal on T2-weighted MR images and enhances markedly with contrast (see **Fig. 7**).

Neoplastic processes tend to produce bulkier and more confluent mass-like adenopathy than infectious causes although the underlying etiology may be difficult to predict. Lymphoma, both Hodgkin and non-Hodgkin types, may occur in the middle mediastinum. Intrapulmonary malignancies may be associated with hilar and mediastinal adenopathy, often ipsilateral. Although intrapulmonary metastases are more common, metastatic mediastinal adenopathy does occur, especially with osteosarcoma and other sarcomas as well as neuroblastoma and Wilms tumor (**Fig. 8**).

Posterior Mediastinum

The posterior mediastinum is predominantly the domain of the neurogenic lesions, including neurogenic cyst, anterior meningocele, and neurogenic tumors of sympathetic ganglion origin (ganglioneuroma, ganglioneuroblastoma, and neuroblastoma)

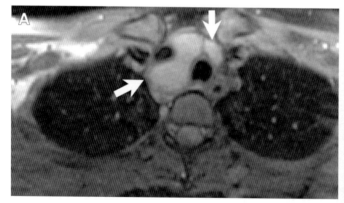
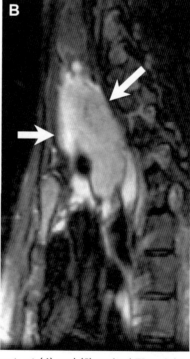

Fig. 7. A 16-year-old boy—Castleman disease. Axial T1-weighted postcontrast (*A*) and (*B*) sagittal T2-weighted MR images demonstrate confluent bright T2 signal with prominent enhancement of a nodal mass (*arrows*) in the middle and anterior mediastinum displacing airway and vessels.

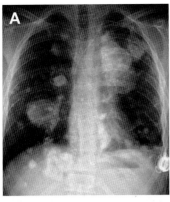
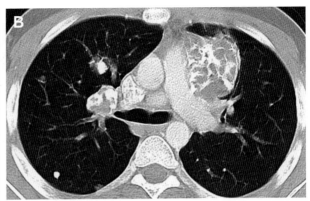

Fig. 8. A 16-year-old boy. (*A*) Chest radiograph to follow-up osteogenic sarcoma. Note multiple calcified small and large pulmonary metastases. (*B*) CT scan demonstrates multiple intrapulmonary metastatic lesions, some of which are densely calcified as well as large middle mediastinal masses/nodal tumor metastases. (*Reprinted from* Newman B, Effmann EL. Lung masses. In: Slovis T, editor. Caffey's pediatric diagnostic imaging, vol. 1. 11th edition. Philadelphia: Mosby Elsevier; 2008:1294–323; with permission.)

(**Fig. 9**), peripheral nerve origin (neurofibroma and schwannoma), or paraganglia cells (paraganglioma).[9] Other lesions may include esophageal masses (eg, esophageal duplication cyst or leiomyoma/leomyosarcoma), vascular abnormalities (aneurysm and vascular/lymphatic malformation) (**Fig. 10**), and vertebral/paravertebral lesions (extramedullary hematopoiesis (**Fig. 11**), lipomatosis, diskitis, osteomyelitis, LCH, osteosarcoma, and Ewing sarcoma). Mimickers of a posterior mediastinal mass include the normal right-sided paraspinal shadow of the confluence of pulmonary veins and rounded left lower lobe atelectasis medial to the pulmonary ligament.

Among the neurogenic tumors, neuroblastoma predominates, especially in young children. Less-aggressive forms of the ganglioneuroma neuroblastoma spectrum are more common in older children and may represent maturation of neuroblastoma. The lesions commonly contain speckled calcification, are typically bright on T2-weighted imaging, and enhance moderately (see **Fig. 9**). Local extent and distant metastases are often well shown on MIBG scintigraphic scans (**Fig. 12**).[7,9]

Neuroblastoma may present with a paraneoplastic syndrome,[9] including opsoclonus myoclonus, profuse watery diarrhea (vasoactive intestinal polypeptide), and pheochromocytoma-like syndrome (catecholamines), prompting a search for an underlying tumor, sometimes quite occult. The majority of neuroblastoma tumors occur in the abdomen in the region of the adrenal glands; these can occasionally spread to the chest contiguously through the retrocrural nodes. Only approximately 10% to 15% are primarily located in the chest and may coexist with one or more tumors elsewhere. Neuroblastoma in the chest may have a better prognosis,

perhaps because of earlier diagnosis and lower stage at the time of presentation. There is typically a paraspinal posterior mediastinal mass that may infiltrate the posterior soft tissues, can spread to nodes and vessels, or be large enough to compromise the airway. There is often a dumbbell lesion extending into multiple intervertebral foramina and the extradural space (see **Fig. 9**). For this reason, MR imaging is considered the best imaging modality to optimally visualize spinal involvement.[6] Other tumors may take on a dumbbell appearance, including Ewing sarcoma/primitive neurectodermal tumor (PNET), rhabdomyosarcoma, lipoblastoma, and vascular masses.[7]

Neurofibromas are usually associated with neurofibromatosis type 1; the lesions may be multiple and discrete, often at multiple foraminal levels, or may be large and extend into the middle mediastinum, especially as a plexiform neurofibroma. Extensive infiltration may occur along neurovascular bundles, including into the lung hila as well as along the pleura. They may be confused with other more aggressive tumors, such as lymphoma. Neurofibromas, however, tend to be hypodense with modest enhancement postcontrast. Other chest stigmata of neurofibromatosis, such as skin lesions, dural ectasia, scoliosis, and ribbon rib deformities, may be helpful.

CARDIAC NEOPLASMS

- Cardiac lesions may be intracavitary attached to the endocardium, within the myocardium, or pericardial (**Box 2**).
- Cardiac neoplasms are rare in children; most are benign.

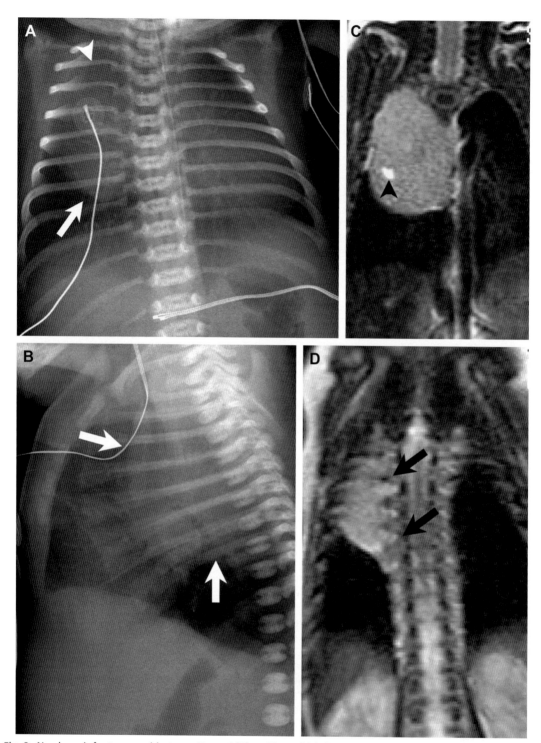

Fig. 9. Newborn infant—neuroblastoma. Frontal (*A*) and lateral (*B*) chest radiographs. There is a large mass in the right chest posteriorly (*arrows*). Thinning and splaying of the right posterior upper ribs (*arrowhead*) suggest a posterior mediastinal location, confirmed on the lateral view. Coronal T1-weighted postcontrast MR images (*C, D*) demonstrate a large moderately enhancing right posterior mass with vertebral foraminal extension at multiple levels (*arrows*). The punctate bright focus within the mass (*arrowhead*) is probably calcification.

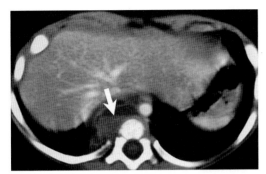

Fig. 10. Posterior mediastinal lymphangioma. Axial contrasted CT shows fluid/fluid levels (*arrow*) in the mass and no bone or spine involvement.

- Malignant cardiac or pericardial tumors are more likely to be metastatic than primary.
- Many childhood cardiac tumors are associated with specific syndromes or systemic diseases.
- Non-neoplastic entities may simulate and be difficult to distinguish from a cardiac neoplasm.

Cardiac tumors are included in the differential considerations for a middle mediastinal mass. Cardiac tumors may manifest on chest radiographs as cardiomegaly, abnormal cardiac contour, or pulmonary edema.[14] Other entities may simulate a cardiac mass, including normal variants, cardiomyopathy, other mediastinal masses, postsurgical changes, myocardial or arterial aneurysm, venous varix, abscess, diaphragmatic hernia, and pericardial abnormalities.

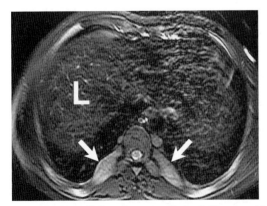

Fig. 11. Extramedullary hematopoiesis. A 22 year old with thallassemia post–multiple blood transfusions. Axial T2-weighted MR scan. Note the T2 dark signal in the liver (L) due to iron overload and T2 bright bilateral posterior paraspinal soft tissue masses (*arrows*) consistent with extramedullary hematopoiesis.

The most common intracardiac neoplasms in children are rhabdomyoma, myxoma and fibroma (**Figs. 13–16**).[14] Other benign entities include hamartoma, lipoma, fibroelastoma, hemangioma, fibrous histiocytoma, and inflammatory pseudotumor. Asymmetric septal or focal myocardial hypertrophy in hypertrophic cardiomyopathy (idiopathic, familial, or associated with maternal diabetes) may simulate an intracardiac mass. MR imaging features that serve to identify hypertrophied myocardium include similar signal, contractility, and enhancement characteristics as normal myocardium on multiple sequences.

Rhabdomyomas are hamartomas of the heart that have a strong association with tuberous sclerosis.[15,16] The tumors may be large or small, typically multiple rather than single.[17] The presence of multiple myocardial masses in a fetus or newborn infant is essentially diagnostic of tuberous sclerosis. These are rounded, well-defined intramyocardial masses on US. They are usually somewhat hyperintense on proton density MR images and enhance less than normal myocardium on postcontrast MR images as well as CT images (see **Fig. 13**). They may disrupt the conduction system of the heart or distort or obstruct the cavity or valves.[17] The neonatal rhabdomyomas associated with tuberous sclerosis tend to decrease in size over time usually completely regressing by age 6 years with no malignant potential.[14]

The second most common cardiac tumor in childhood is a cardiac fibroma. This tumor is usually solitary, often large, and although benign may cause significant cardiac dysfunction. It is typified by lower signal than normal myocardium especially on T2-weighted images with characteristic delayed contrast enhancement (see **Fig. 14**). Calcifications are common within the tumor, better appreciated on CT than MR imaging.[14] Cardiac fibroma has an association with Gorlin syndrome (basal cell nevi and multiple other tumors) and Beckwith-Wiedemann syndrome (better known for association with macroglossia, ompahlocele, hemihypertrophy, and abdominal tumors, especially Wilms tumor).[15,16]

Cardiac myxoma, usually in the left atrium, is the most common cardiac tumor in adults but uncommon in children. Cardiac myxomas in childhood have a syndromic association with the Carney complex (myxomas, endocrine lesions, and pigmented skin lesions) (see **Figs. 15** and **16**).[15,16,18] The cardiac myxomas may be multiple and widely distributed in both atria and ventricles (see **Fig. 16**). On MR imaging, atrial myxomas may have foci of low signal due to hemorrhage or calcification, most evident on gradient-echo

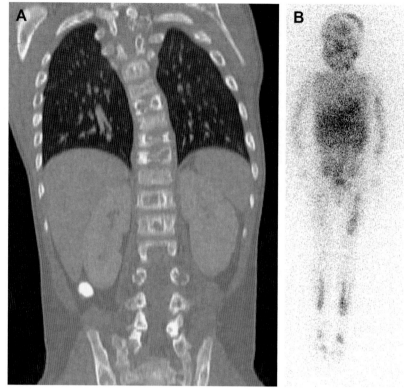

Fig. 12. Metastatic neuroblastoma in a 5-year-old boy. (*A*) Coronal CT reformat with diffuse lytic and sclerotic bony metastases, including spine, skull, scapulae, ribs, and pelvis. (*B*) MIBG scan—anterior view with diffuse and patchy bony uptake of radiotracer. There is physiologic uptake in salivary glands, myocardium, liver, and bladder.

images (see **Fig. 16**). They are usually attached to the atrial septum or other endocardium by a stalk and may be mobile and cause inflow or outflow obstruction of the ventricles or valvular dysfunction.

Primary malignant cardiac tumors are rare and include lymphoma, germ cell tumor, rhabdomyosarcoma, fibrosarcoma, angiosarcoma, and leiomyosarcoma.[14] Secondary cardiac involvement is more common than primary cardiac malignancy. This is usually associated with venous tumor thrombus extension or embolization, most likely in Wilms tumor, hepatoblastoma, and neuroblastoma (**Fig. 17**). Other tumors, such as osteosarcoma, Ewing sarcoma, and leukemia/lymphoma, can involve the heart by direct contiguous spread. Hematogenous metastases to the heart are rare.

Intracardiac thrombus may be difficult to differentiate from a tumor. Useful sequences include gradient-echo and T2 images, where thrombus is typically low and most tumors high in signal

relative to normal myocardium, as well as post-contrast images, where tumors usually enhance and thrombus (unless chronic and organized) does not (**Fig. 18**).

Pericardial masses include pericardial cyst, teratoma, hemangioma, and lymphangioma. A range of other lesions may simulate a pericardial neoplasm, including irregular pericardial thickening/calcification, pericardial hemorrhagic effusion/hematoma (see **Fig. 18**), intrapericardial extension of a diaphragmatic hernia, myocardial diverticulum, and partial absence of the pericardium.[19] CT or MR imaging is often helpful in defining the location and likely nature of the mass and may occasionally be able to suggest a specific diagnosis (eg, the presence of both fat and calcification strongly suggests a teratoma). Primary malignant tumors and hematogenous metastases to the pericardium are rare.[19] More likely is contiguous spread of a mediastinal mass such as lymphoma (**Fig. 19**) or thymoma to involve the pericardium; these may result in constrictive pericarditis.

Cardiac

1. Benign

   a. Rhabdomyoma
   b. Myxoma
   c. Fibroma
   d. Hemangioma
   e. Hamartoma
   f. Lipoma
   g. Fibroelastoma
   h. Fibrous histiocytoma
   i. Inflammatory pseudotumor

2. Malignant

   a. Primary
      i. Lymphoma
      ii. Germ cell tumor
      iii. Rhabdomyosarcoma, fibrosarcoma, angiosarcoma, and leiomyosarcoma

   b. Metastatic
      i. Contiguous—ostesarcoma, Ewing sarcoma, rhabdomyosarcoma, and leukemia/lymphoma
      ii. Venous thrombus/hematogenous—Wilms, neuroblastoma, hepatoblastoma, and rhabdomyosarcoma

Pericardial

1. Benign
   a. Teratoma
   b. Hemangioma/lymphangioma

2. Malignant
   a. Germ cell tumor
   b. Contiguous/metastatic spread (eg, lymphoma and thymoma)

INTRAPULMONARY NEOPLASMS

- Pulmonary masses are less common than mediastinal masses in children (**Box 3**).[20]
- The majority are non-neoplastic congenital or inflammatory lesions.
- Neoplastic intrapulmonary lesions are more likely malignant than benign.
- Malignant lesions are more likely metastatic than primary.
- It may be difficult to determine the origin of large pleural, mediastinal, or chest wall tumors that spread contiguously to involve the lung (**Fig. 20**).

Several extrinsic densities may simulate an intrapulmonary mass. These include skin lesions, breast buds, rib and other chest wall abnormalities, diaphragmatic hernia or eventration, and hair braids.[21] Rounded intrapulmonary lesions can also masquerade as pulmonary neoplasms, including round pneumonia, rounded atelectasis, lung abscess, fungal or granulomatous nodules, loculated pleural fluid, hematoma, and vasculitic lesions.[20,21]

Bronchopulmonary malformations are common congenital non-neoplastic lung masses that need to be differentiated from other pulmonary tumors. These are frequently found prenatally as large solid or cystic or combined T2 bright lesions in utero. Often they are largest in the second trimester and progressively decrease in size and conspicuity later in pregnancy. They may be small or not visible on postnatal chest radiographs but are usually apparent on CT imaging.[22] There is considerable overlap of the lesions, with features of multiple entities common rather than exceptional. The bronchopulomonary malformations are thought to represent the spectrum of underlying airway obstruction in utero with consequent lung malformation.[23] The histologic nature of the lesion may depend on the timing and severity of this obstruction malformation sequence.[23] In many cases, careful pathologic evaluation has revealed bronchial atresia to be the underlying obstructive lesion.[22,24] Typical findings that may be identified both prenatally and postnatally include lobar or segmental hyperinflation (congenital lobar/segmental overinflation); central bronchial mucoid impaction (bronchial atresia); single (bronchogenic cyst) or multiple cysts (congenital pulmonary airway malformation [CPAM]), and systemic arterial supply to the lung (pulmonary sequestration).[22] Other prenatal pulmonary masses occur but are uncommon (**Fig. 21**).

Benign lung neoplasms encountered in children include hamartoma, chondroma, vascular/lymphatic lesions, LCH, respiratory papillomatosis, granular cell tumor, neurofibroma, schwannoma, teratoma, and benign lymphoproliferative lesions.[25]

Hamartomas and chondromas are uncommon in children. The presence of typical popcorn calcification in a lesion may help in suggesting the diagnosis of a hamartoma; however, many other benign and malignant neoplasms, including metastases, can calcify.[20] Similarly, non-neoplastic lesions, such as infections or infarcts, may also calcify. Pulmonary chondroma is uncommon, tends to be densely calcified, and is difficult to differentiate from hamartoma both on imaging and pathology. The presence of pulmonary chondroma, especially multiple lesions in a young woman, should raise suspicion for Carney triad. This triad describes the synchronous or metachronous occurrence of pulmonary chondroma, gastric stromal tumor, and extradrenal paraganglioma.[25,26] Additional tumors are also

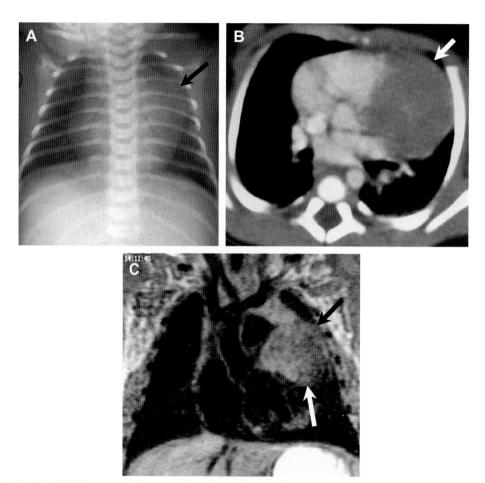

Fig. 13. Cardiac rhabdomyoma. Tuberous sclerosis, newborn infant. (*A*) Chest radiograph, there is an unusual cardiac contour with bulging of the left superior heart border (*arrow*). (*B*) Axial postcontrast CT. (*C*) Coronal T2-weighted MR imaging. There is a large bulging myocardial mass (*arrows*), moderately T2 bright with slight enhancement with contrast. (*Reprinted from* Towbin AJ, Newman B. Cardiac involvement by systemic diseases. In: Slovis T, editor. Caffey's pediatric diagnostic imaging, vol. 1. 11th edition. Philadelphia: Mosby Elsevier; 2008. p. 1687–706; with permission.)

associated, including adrenal adenoma and esophageal leiomyoma.[27]

Vascular lesions include non-neoplastic entities that can mimic tumor, encompassing arterial aneurysm, venous varix, arteriovenous malformation (AVM), and vasculitic lesions, such as Wegener granulomatosis and Takayasu disease. AVMs are the most common intrapulmonary vascular lesion; 70% of these are associated with hereditary hemorrhagic telangiectasia, although the lesions are usually not clinically manifest until later childhood or adulthood.[20] There may be 1 or more large or small AVMs or diffuse tiny AVMs predominantly in the lower lobes. Location, size, and number can often be determined noninvasively with CTA, although diffuse microscopic lesions may be more difficult to appreciate on CTA

compared with conventional angiography. There are frequently soft tissue and visceral AVM's present elsewhere in the body.

Diffuse arteriocapillary dilatation and ultimately diffuse AVMs are also encountered in hepatopulmonary and portopulmonary syndrome and after superior cavopulmonary anastomosis with exclusion of hepatic venous blood from the lungs; the cause of this is poorly understood. Diffuse pulmonary arteriovenous shunting in these conditions results in hypoxemia and pulmonary hypertension.[28]

Benign vascular neoplasms include intrapulmonary lymphangioma (**Fig. 22**)[29] and hemangioma. Intrapulmonary lymphangioma can be extensive, involving lung, pleura, and mediastinum (see **Fig. 22**); as such, it may be difficult to distinguish

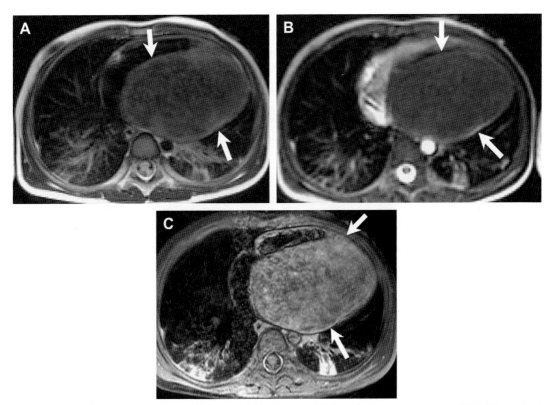

Fig. 14. Cardiac fibroma in a 3-year-old girl. Axial MR images. (A) Double inversion recovery (T1), (B) gradient-echo T2, and (C) delayed T1 postcontrast show a large mildly heterogeneous intracardiac mass (arrows) that is dark on both T1 and especially T2 sequences with moderate contrast enhancement on delayed (not early) post-contrast images (C). Despite the large size of the mass with some impingement on both ventricular cavities, there was no obstruction or cardiac dysfunction.

from a diffusely infiltrating malignant tumor, such as pleuropulmonary blastoma (PPB).[20] PPB tends, however, to be more heterogeneous with some solid nodular components. Pulmonary lymphangiomatosis or hemangiomatosis may be part of a more generalized diffuse entity that may involve multiple other organs, including liver, soft tissues, mediastinum, bone, spleen, intestine, and kidneys.[10,20,30] Lymphangioleiomyomatosis with diffuse thin-walled cysts in the lungs is most

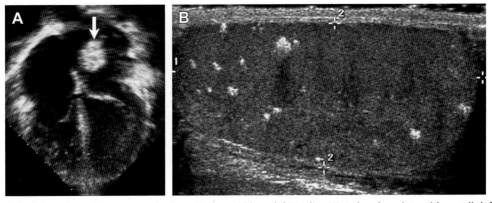

Fig. 15. Atrial myxoma, Carney complex in a 12-year-old boy. (A) Cardiac US 4-chamber view with a well defined hyperechoic mass in the left atrium (arrow). (B) Testicular US with multiple small calcified Sertoli cell tumors. (Reprinted from Towbin AJ, Newman B. Cardiac involvement by systemic diseases. In: Slovis T, editor. Caffey's pediatric diagnostic imaging, vol. 1. 11th edition. Philadelphia: Mosby Elsevier; 2008. p. 1687–706; with permission.)

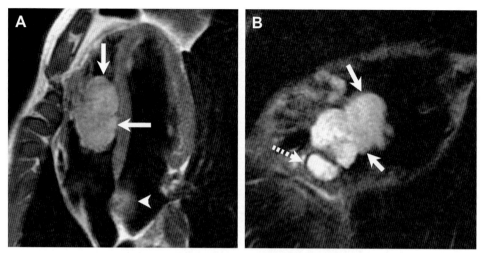

Fig. 16. Multiple atrial myxomas, Carney complex. A 17-year-old boy, status post orchiectomy for Sertoli-Leydig cell tumor. (*A*) Double inversion recovery (T1) 4-chamber and (*B*) Triple inversion recovery (T2) right ventricular 2-chamber images showing multiple T2 bright intracavitary myxomas including left atrium adjacent to the septum (*arrowhead*) and a large lobulated mass in the right ventricle (*arrows*). Note the dark rim around the proximal portion of the right ventricular mass (*broken arrow*), likely due to hemorrhage and hemosiderin deposition.

commonly seen in young adult women in association with tuberous sclerosis and occasionally encountered in older adolescents.

The lung is affected in approximately 50% of children with systemic LCH; approximately 11% have lung involvement at the time of initial diagnosis.[20,31] There may be focal or diffuse lung involvement (upper lobe predominance) with solid (**Fig. 23**) and cavitating nodules that form small and large cysts. A cyst that is peripheral in location may break through to the pleural space, presenting as an acute pneumothorax (approximately 10%).

The lesions of respiratory papillomatosis are a neoplastic proliferation caused by the papillomavirus acquired in the maternal birth canal during delivery. The disease is usually confined to the larynx and upper tracheal airway with spread to the lung in less than 1% of cases (**Fig. 24**).[20,32] Intrapulmonary spread is thought possibly related to surgical/laser spillage during treatment of the upper airway lesions. Proliferation in the lung produces solid and cavitating cystic pulmonary masses (see **Fig. 24**). The ultimate prognosis is poor, treatment is difficult, recurrence common

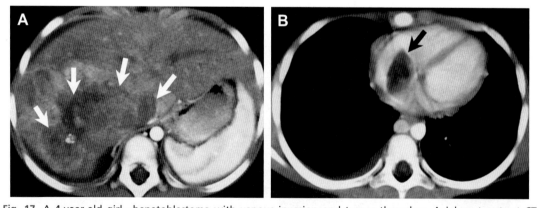

Fig. 17. A 4-year-old girl—hepatoblastoma with venous invasion and tumor thrombus. Axial postcontrast CT images. (*A*) Upper liver—there is a large heterogeneous right hepatic mass with expanding enhancing tumor thrombus in the right hepatic vein and inferior vena cava (*arrows*) extending into the (*B*) right atrium (*arrow*). (*Reprinted from* Towbin AJ, Newman B. Cardiac Involvement by systemic diseases. In: Slovis T, editor. Caffey's pediatric diagnostic imaging, vol. 1. 11th edition. Philadelphia: Mosby Elsevier; 2008. p. 1687–706; with permission.)

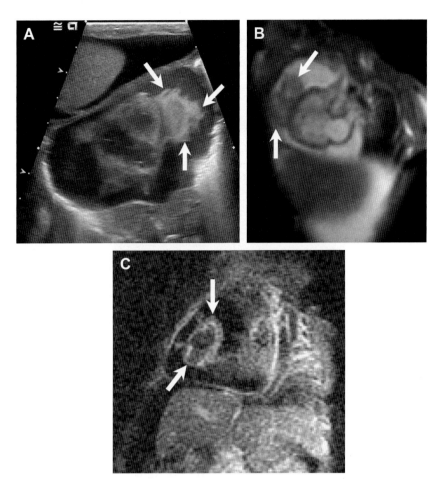

Fig. 18. Pericardial effusion with organized thrombus simulating a pericardial mass. A 1-day-old girl. (A) US sub-costal view shows large ascites and pericardial effusion with an irregular inhomogeneously echogenic mass that appears attached to the visceral pericardium (arrows). (B) Right ventricle 3-chamber fast imaging employing steady state (FIESTA) single shot fast field echo image. (C) Delayed postcontrast image show ascites, large pericar-dial effusion, and an inhomogeneous pericardial mass (arrows) that appears to have both solid and cystic compo-nents with moderate patchy delayed enhancement peripherally. There is a dark signal rim and some central dark signal (B) thought to represent hemorrhage. Pericardial teratoma was thought the most likely diagnosis based on imaging. Only organized thrombus was found at surgery and pathologic examination.

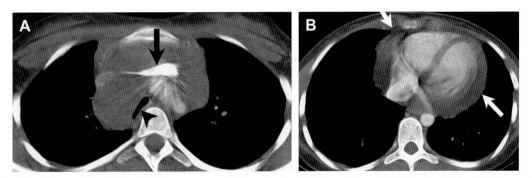

Fig. 19. A 7 year old with Hodgkin lymphoma. Axial contrasted CT slices. There is bulky tumor in the anterior and middle mediastinum with marked compression and displacement of the (A) innominate vein (arrow) and airway (arrowhead) and inferior extension of the tumor to involve the (B) pericardium (arrows). (Reprinted from Towbin AJ, Newman B. Cardiac involvement by systemic diseases. In: Slovis T, editor. Caffey's pediatric diagnostic imaging, vol. 1. 11th edition. Philadelphia: Mosby Elsevier; 2008. p. 1687–706; with permission.)

Box 3
Lung neoplasms in children

Benign

1. Inflammatory myofibroblastic tumor
2. Hamartoma
3. Lymphangioma/hemangioma
4. Chondroma
5. Papillomatosis
6. LCH
7. Neurogenic tumors
8. Lymphoproliferative lesions; post-transplant lymphoproliferative disorder (PTLD), smooth muscle cell proliferation, and lymphomatoid granulomatosis
9. Congenital peribronchial myofibroblastic tumor

Malignant

1. Amine precursor uptake and decarboxylation (APUD) carcinoid tumors
2. Pleuropulmonary blastoma
3. Bronchogenic carcinoma
4. Sarcomas
5. Lymphoma
6. Metastatic tumor: osteosarcoma, Ewing sarcoma, rhabdomyosarcoma, Wilms tumor, germ cell tumor, lymphoma, and so forth

with high morbidity, and there is approximately 10% long-term risk of conversion of the lesions to squamous cell carcinoma.[20,25,32]

Benign reactive lymphoproliferative lesions in the lung consist of a variety of entities, most uncommon. The spectrum includes inflammatory myofibroblastic tumor; mucosal-associated lymphoproliferation, also known as pseudolymphoma; bronchus-associated lymphoproliferation, subdivided into lymphoid interstitial pneumonitis and follicular bronchiolitis; lymphomatoid granulomatosis; and PTLD.

Inflammatory myofibroblastic tumor (also known as plasma cell granuloma or inflammatory pseudotumor) is the most common benign intrapulmonary neoplastic lesion in children.[33–35] It is still controversial as to whether this entity represents an atypical reaction to prior infection versus a low-grade neoplasm.[34] There are single or multiple small to large poorly enhancing rounded masses in the lung (**Fig. 25**) with calcification present in approximately 20% of lesions. Support for the possible neoplastic nature of this lesion is occasional aggressive and invasive behavior.[33,36]

An uncommon solid tumor that may be discovered prenatally or in newborn infants is the congenital peribronchial myofibroblastic tumor (also known as congenital fibrosarcoma).[25] This

lesion is thought to be benign in behavior but is typically large in size and may be difficult to resect (see **Fig. 21**).[25] Similar to other large chest masses in utero, there is an increased risk of development of hydrops fetalis with high fetal mortality,[25] so there should be careful follow-up in utero with US and/or MR imaging.

Lymphomatoid granulomatosis is an angiocentric destructive lesion with the lung as the primary site of occurrence. There is a basal predominance of nodular and less well-defined larger confluent lesions that tend to cavitate and may sometimes resemble confluent pneumonia or empyema. Lymphomatoid granulomatosis and PTLD are similar entities, both being related to B-cell lymphoproliferation associated with Epstein-Barr virus in immunocompromised individuals. There is a spectrum of lymphoproliferation from benign to frank B-cell lymphoma.[20]

PTLD is more common in pediatric than adult transplant patients, with the highest frequency in lung or heart-lung transplants.[20] PTLD has a predilection for the allograft site (with the exception of the heart) in addition to a variety of other locations, including tonsils, lymphoid tissue in the neck, lung, gastrointestinal tract, and central nervous system.[20,37] Lesions in the lung consist of single or multiple small or large nodules or areas of consolidation simulating pneumonia (**Fig. 26**).[37] Larger lesions tend to cavitate (see **Fig. 26**); associated hilar or mediastinal adenopathy may be present. Diagnosis of PTLD is made by biopsy of the most easily accessible site, usually not the lung. Decreasing the dose of immunosuppressive drugs is usually effective treatment for PTLD but it may be difficult to find a balance between PTLD and organ rejection.[37] Occasionally, especially with longstanding lesions or delayed diagnosis, PTLD may become a monoclonal lymphoma requiring aggressive chemotherapy.

Spindle/smooth muscle cell tumors are a less common but similar neoplastic cell proliferation to PTLD. Like PTLD, smooth muscle cell tumors are Epstein-Barr virus driven in immunocompromised individuals (HIV and post-transplant), but are histologically distinct from PTLD with a less favorable prognosis.[20,38] Spindle/smooth muscle cell tumors are usually discrete masses most often in the chest or abdomen. An endobronchial location of this lesion may also occur.

Pulmonary lymphoma is most commonly associated with mediastinal tumor involvement but primary pulmonary lymphoma occurs on occasion; 12% of children with Hodgkin disease and 10% of non Hodgkin-lymphoma have lung involvement, most at initial diagnosis.[20] The appearance of pulmonary lymphoma can be widely varied

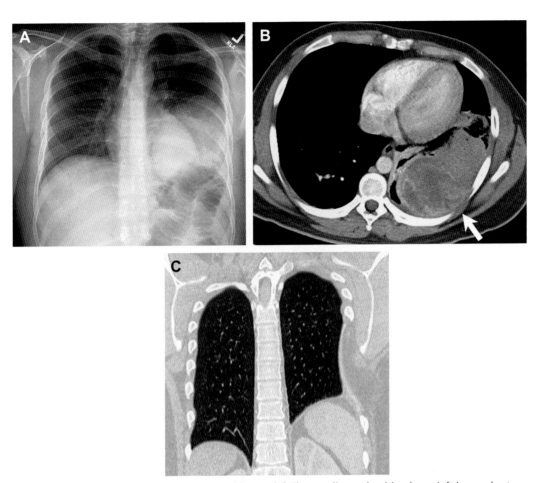

Fig. 20. Pleural synovial sarcoma in an 18-year-old man. (*A*) Chest radiograph with a large left lower chest mass. The origin of the mass (intrapulmonary versus chest wall) is uncertain. (*B*) Contrasted chest CT (mediastinal window) shows a heterogeneous enhancing mass, probably pleural in origin, projecting into the left lower lung with adjacent atelectasis. There is subtle involvement of the left posterior chest wall (*arrow*). (*C*) Postoperative coronal CT reformat (bone window). There has been surgical removal of the mass, left lower lobe and several ribs with graft placement. There is resultant deformity of the chest wall. No residual or recurrent mass was seen.

similar to benign lymphoproliferative disorders. The most common appearance is the presence of pulmonary nodules that may cavitate (see **Fig. 5**). Less common are alveolar infiltration (**Fig. 27**), lymphangitic tumor spread, and endobronchial tumor spread.[20]

Pulmonary metastases are considerably more common than primary pulmonary malignant lesions.[33,39] The most common hematogenous metastases are from osteosarcoma, Wilms tumor, and other sarcomas (see **Fig. 8**).[20] Pulmonary metastases are most commonly located in the peripheral and basilar lungs. They are typically multiple, occasionally single, well-defined rounded pulmonary nodules or masses that can become large. Some tend to calcify (osteogenic sarcoma) (see **Fig. 8**) or cavitate (**Fig. 28**) (sarcomas,

lymphoma, and occasionally Wilms tumor).[20] Approximately one-third of lung nodules in children with a known underlying malignancy are non-metastatic. On biopsy, alternative pathologic diagnoses include intrapulmonary lymph nodes, infection, scar, drug reaction, myofibroblastic tumor, lipid nodules, vasculitis, and occasionally a second malignancy (see **Fig. 25**).[20,21,40] Lesions larger than 5 mm are more likely to be metastases.[20] Accurate and early recognition of possible pulmonary metastases is important because long-term survival in osteogenic tumors as well as other sarcomas is significantly improved after metastectomy.[33,41,42]

Pulmonary malignancy may also involve the lung contiguously from adjacent mediastinum, hilar, or pleural tumor. Spread via lymphatic channels

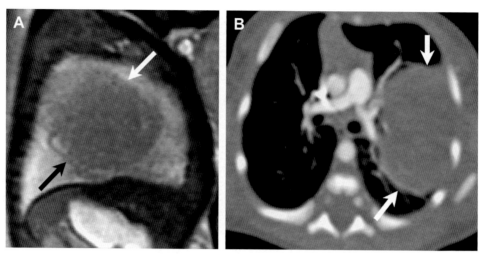

Fig. 21. Congenital peribronchial myofibroblastic tumor. (*A*) Prenatal T2-weighted sagittal MR image at 32 weeks' gestation with a large low signal mass in the left lung (*arrows*). This has a different appearance from that of the more common bronchopulmonary malformations, which are bright on T2. The correct diagnosis was suggested on the basis of the prenatal appearance of the mass. (*B*) Axial postcontrast newborn CT confirms the large low attenuation poorly enhancing mass in the left lung (*arrows*).

(lymphangitic metastases, most common in rhabdomyosarcoma, neuroblastoma, and lymphoma) or along the airway is an occasional method of intrapulmonary tumoral involvement.

Primary pulmonary malignant neoplasms are rare in children. The most common of these are the spectrum of APUD neurendocrine tumors; these are responsible for approximately 45% of primary pediatric lung tumors. Bronchogenic carcinomas and mesenchymal tumors account

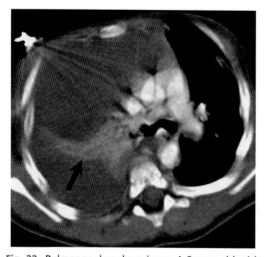

Fig. 22. Pulmonary lymphangioma. A 2 year old with whiteout of the right lung on chest radiograph. CT shows atelectatic right lower lung (*arrow*) surrounded by a large low attenuation infiltrating intrapulmonary mass extending into the anterior mediastinum with leftward shift of midline structures.

for an additional 25% each[20]; 80% of the APUD tumors in children are low-grade carcinoid tumors[20,33] (**Fig. 29**); less common tumors include mucoepidermoid tumor, cylindroma, and mucous gland adenoma. These are usually endobronchial lesions, most commonly in the lobar bronchi, and may spread contiguously to involve adjacent nodes or lung.[20,43] The lung distal to the lesion shows findings of partial (air trapping) or more commonly complete airway obstruction (atelectasis/recurrent infection of the affected lobe or segment). Contrast CT with particular attention to 2-D and 3-D and virtual bronchoscopic reconstructions is helpful in identifying these lesions (see **Fig. 29**). Carcinoid tumors infrequently present with Cushing syndrome or carcinoid syndrome (generally implies metastases) and are occasionally encountered as part of a multiple endocrine neoplasia syndrome.[33]

Bronchogenic carcinomas are unusual in childhood. Approximately half of these are bronchoalveoalar carcinoma (BAC) with a smaller number of squamous cell carcinomas.[20] The squamous cell tumors are usually large at the time of diagnosis and aggressive, with a poor prognosis (**Fig. 30**). Although the incidence is small (approximately 1%), BAC seems to arise in some cases in or adjacent to an underlying bronchopulmonary malformation, principally large cyst CPAM.[44,45] This relationship can apparently persist even when the underlying lesion has been previously surgically excised. This has been variably suggested to be due to incomplete surgical removal versus an oncogenic potential related to the

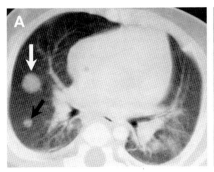
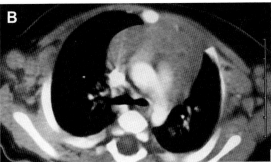

Fig. 23. Langerhans cell histiocytosis in a 3-month-old boy. (A) Chest CT lung window - there are multiple well-defined pulmonary nodules (*arrows*). (B) Contrasted CT, mediastinal window at the level of the aortic arch. The thymus is enlarged with heterogeneous low attenuation foci. These subsequently calcified after treatment (not shown). Note also bilateral axillary adenopathy.

presence of abnormal mucigenic cells in large cyst CPAM.[45,46] BAC is usually confined to a segment or lobe, is not aggressive in its spread, and rarely is metastatic. Recognition and differentiation from infection may be difficult.

Mesenchymal tumors in children are mostly sarcomas, now recognized as predominantly PPB (**Fig. 31**) with occasional other sarcomas, such as rhabdomyosarcoma, leiomyosarcoma, synovial cell sarcoma, or liposarcoma.[25]

PPB is a dysontogenetic anlage of Wilms tumor, neuroblastoma, and hepatoblastoma.[20] PPB consists of malignant blastema with frequent mesenchymal sarcomatous components, especially rhabdosarcoma and chondrosarcoma[25]; 90% are identified in children less than 6 years old with the cystic form almost invariably in children less than 3 years of age.[47] There are 3 types representing a progression from cystic to solid along with increasing age and tumor aggression: type 1 is cystic, type 2 is cystic and solid, and type 3 is solid (see **Fig. 31**).[25,47,48] Type 1 has an 82% 5-year survival with only 42% in type 3, with both aggressive local spread and recurrence as well as distant metastases.[20,44,47,48] Lesions may consist of a small nodule or single cyst or a huge cystic or solid mass that can involve lung parenchyma, pleura, and mediastinum.[20,48]

PPB has a hereditary tumor predisposition with an association with cystic nephroma in particular as well as other tumors including rhabdomyosarcoma, medulloblastoma, thyroid, Hodgkin lymphoma, leukemia, and germ cell tumors.[20,25,47,48] PPB is unusual prenatal but has been described as early as 19 to 21 weeks, progressively increasing in size with advancing gestation, different from the typical pattern of bronchopulmonary malformations (BPMs).[44] PPB lesions are frequently multiple or bilateral (49%), occurring both synchronously or metachronously.[44] Therefore, surgical removal does not obviate ongoing surveillance. A DICER 1 gene mutation on

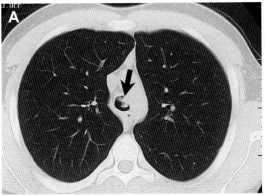
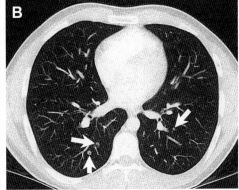

Fig. 24. Respiratory papillomatosis in a 16-year-old boy. History of asthma since infancy. (A) Initial CT shows a lobulated intratracheal soft tissue mass (*arrow*). These were present at multiple levels. No pulmonary abnormality was appreciated. (B) Eight months after surgical extirpation of the tracheal lesions, there are multiple small solid and cavitating intrapulmonary nodules (*arrows*) consistent with intrapulmonary spread of the papillomatosis.

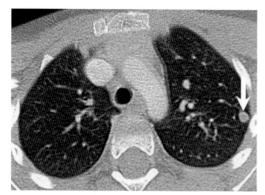

Fig. 25. A 5 year old. Inflammatory myofibroblastic tumors. Several new lung nodules (*arrow*) were found on this routine follow-up CT for neuroblastoma. They were removed surgically because of concern for metastases.

chromosome 14 in airway epithelial cells has recently been identified in familial cases of PPB.[49]

Although not universally accepted, current pathologic literature suggests that PPB arises de novo and is not a complication of congenital bronchopulmonary malformations and that prior reports linking the two originally misidentified the lesion and missed the correct diagnosis of PPB.[48,50] Cystic PPB is difficult to separate from other cystic lung lesions, especially the large cyst CPAM (type 1) on imaging and many cases subsequently identified as PPB are initially diagnosed as CPAM lesions.[20,48,50] Correct pathologic diagnosis also may be subtle.[25] Features that suggest PPB rather than CPAM include atypical in utero growth pattern (BPMs present and are often largest in second trimester; PPB unlikely to be present early and progressively enlarges), presence or development of solid nodules, multiple lesions, pneumothorax (uncommon in CPAM; PPB a more

peripheral lesion), known familial tumor predisposition, or family history of childhood cancer.[20,48]

Malignant intrapulmonary vascular neoplasms, such as hemangiopericytoma and angiosarcoma, are uncommon in children.[20] Epithelioid hemangioendothelioma (also known as intravascular bronchoalveolar tumor) is a low-grade rare intrapulmonary vascular malignancy, more common in young women with findings of single or multiple (including bilateral) pulmonary nodules and occasionally hemorrhagic pleural effusion (a poor prognostic feature).[51] This tumor is rarely diagnosed before biopsy and more commonly occurs in liver rather than lung.

MASSES AFFECTING THE INTRATHORACIC AIRWAY

- Masses obstructing the airway may be intrinsic (intraluminal or intramural) or extrinsic.
- The airway may be affected at any level from the trachea to smaller intrapulmonary bronchi.
- Incomplete intrathoracic airway obstruction produces air trapping of the affected distal lung, bilateral in the case of tracheal obstruction, and unilateral, lobar, or segmental when more distal airways are involved.
- Complete airway obstruction results in distal atelectasis of the affected lung, frequently with superimposed infection.

Masses affecting the airway arise in any thoracic region, including mediastinal, intrapulmonary, and occasionally chest wall. Ectopic thymic or thyroid tissue is a rare cause of an intratracheal mass in children.[52]

A foreign body, granulation tissue, or infectious/inflammatory debris in the airway may sometimes be difficult to distinguish from a neoplasm. An

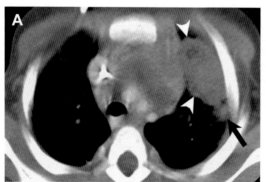
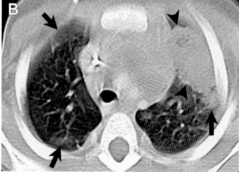

Fig. 26. A 4-year-old boy post–liver transplant with post transplant lymphoproliferative disease (PTLD). (*A, B*) Contrasted axial CT scan, mediastinal window (*A*) and lung window (*B*) with a large cavitating lesion in the left upper lobe (*arrowheads*). There are also multiple smaller ill-defined ground glass nodules in both lungs (*arrows*).

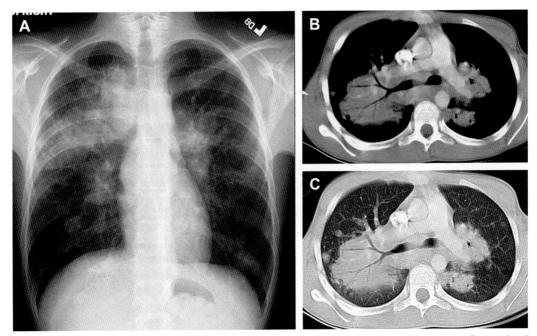

Fig. 27. Hodgkin lymphoma in a 15 year old. (*A*) Chest radiograph. There are large bilateral confluent alveolar opacities as well as some scattered nodules. (*B*) Contrasted CT scan (mediastinal window) and (*C*) (lung window). Note prominent hilar nodes and contiguous adjacent consolidated lungs as well as several scattered nodules. Air bronchograms and intact vessels within the mass are a characteristic pulmonary appearance of lymphoma. (*A* and *C, Reprinted from* Newman B, Effmann EL. Lung masses. In: Slovis T, editor. Caffey's pediatric diagnostic imaging, vol. 1. 11th edition. Philadelphia: Mosby Elsevier; 2008:1294–323; with permission.)

aggressive intrinsic airway neoplasm is more likely to produce complete airway obstruction with distal atelectasis/infection, whereas acute foreign bodies are more likely associated with partial airway obstruction and air trapping.

Benign intrinsic airway lesions include hemangioma and respiratory papillomatosis (see **Fig. 24**)

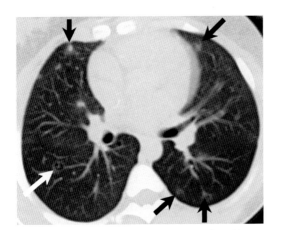

Fig. 28. Cavitating pulmonary metastases in a 14-year-old girl with chordoma. The CT (lung window) image shows multiple well-defined small pulmonary nodules both solid (*arrows*), with central cavitation and cystic (*white arrow*).

as well as PTLD, leiomyoma, granular cell tumor, hamartoma, and inflammatory pseudotumor.[20,35,53] The APUD tumors, especially carcinoid tumor (see **Fig. 29**), are the most common intrinsic airway malignancy; bronchogenic carcinomas and primary bronchial fibrosarcoma are rare in childhood (see **Fig. 30**).[25,43] Extrinsic lesions that commonly cause airway compression include benign lesions, such as congenital cysts and cystic hygroma. These may present with sudden airway symptoms as a result of acute hemorrhage and enlargement. Extrinsic malignant neoplasms that tend to compress the airway include lymphoma/leukemia (see **Fig. 19**), other causes of adenopathy (see **Fig. 7**), germ cell tumors, and occasionally neurogenic tumors. Any large aggressive chest neoplasm can displace, distort, compress, or even infiltrate the airway. Specific lesions have been discussed earlier.

PLEURAL, DIAPHRAGM, AND CHEST WALL MASSES

- Pleural masses are often due to direct contiguous spread from intrapulmonary, mediastinal or chest wall lesions (**Box 4**).
- Chest wall masses are relatively uncommon in children.

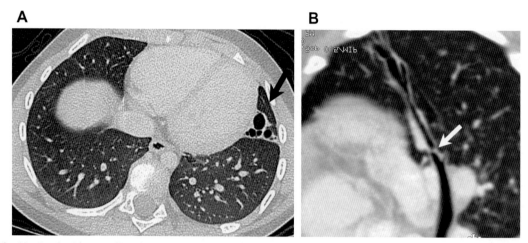

Fig. 29. Carcinoid tumor lingula bronchus. A 6-year-old girl with history of recurrent pneumonia. (*A*) Axial CT slice (lung window). There is focal bronchiectasis in the inferior lingula (*arrow*). (*B*) Curved reformat of the lingula bronchus shows narrowing of the bronchus with small intraluminal enhancing soft tissue (*arrow*) as well as extraluminal mass with distal bronchiectasis. Both intraluminal and extraluminal masses were carcinoid tumor.

- Most asymptomatic chest wall lumps are due to benign anatomic variations of the chest wall.
- Many benign lesions can appear infiltrative whereas malignant lesions may appear well circumscribed.
- Metastatic tumor is more common than primary chest wall malignancy.
- MR imaging is typically the best method for detailed imaging evaluation of chest wall neoplasms.

Contiguous involvement of the pleura from adjacent intrapulmonary, mediastinal, or chest wall lesions is common.[54] Inflammatory pleural thickening or loculated fluid may be difficult to differentiate from pleural tumor although the latter tends to have a more irregular lumpy configuration. Pleural effusion is associated with a large number of infectious, inflammatory, and neoplastic causes. Thoracic tumors, including pleuropulmonary blastoma, teratoma, leukemia/lymphoma, and PNET, can clinically mimic infectious empyema with

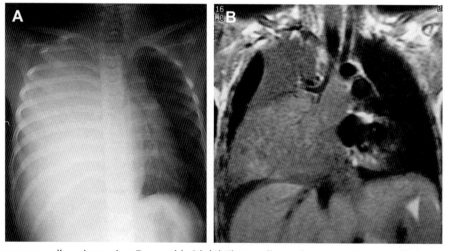

Fig. 30. Squamous cell carcinoma in a 7-year-old girl. (*A*) Chest radiograph. Large right mass obscuring right lung and extending across the midline with contralateral mediastinal shift. (*B*) Coronal MR image, T1 postcontrast. There is a large infiltrating intrapulmonary mass encasing the right lower bronchi and extending into the mediastinum. Moderate right pleural effusion is present. (*Reprinted from* Newman B, Effmann EL. Lung masses. In: Slovis T, editor. Caffey's pediatric diagnostic imaging, vol. 1. 11th edition. Philadelphia: Mosby Elsevier; 2008:1294–323; with permission.)

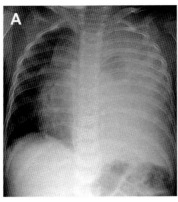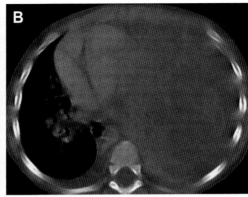

Fig. 31. A 2 year old—pleuropulmonary blastoma. (*A*) Chest radiograph. There is almost complete opacification of the left hemithorax with rightward cardiomedistinal shift. (*B*) CT axial postcontrast image. There is a heterogeneous mass replacing the left lung and extending to the posterior mediastinum with contralateral midline shift. There are bilateral moderate pleural effusions. (*Reprinted from* Newman B, Effmann EL. Lung masses. In: Slovis T, editor. Caffey's pediatric diagnostic imaging, vol. 1. 11th edition. Philadelphia: Mosby Elsevier; 2008:1294–323; with permission.)

or without an actual pleural effusion (see **Fig. 31**).[54,55]

Benign pleural tumors include hemangioma, lymphangioma (**Fig. 32**), neurofibromas, and lipomas. Malignant tumors may arise in or spread to the pleura. These include PPB (see **Fig. 31**), PNET, sarcomas (see **Fig. 20**), mesothelioma, thymic carcinoma (see **Fig. 6**), metastatic Wilms, and neuroblastoma. Large effusions frequently accompany and may obscure pleural tumor.[56]

Non-neoplastic lesions of the diaphragm may simulate a mediastinal or intrapulmonary mass. These include diaphragmatic hernias, eventration, and paresis or paralysis of the diaphragm. Neoplasms of the diaphragm are rare in children.[54,57] Rhabdomyosarcoma is the expected primary malignant neoplasm; inflammatory pseudotumor has been described as a benign neoplasm arising in the diaphragm.[54,57] Intrathoracic masses may displace, evert, and occasionally infiltrate the diaphragm. Abdominal tumors, such as hepatoblastoma and neuroblastoma, can extend to and occasionally invade the diaphragm. Retrocrural extension of tumors, such as lymphoma and neuroblastoma, are not uncommon. Juxtadiaphragmatic masses include lipoma, hemangio/lymphangioma, rhabdomyosarcoma, and esophagogastric tumors.

Chest wall tumors are uncommon in children, and although many lesions are benign, the appearance of the lesion can be deceptive. A highly aggressive malignant tumor, such as synovial sarcoma, can appear to be well circumscribed (see **Fig. 20**) although a benign vascular malformation may have a diffusely infiltrative appearance (see **Fig. 32**).[1,54] When needed, CT or MR imaging

is helpful for defining the location, extent, and internal characteristics of these lesions. MR imaging is generally preferable for most chest wall masses. CT may be preferred when lung detail is needed.

Several anatomic variations of the chest wall can masquerade as a chest wall neoplasm. The most common of these is a congenital abnormality of clavicle, sternum, rib, or costal cartilage, which results in asymmetry of the chest wall or a hard focal lump. The abnormalities seen most often are sternal tilt, fusion or pectus, sternoclavicular subluxation, bifid rib/cartilage, and parachondral node (**Fig. 33**). When the lesion is asymptomatic, it is most likely due to an incidental chest wall anomaly, and imaging beyond a chest radiograph is usually unnecessary.[58] The benign nature of these lesions can be further elucidated if needed by US or low-dose CT.[59] Appreciating the nature of the abnormality is often difficult on plain radiographs and even axial CT, especially in young children. 3-D reconstructions of the CT data are often helpful (see **Fig. 33**).[59] Other non-neoplastic chest wall masses include trauma (bony fracture or healing and soft tissue hematoma) and infection, including adenopathy, cellulitis, soft tissue abscess, and osteomyelitis. Chest wall extension of pulmonary infections, such as tuberculosis, aspergillus, and actinomycosis, can be difficult to differentiate from an aggressive neoplasm. Pathologic fractures may occur with both benign or malignant bone lesions, and the nature of the underlying lesion may be difficult to assess acutely.

Benign lesions of bone that masquerade as chest wall masses may involve the sternum, clavicle,

Box 4
Pleural and chest wall masses in children

Pleural

1. Benign
   a. Hemangioma
   b. Lymphangioma
   c. Neurofibromas
   d. Lipomas

2. Malignant
   a. Pleuropulmonary blastoma
   b. Contiguous or metastatic tumor: Wilms tumor, neuroblastoma, sarcoma, thymoma, and thymic carcinoma
   c. Pleural lipoma/liposarcoma, other sarcoma, PNET
   d. Neurofibrosarcoma
   e. Mesothelioma

Chest wall

1. Benign
   a. Soft tissue origin
      i. Hemangioma/vascular malformation
      ii. Lymphangioma
      iii. Lipoma/lipoblastoma
      iv. Hamartoma (including infantile mesenchymal hamartoma)
      v. Neurofibroma and ganglion cell tumor
      vi. Fibroma/fibromatosis/desmoid
   b. Bone origin
      i. Osteochondroma, osteoid osteoma, osteoblastoma, and aneurysmal bone cyst
      ii. Fibrous dysplasia
      iii. LCH

2. Malignant
   a. Ewing sarcoma/PNET
   b. Rhabdomyosarcoma, osteosarcoma, synovial sarcoma, chondrosarcoma, liposarcoma, leiomyosarcoma, dermatofibrosarcoma, and epithelioid sarcoma
   c. Malignant fibrous histiocytoma
   d. Lymphoma/leukemia
   e. Malignant peripheral nerve cell tumor
   f. Bone and soft tissue metastases (neuroblastoma, hepatoblastoma, and leukemia/lymphoma)

Breast

1. Benign
   a. Hemangioma
   b. Fibroadenoma/giant fibroadenoma

2. Malignant
   a. Cystosarcoma phylloides
   b. Metastases—lymphoma/leukemia and rhabdomyosarcoma
   c. Secondary malignancy—ductal carcinoma

scapula, or ribs; be expansile, lytic, or sclerotic; or project from the bone surface. These include exostoses, enchondroma, fibrous dysplasia, and aneurysmal bone cysts.[54,60] Some of the lesions (eg, exostoses or fibrous dysplasia) may be clearly characterized on plain films and not require additional imaging. LCH may involve one or more sites in the chest with an expansile destructive bony lesion and soft tissue mass that may be difficult to separate from an aggressive lesion, such as Ewing sarcoma, on imaging. Similarly, osteoblastoma, hemangiomas, or lymphangiomas of bone may simulate a more aggressive lesion.[54]

Chest wall tumors arise from any of the tissue components that make up the chest wall including blood vessels, nerves, bone, cartilage, muscle, and fat. The most common benign soft tissue chest wall neoplasms are vascular lesions. These range from single or mutiple focal small subcutaneous lesions to large extensive infiltrative masses; they can also be intrapulmonary or mediastinal in location.[6,20] They are divided into high-flow or low-flow lesions.

In infants, hemangiomas are the most common high-flow vascular lesions. They are typified by high T2 signal on MR imaging and marked contrast enhancement with an early peripheral to later central enhancement pattern on dynamic imaging. There may be tubular signal voids from large vessels on noncontrast images.[4] They tend to grow rapidly in the first year of life and then gradually involute and become infiltrated with fibrofatty tissue. Subcutaneous lesions may be associated with visceral lesions especially in the liver or lung.

In older children, high-flow lesions include atypical hemangiomas as well as arterial vascular malformations, and arteriovenous fistulae. Especially in infants, the rapid-flow lesions may present clinically with high output cardiac failure due to large shunting or thrombocytopenic bleeding associated with platelet sequestration in the mass.[1] Multiphasic magnetic resonance angiography (MRA) is useful in defining the flow pattern and presence of arteriovenous connections. A rapid time resolved MRA sequence (fat-suppressed, T1-weighted, volumetric, spoiled gradient echo) allows for rapidly repeating sequences affording improved temporal resolution at the expense of spatial resolution.[4] Differentiating the flow pattern of a vascular lesion often helps with management decisions and may obviate biopsy, which could be hazardous. High-flow lesions may be managed (alone or in conjunction with surgery) with arterial embolization whereas venolymphatic malformations can be injected percutaneously with sclerosing agents.

Low-flow lesions include venocapillary and lymphatic malformations. The nature and extent

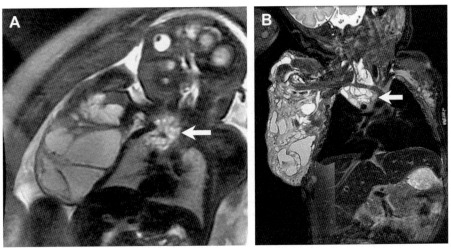

Fig. 32. Lymphangioma (*A*) Thirty weeks' gestation prenatal coronal T2-weighted image. (*B*) Coronal T2 image at 10 days of age. Both studies show a large right multicystic chest wall mass extending into the right neck and mediastinum (*arrows*).

of these lesions are also well defined by MR imaging (see **Fig. 32**). Venocapillary lesions are characterized by slow flow, dilated veins, and phleboliths (bright on T2, diffuse venous phase enhancement with phleboliths appearing as signal voids). The macrocystic lymphatic lesion is recognized by large or small T2 bright cystic spaces with enhancing walls.[1] Microcystic lymphangioma may appear to be a diffusely enhancing soft tissue mass because of the closely packed small cyst walls.[4] Protein or blood products within the cysts may be bright on T1-weighted MR images and dense on CT images and produce fluid-fluid levels

(see **Fig. 10**).[4] Lymphatic malformations (also known as cystic hygromas) can be large and extensive and may be initially recognized on prenatal US or MR imaging (see **Fig. 32**). Involvement of the soft tissues of the neck, axilla, and upper extremity are most common with spread to the chest wall and mediastinum usually secondary (see **Fig. 32**).[4,10,30] Lymphangiomas are particularly associated with Turner syndrome and Noonan syndrome.[18]

Careful fetal evaluation and follow-up are needed, particularly to assess whether a lesion compromises the airway, so that time, location,

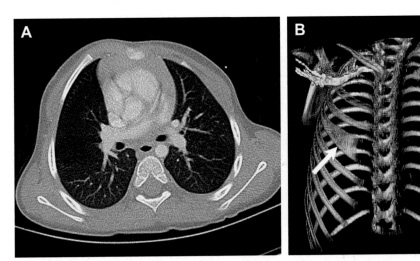

Fig. 33. Rib anomaly simulating a chest wall mass. A 2 year old with a hard palpable mass in the right anterior chest wall. (*A*) Axial CT slice (lung window) shows assymmetry of the anterior chest wall with bulging of the right side with prominent costal cartilage and sternal tilting. Specific rib abnormality was difficult to appreciate on the axial images. (*B*) Oblique coronal 3-D reconstruction clearly depicts a bifid right anterior 4th rib as the cause of the palpable mass (*arrow*).

and mode of delivery can be planned. If the airway is at risk from this or other lesions, an ex utero intrapartum treatment (EXIT) procedure may be needed to safely deliver the baby while maintaining the placental circulation, providing extra time to secure the airway.

Other benign chest wall neoplasms include fatty tumors, such as lipoma (**Fig. 34**) and lipoblastoma (may be locally aggressive); fibrous lesions, such as fibromas, desmoid tumors, and fibromatosis; and neural origin tumors, such as neurofibromas and ganglion cell tumors.[1,54,60] Although these lesions are benign in that they do not metastasize; they may be extensive and difficult to eradicate locally, with recurrence. The fatty nature of lipomas and the fatty components of lipoblastoma follow the readily recognizable imaging characteristics of normal fat on both MR images (bright on T1, dark on short T1 inversion recovery (STIR) and fat saturation images) and CT images (low attenuation) (see **Fig. 34**). Fibrous lesions are less specific but generally are of low signal on T2-weighted MR images with mild enhancement postcontrast. Neural origin tumors tend to be bright on T2-weighted MR imaging. Neurofibromas are often associated with neurofibromatosis type 1; they are well defined and often multiple or lobulated with a typical target-like appearance on T2-weighted and postcontrast images. The target appearance consists of lower signal centrally on T2 with increased central enhancement, thought to be due to the more densely cellular central portion of the tumor.[60] Soft tissue and other desmoid tumors are associated with Gardner syndrome (familial adenomatous polyposis) or may occur at sites of prior surgery or trauma.[61] Mutiple or diffuse soft tissue tumors accompany several systemic syndromes, such as neurofibromatosis type 1 (neurofibromas, nevi, hemangiomas, and xanthogranulomas); proteus syndrome (lipomas/lipomatosis, hemangiomas, lymphangiomas, hamartomas, and hyperkeratosis); and PTEN mutation syndromes (Bannayan-Riley-Ruvalcaba syndrome [lipoma/lipomatosis, hemangiomas, and lymphangiomas]) and Cowden syndrome (lipomas, fibroangiomas, hamartomas, breast fibroadenoma, oral papillomas) (see **Fig. 34**). Many of these entities are also associated with an increased incidence of malignancy.[18,62]

Mesenchmal hamartoma of the chest wall is a unique benign entity in infants characterized by focal overgrowth of skeletal elements of the chest wall with no malignant propensity. A large usually unilateral mass distorting the chest wall is the typical appearance; it is occasionally mutifocal.[1,63] Heterogeneous high-signal T1 areas are thought to be due to hemorrhage and high signal regions on T2 due to cartilage; there are typically multiple fluid/fluid levels suggestive of secondary aneurysmal bone cyst formation.[63,64] The CT appearance is that of rib expansion and destruction and a large lobulated soft tissue mass with chondroid calcification.[64]

Malignant chest wall masses may be difficult to differentiate from their benign counterparts. LCH in particular should be considered in the differential diagnosis of Ewing sarcoma/PNET especially when there is both bone destruction and an adjacent soft tissue mass. Pretreatment biopsy is usually required.[54]

Metastases to bone or occasionally soft tissues of the chest wall are more common than primary chest wall malignant tumors.[59] Chest wall metastatic lesions (see **Fig. 12**) are most often due to neuroblastoma, hepatoblastoma, and leukemia/lymphoma.

Ewings sarcoma/PNET family of tumors and rhabdomyosarcoma, although uncommon, are the most frequently encountered malignant chest wall neoplasms in children, with a high rate of local recurrence and distant metastases (**Fig. 35**).[54,65] Rhabdomyosarcoma of the chest wall is usually of the alveolar (most aggressive form) or embryonal type; the tumor may be heterogeneous with

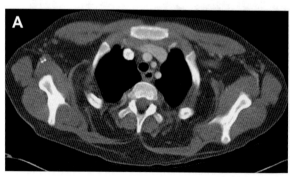
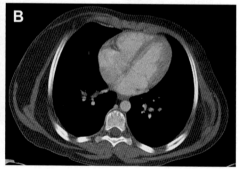

Fig. 34. Chest wall lipomatosis. An 11 year old with PTEN mutation syndrome. (*A, B*) Axial contrasted CT images with extensive low attenuation fatty masses and fatty infiltration of the soft tissues of the chest wall.

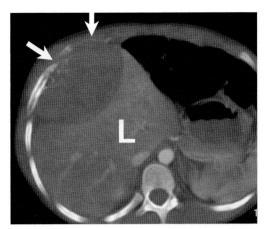

Fig. 35. Ewing sarcoma—8-year-old girl. CT contrasted image at the thoracoabdominal junction shows a large slightly heterogeneous chest wall soft tissue mass centered around the anterior rib with bony destructive changes (*arrows*). The posterior component of the soft tissue mass exerts external mass effect on the liver (L).

multiple areas of necrosis.[66] The chest wall is a site of predilection for Ewing and PNET (also known as Askin tumor)[1,4]; the tumor may originate in bone, soft tissue, or pleura or rarely may be intrapulmonary.[65,67] Imaging helps define the location, possible origin, and extent (see **Fig. 35**). The chest wall is a difficult region to obtain an adequate tumor resection with clear margins without marked deformity and respiratory compromise (see **Fig. 20**).[65]

Other primary chest wall malignant lesions in childhood include osteogenic sarcoma, chondrosarcoma, synovial sarcoma (see **Fig. 20**), malignant peripheral nerve sheath tumors, liposarcoma, leiomyosarcoma, malignant fibrous histiocytoma, epithelioid sarcoma, dermatofibrosarcoma, and

lymphoma/leukemia (**Fig. 36**). Degeneration into chondrosarcoma is of particular concern in multiple hereditary exostoses, most often occurring in adulthood. Malignancy is more common in the axial rather than the appendicular skeleton. Malignant transformation of an osteochondroma may be difficult to recognize. Thickening and irregularity of the cartilaginous cap, lesion enlargement, development of a soft tissue mass, and heterogeneous enhancement are concerning features.[4,66]

Tumors of the breast are uncommon in children and are usually benign; these are most often evaluated by US; occasionally, MR imaging may be obtained (**Fig. 37**). Sonographic evaluation identifies normal breast tissue and differentiates cystic, mixed, or solid lesions and their vascularity. Mammography or CT is usually unnecessary and unhelpful.[54] It is important to recognize an enlarged breast bud from a mass when imaging an infant or child with unilateral or bilateral breast enlargement. Hemangioma is the most common benign lesion of the breast in infants and fibroadenoma in older children (see **Fig. 37**).[54] The giant fibroadenoma of adolescents is typically larger than 10 cm. These are well-defined, uniform rounded large hypoechoic masses on US.[3] Other benign lesions include papilloma, lipoma, and lymphangioma.[3] Primary breast malignancies are unusual in childhood; the most common tumor is cystosarcoma phylloides.[54] Metastases to the breast may occur with lymphoma, leukemia, and rhabdomyosarcoma.

LONG-TERM EFFECTS OF CHILDHOOD CANCER

Late effects of treatment of childhood cancer are increasingly recognized as common and important.[68,69] Long-term morbidity, often at an early age, is present in more than half of childhood

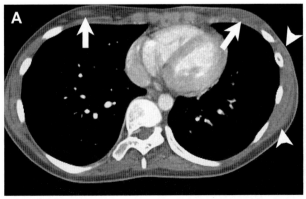
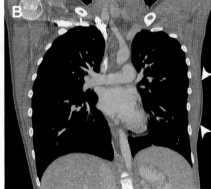

Fig. 36. A 15-year-old girl with cutaneous/subcutaneous T cell lymphoma. Axial (*A*) and coronal (*B*) postcontrast CT images with plaque like superficial lesions (*arrows*) as well as a larger infiltrating lesion of the chest wall soft tissues on the left (*arrowheads*) with loss of normal muscle/fat planes.

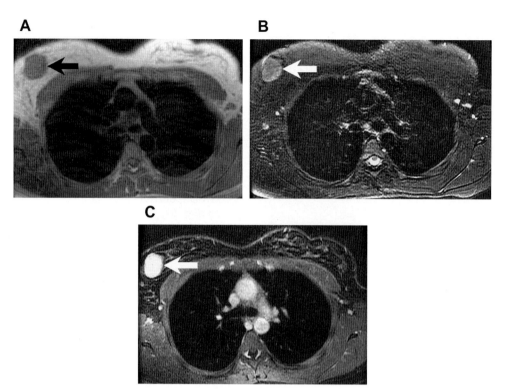

Fig. 37. An 18-year-old woman. Right breast fibroadenoma. (*A*) Axial T1-weighted, (*B*) axial T2-weighted, and (*C*) axial postcontrast MR images. There is a 4.5-cm well-defined sharply marginated solid enhancing mass in the right breast (*arrows*). This was an incidental finding on this MR, obtained for other reasons. The MR imaging characteristics (T2 bright with enhancement) suggest that this is an adenomatous or myxomatous rather than fibrous histologic tumor type. This MR imaging appearance does not distinguish fibroadenoma from malignant tumors.

cancer survivors. These include joint disease, osteoporsosis, scoliosis, congestive heart failure, restrictive/obstructive lung disease/pulmonary fibrosis, second cancers, cognitive dysfunction, coronary artery disease, cerebrovascular accident, renal failure, cystitis/bladder fibrosis, asplenia (infection risk), hepatic cirrhosis, bowel fibrosis/obstruction, hearing and vision loss, growth failure, and gonadal failure.[68]

Resection of thoracic tumors both benign and malignant may have significant prolonged effects in terms of thoracic deformity (see **Fig. 20**) with distortion of vessels and airways and lung restriction as well as affecting overall well-being and self-image.

With regard to the thorax, breast and thyroid cancer are the most common second malignancies. Breast cancer is usually invasive ductal carcinoma or ductal carcinoma in situ and is most common after radiation for Hodgkin lymphoma in girls between 10 and 20 years of age.[68,69] Papillary thyroid cancer is correlated with head, neck, and chest irradiation in children less than 10 years of age.[68] This tumor carries a good prognosis even when metastases are present. Benign and

malignant bone tumors and soft tissue sarcomas as well as leukemia/lymphoma and bronchogenic carcinoma, including bronchoalveolar carcinoma, are concerns for second tumors after radiation/chemotherapy.[40,68,69] Even though treatment regimens have changed, radiation therapy, in particular, is used less and at lower, more directed doses, close follow-up of childhood cancer survivors is needed. Radiologists as well as clinicians need to be aware of and vigilant for secondary complications of prior malignancies.

REFERENCES

1. Watt AJ. Chest wall lesions. Paediatr Respir Rev 2002;3(4):328–38.
2. Ben-Ami TE, O'Donovan JC, Yousefzadeh DK. Sonography of the chest in children. Radiol Clin North Am 1993;31(3):517–31.
3. Siegel MJ. Chest. In: Siegel MJ, editor. Pediatric sonography. 3rd edition. Philadelphia: Lippincott Williams & Wilkins; 2002.
4. Fefferman NR, Pinkney LP. Imaging evaluation of chest wall disorders in children. Radiol Clin North Am 2005;43(2):355–70.

5. Merten DF. Diagnostic imaging of mediastinal masses in children. AJR Am J Roentgenol 1992; 158(4):825–32.

6. Arcement C, Newman B. Practical imaging of mediastinal and pulmonary masses in children. Contemporary Diagnostic Radiology 1998;21(21):1–6.

7. Binkovitz LA, Binkovitz I, Kuhn JP. The mediastinum. In: Slovis T, editor. Caffey's pediatric diagnostic imaging, vol. 1. 11th edition. Philadelphia: Mosby Elsevier; 2008. p. 1324–88.

8. Gielda BT, Peng R, Coleman JL, et al. Treatment of early stage thymic tumors: surgery and radiation therapy. Curr Treat Options Oncol 2008;9(4–6):259–68.

9. Jaggers J, Balsara K. Mediastinal masses in children. Semin Thorac Cardiovasc Surg 2004;16(3):201–8.

10. Strollo DC, Rosado de Christenson ML, Jett JR. Primary mediastinal tumors. Part 1: tumors of the anterior mediastinum. Chest 1997;112(2):511–22.

11. Yaris N, Nas Y, Cobanoglu U, et al. Thymic carcinoma in children. Pediatr Blood Cancer 2006; 47(2):224–7.

12. Orki A, Patlakoglu MS, Tahaoglu C, et al. Malignant invasive thymoma in the posterior mediastinum. Ann Thorac Surg 2009;87(4):1274–5.

13. Flieder DB, Suster S, Moran CA. Idiopathic fibroinflammatory (fibrosing/sclerosing) lesions of the mediastinum: a study of 30 cases with emphasis on morphologic heterogeneity. Mod Pathol 1999; 12(3):257–64.

14. Greenberg SB, MacDonald C. Cardiac tumors. In: Slovis T, editor. Caffey's pediatric diagnostic imaging, vol. 2. 11th edition. Philadelphia: Mosby Elsevier; 2008. p. 1707–12.

15. Towbin AJ, Newman B. Syndromes and chromosomal anomalies. In: Slovis T, editor. Caffey's pediatric diagnostic imaging, vol. 1. 11th edition. Philadelphia: Mosby Elsevier; 2008. p. 1605–32.

16. Towbin AJ, Newman B. Cardiac involvement by systemic diseases. In: Slovis T, editor. Caffey's pediatric diagnostic imaging, vol. 1. 11th edition. Philadelphia: Mosby Elsevier; 2008. p. 1687–706.

17. Isaacs H. Perinatal (fetal and neonatal) tuberous sclerosis: a review. Am J Perinatol 2009;26(10):755–60.

18. Taybi H, Lachman RS. Syndromes. Radiology of syndromes, metabolic disorders, and skeletal dysplasias. St Louis: Mosby Year Book Inc; 1996. p. 66–7, 352–5, 504–7.

19. Wang ZJ, Reddy GP, Gotway MB, et al. CT and MR imaging of pericardial disease. Radiographics 2003; 23:S167–80.

20. Newman B, Effmann EL. Lung masses. In: Slovis T, editor. Caffey's pediatric diagnostic imaging, vol. 1. 11th edition. Philadelphia: Mosby Elsevier; 2008. p. 1294–323.

21. Eggli KD, Newman B. Nodules, masses, and pseudomasses in the pediatric lung. Radiol Clin North Am 1993;31(3):651–66.

22. Newman B. Congenital bronchopulmonary foregut malformations: concepts and controversies. Pediatr Radiol 2006;36(8):773–91.

23. Langston C. New concepts in the pathology of congenital lung malformations. Semin Pediatr Surg 2003;12(1):17–37.

24. Kunisaki SM, Fauza DO, Nemes LP, et al. Bronchial atresia: the hidden pathology within a spectrum of prenatally diagnosed lung masses. J Pediatr Surg 2006;41(1):61–5.

25. Dishop MK, Kuruvilla S. Primary and metastatic lung tumors in the pediatric population: a review and 25-year experience at a large children's hospital. Arch Pathol Lab Med 2008;132(7):1079–103.

26. Qiao GB, Zeng WS, Peng LJ, et al. Multiple pulmonary chondromas in a young female patient: a component of Carney triad. J Thorac Oncol 2009;4(6):751–2.

27. Carney JA. Carney triad: a syndrome featuring paraganglionic, adrenocortical, and possibly other endocrine tumors. J Clin Endocrinol Metab 2009;94(10): 3656–62.

28. Newman B, Feinstein JA, Cohen RA, et al. Congenital extrahepatic portosystemic shunt associated with heterotaxy and polysplenia. Pediatr Radiol 2010;40(7):1222–30.

29. Faul JL, Berry GJ, Colby TV, et al. Thoracic lymphangiomas, lymphangiectasis, lymphangiomatosis, and lymphatic dysplasia syndrome. Am J Respir Crit Care Med 2000;161:1037–46.

30. Alvarez OA, Kjellin I, Zuppan CW. Thoracic lymphangiomatosis in a child. J Pediatr Hematol Oncol 2004;26(2):136–41.

31. Braier J, Chantada G, Rosso D, et al. Langerhans cell histiocytosis: retrospective evaluation of 123 patients at a single institution. Pediatr Hematol Oncol 1999;16(5):377–85.

32. Marchiori E, Araujo Neto C, Meirelles GS, et al. Laryngotracheobronchial papillomatosis: findings on computed tomography scans of the chest. J Bras Pneumol 2008;34(12):1084–9.

33. Weldon CB, Shamberger RC. Pediatric pulmonary tumors: primary and metastatic. Semin Pediatr Surg 2008;17(1):17–29.

34. DasNarla L, Newman B, Spottswood SS, et al. Inflammatory pseudotumor. Radiographics 2003; 23(3):719–29.

35. Al-Qahtani AR, Di Lorenzo M, Yazbeck S. Endobronchial tumors in children: Institutional experience and literature review. J Pediatr Surg 2003; 38(5):733–6.

36. Hedlund GL, Navoy JF, Galliani CA, et al. Aggressive manifestations of inflammatory pulmonary pseudotumor in children. Pediatr Radiol 1999;29(2):112–6.

37. Lim GY, Newman B, Kurland G, et al. Posttransplantation lymphoproliferative disorder: manifestations in pediatric thoracic organ recipients. Radiology 2002; 222(3):699–708.

38. Pollock AN, Newman B, Putnam PE, et al. Imaging of post-transplant spindle cell tumors. Pediatr Radiol 1995;25(Suppl 1):S118–21.

39. Neville HL, Hogan AR, Zhuge Y, et al. Incidence and outcomes of malignant pediatric lung neoplasms. J Surg Res 2009;156(2):224–30.

40. Lebensburger J, Katzenstein H, Jenkins JJ, et al. Bronchioloalveolar carcinoma as a second malignancy in osteosarcoma survivors. Pediatr Blood Cancer 2009;53(3):499–501.

41. Chen F, Miyahara R, Bando T, et al. Repeat resection of pulmonary metastasis is beneficial for patients with osteosarcoma of the extremities. Interact Cardiovasc Thorac Surg 2009;9(4):649–53.

42. Blackmon SH, Shah N, Roth JA, et al. Resection of pulmonary and extrapulmonary sarcomatous metastases is associated with long-term survival. Ann Thorac Surg 2009;88(3):877–84.

43. Kunst PW, Sutedja G, Golding RP, et al. Unusual Pulmonary Lesions: Case 1. A Juvenile Bronchopulmonary Fibrosarcoma. J Clin Oncol 2002;20(11):2745–51.

44. Miniati DN, Chintagumpala M, Langston C, et al. Prenatal presentation and outcome of children with pleuropulmonary blastoma. J Pediatr Surg 2006; 41(1):66–71.

45. Granata C, Gambini C, Balducci T, et al. Bronchioloalveolar carcinoma arising in congenital cystic adenomatoid malformation in a child: a case report and review on malignancies originating in congenital cystic adenomatoid malformation. Pediatr Pulmonol 1998;25(1):62–6.

46. Epelman M, Kreiger PA, Servaes S, et al. Current imaging of prenatally diagnosed congenital lung lesions. Semin Ultrasound CT MR 2010;31(2):141–57.

47. Priest JR, Watterson J, Strong L, et al. Pleuropulmonary blastoma: a marker for familial disease. J Pediatr 1996;128(2):220–4.

48. Hill DA, Jarzembowski JA, Priest JR, et al. Type I pleuropulmonary blastoma: pathology and biology study of 51 cases from the international pleuropulmonary blastoma registry. Am J Surg Pathol 2008; 32(2):282–95.

49. Hill DA, Ivanovich J, Priest JR, et al. DICER1 mutations in familial pleuropulmonary blastoma. Science 2009;325(5943):965. DOI:10.1126/science.1174334.

50. Dehner LP. Beware of "degenerating" congenital pulmonary cysts. Pediatr Surg Int 2005;21(2):123–4.

51. Bagan P, Hassan M, Le Pimpec Barthes F, et al. Prognostic factors and surgical indications of pulmonary epithelioid hemangioendothelioma: a review of the literature. Ann Thorac Surg 2006;82(6):2010–3.

52. Long FR, Druhan SM, Kuhn JP. Disease of the bronchi and pulmonary aeration. In: Slovis T, editor. 11th edition, Caffey's pediatric diagnostic imaging, vol. 1. Philadelphia: Mosby Elsevier; 2008. p. 1121–76.

53. Abdulhamid I, Rabah R. Granular cell tumor of the bronchus. Pediatr Pulmonol 2000;30(5):425–8.

54. Dwek JR, Effman EL. Chest wall. In: Slovis T, editor. Caffey's pediatric diagnostic imaging, vol. 1. 11th edition. Philadelphia: Mosby Elsevier; 2008. p. 1389–430.

55. Sharif K, Alton H, Clarke J, et al. Paediatric thoracic tumours presenting as empyema. Pediatr Surg Int 2006;22(12):1009–14.

56. Dwek JR, Kuhn JP. Pleura. In: Slovis T, editor. Caffey's pediatric diagnostic imaging, vol. 1. 11th edition. Philadelphia: Mosby Elsevier; 2008. p. 1431–50.

57. Dwek JR, Kuhn JP. Diaphragm. In: Slovis T, editor. Caffey's pediatric diagnostic imaging, vol. 1. 11th edition. Philadelphia: Mosby Elsevier; 2008. p. 1451–62.

58. Donnelly LF, Taylor CN, Emery KH, et al. Asymptomatic, palpable, anterior chest wall lesions in children: is cross-sectional imaging necessary? Radiology 1997;202(3):829–31.

59. Donnelly LF. Use of three-dimensional reconstructed helical CT images in recognition and communication of chest wall anomalies in children. AJR Am J Roentgenol 2001;177(2):441–5.

60. Tateishi U, Gladish GW, Kusumoto M, et al. Chest wall tumors: radiologic findings and pathologic correlation: part 1. Benign tumors. Radiographics 2003;23(6):1477–90.

61. Bolke E, Krasniqi H, Lammering G, et al. Chest wall and intrathoracic desmoid tumors: surgical experience and review of the literature. Eur J Med Res 2009;14(6):240–3.

62. Marsh DJ, Kum JB, Lunetta KL, et al. PTEN mutation spectrum and genotype-phenotype correlations in Bannayan-Riley-Ruvalcaba syndrome suggest a single entity with Cowden syndrome. Hum Mol Genet 1999;8(8):1461–72.

63. Lisle DA, Ault DJ, Earwaker JW, et al. Mesenchymal hamartoma of the chest wall in infants: report of three cases and literature review. Australas Radiol 2003;47(1):78–82.

64. Subramanian S, Seith A, Abhey P, et al. Answer to case of the month #143 mesenchymal hamartoma of the chest wall. Can Assoc Radiol J 2009;60(1):47–9.

65. Demir A, Gunluoglu MZ, Dagoglu N, et al. Surgical treatment and prognosis of primitive neuroectodermal tumors of the thorax. J Thorac Oncol 2009; 4(2):185–92.

66. Tateishi U, Gladish GW, Kusumoto M, et al. Chest wall tumors: radiologic findings and pathologic correlation: part 2. Malignant tumors. Radiographics 2003;23(6):1491–508.

67. Takahashi D, Nagayama J, Nagatoshi Y, et al. Primary Ewing's sarcoma family tumors of the lung a case report and review of the literature. Jpn J Clin Oncol 2007;37(11):874–7.

68. Dickerman JD. The late effects of childhood cancer therapy. Pediatrics 2007;119(3):554–68.

69. Ng AK, Kenney LB, Gilbert ES, et al. Secondary malignancies across the age spectrum. Semin Radiat Oncol 2010;20(1):67–78.

Gastrointestinal Tumors in Children

Maria F. Ladino-Torres, MD[a],*, Peter J. Strouse, MD[b]

KEYWORDS
- Pancreas • Spleen • Gastrointestinal
- Neoplasm • Pediatric

This article focuses on the neoplasms arising from the pancreas, spleen, and the gastrointestinal tract in children. Tumors of the liver are discussed in another article elsewhere in this issue. Clinical presentation and imaging features depend on patient age and the organ of origin. Children may present with an abdominal mass, increased abdominal girth, constipation, decreased appetite, abdominal pain, or rectal bleeding. Pallor or weakness may also be present related to anemia. Initial imaging with abdominal radiograph contributes to the evaluation for intestinal obstruction, constipation, and mass effect, and sometimes may reveal areas of calcification.[1,2]

Ultrasound is the preferred study in the initial assessment of most suspected abdominal masses to determine the organ of origin and intrinsic characteristics without the need for ionizing radiation or sedation in young patients. Assessment for intrinsic vascularity or relation with the major vascular structures may be accomplished with Doppler imaging.[3] Ultrasound also guides further workup and therapy. Assessment with CT, MR imaging, or nuclear medicine may be required for further characterization, assessing involvement of adjacent organs or vascular structures, and staging of malignant masses. Contrast-enhanced multidetector CT imaging provides detailed anatomic evaluation with rapid acquisition, which allows for minimal need for sedation in young patients and no sedation in older children. A disadvantage of CT is the use of ionizing radiation; however, dedicated pediatric imaging protocols and new CT technologies allow for reduction in radiation dose.

MR imaging also provides an excellent soft tissue characterization and precise anatomic detail. Multiphase post-contrast dynamic MR imaging acquisition is particularly helpful in characterizing solid organ focal lesions. Angiographic information obtained using MR angiography protocols may contribute to surgical planning. Although MR imaging protocols have evolved and the scanning times are shorter than in the past, the disadvantages of MR imaging is the length of the examination and the need for sedation or general anesthesia in the younger pediatric population. Fluoroscopic examinations of the gastrointestinal tract are rarely used to evaluate the suspected neoplasms.

Nonneoplastic conditions may occasionally cause mass effect and mimic a tumor. Differential diagnostic considerations are briefly noted for each organ.

PANCREAS

Pancreatic tumors are rare in children.[4-7] Pancreatoblastoma is an epithelial tumor arising from the acinar cells that occurs almost exclusively in children, and is the most common pancreatic tumor in young children. Solid and papillary epithelial neoplasms (SPENs) affect adolescent girls and young women. Endocrine tumors have been reported in older children, and focal or diffuse neuroendocrine adenomatosis can be present in neonates, causing

---

The authors have nothing to disclose.
a Department of Radiology, C.S. Mott Children's Hospital, University of Michigan, Room F3503, 1500 East Medical Center Drive, Ann Arbor, MI 48109–5252, USA
b Section of Pediatric Radiology, Department of Radiology, C.S. Mott Children's Hospital, University of Michigan Health System, University of Michigan, Room F3503, 1500 East Medical Center Drive, Ann Arbor, MI 48109–5252, USA
* Corresponding author.
E-mail address: marialad@umich.edu

hypoglycemia. Epithelial neoplasms of the pancreas are rare in children, but have been reported. Rarely, lymphoma or metastatic disease may affect the pancreas.

PANCREATOBLASTOMA

Pancreatoblastoma, also called *pancreaticoblastoma*, is a rare neoplasm, with fewer than 75 cases reported in the literature. It is most common in the first decade of life, with a mean age of approximately 5 years and a male to female ratio of 2:1.[4] Congenital cases have been described in association with Beckwith-Wiedemann syndrome.[8] Patients may present with an asymptomatic abdominal mass or with nonspecific abdominal pain, vomiting, or early satiety. As with other embryonal tumors, α-fetoprotein levels may be elevated.[6,9] Pancreatoblastoma usually presents with large abdominal masses ranging from 1.5 to 20 cm, compressing adjacent structures.[10] With larger masses, the organ of origin may be difficult to determine. Half arise from the pancreatic head; however, biliary obstruction is not a frequent presentation. On ultrasound and CT imaging, pancreatoblastomas appear as well-defined, partially circumscribed, heterogeneous masses with both cystic and solid components (**Fig. 1**). On MR imaging, most tumors are heterogeneous with low to intermediate signal intensity on T1-weighted images and high signal intensity on T2-weighted images.[10] Heterogeneous post-contrast enhancement is a common feature. An infiltrative pattern has also been described but

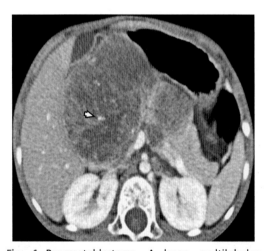

Fig. 1. Pancreatoblastoma. A large, multilobular, mildly heterogeneous soft tissue mass is seen arising from the head and body of the pancreas. Small calcifications are seen within the mass (*arrow*). (*Courtesy of M.J. Callahan, Boston, MA.*)

is uncommon.[10] Small calcifications may be present.[10,11] Invasion of peripancreatic soft tissues and adjacent organs such as the duodenum may occur. Encasement of vascular structures, including the mesenteric vessels and the inferior vena cava, has been described, but vascular invasion is uncommon.[11] Metastatic disease may occur, most commonly affecting the liver, abdominal lymph nodes, and omentum. Prognosis in the absence of metastatic disease with complete surgical resection is good, but recurrence is common.[4,6]

SPEN

SPEN was initially described by Frantz in 1959[12] and is also known by many other terms, including *solid-cystic papillary tumor*, *solid pseudopapillary tumor*, *papillary epithelial neoplasm*, and *Frantz tumor*. It is a distinct tumor of the exocrine pancreas according to the World Health Organization (WHO). This tumor is most frequently reported in adolescent girls and young women with a mean age of 21 years. Approximately 90% of the reported cases are in females.[4] Patients present with abdominal discomfort, pain, or a mass. On imaging, tumors reflect the pathologic components and appear as large, well-circumscribed, usually encapsulated masses, with heterogeneous architecture or mixed solid and cystic elements.[13] Small tumors may appear completely solid. Areas of hemorrhagic necrosis, fluid–fluid levels, and blood products have been described as distinctive features.[14] Areas of hemorrhage and blood degradation products are better depicted on MR imaging.[15] Peripheral calcification may be present in approximately one-third of the cases.[15,16] Post-contrast imaging shows enhancement of the solid component or peripheral rim of enhancement of the fibrous capsule (**Fig. 2**). Early peripheral enhancement and progressive centripetal filling on post-contrast dynamic MR imaging has also been described.[13] Approximately 85% of the cases are limited to the pancreas. Biliary ductal dilatation is uncommon even with large masses. Other uncommon features include parenchymal and extracapsular invasion, and dense calcification have been described.[14]

The course of SPENs is usually benign and tumors are limited to the pancreas in approximately 85% of the cases. Surgery is usually curative but may require a Whipple procedure depending on location of the tumor. Metastatic disease is uncommon but has been reported in older patients and is apparently rare in children. Because of the potential for aggressive behavior (tumor recurrence or metastatic disease), SPENs are usually treated with complete surgical resection.

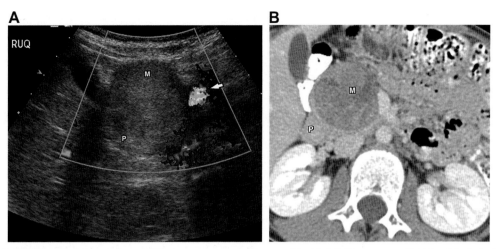

Fig. 2. Solid epithelial neoplasm of the pancreas in a 10-year-old girl. (A) Transverse ultrasound image shows a solid echogenic mass (M) in the head of the pancreas (P) displacing the mesenteric vessels (arrow). (B) Contrast-enhanced CT axial image shows a well-circumscribed mass (M) with heterogeneous enhancing pattern. The mass enhances less than the pancreas (P). No biliary ductal dilatation is seen.

Islet Cell Tumors

Islet cell tumors, also called *neuroendocrine tumors of the pancreas*, may be benign (adenomas) or malignant with metastatic disease (carcinomas). These tumors are most commonly diagnosed in adults but may be seen in children.[17] They may produce hormonally active polypeptide and may present with clinical symptoms. Islet cell tumors are designated as functioning or hyperfunctioning. Hyperfunctioning tumors produce a clinical syndrome. Insulinoma is the most common type of functioning islet cell tumor, followed by gastrinoma.[4] In a series of 224 patients with symptomatic insulinomas published by the Mayo Clinic, only 5% of cases occurred in children, all older than 8 years.[18] In the same case series, patients with multiple endocrine neoplasia type I were younger at diagnosis of insulinoma and had a greater risk of recurrence.

Insulinomas are composed of β cells. Gastrinomas are composed of G cells and may cause Zollinger-Ellison syndrome. All other islet cell tumors are rare in children. Insulinomas are usually seen in the body and tail of the pancreas, and gastrinomas are seen in the pancreatic head.[9] However, gastrinomas may also occur in extrapancreatic locations (eg, duodenum, proximal jejunum, stomach). Multiple pancreatic islet cell tumors may be seen in patients with multiple endocrine neoplasia, type I.

Islet cell tumors are small, usually less than 2 cm, well defined, and homogeneous. Islet cell tumors are usually hypoechoic on ultrasound and may have a hyperechoic rim. On CT, islet cell tumors usually enhance greater than the adjacent normal pancreas but may be difficult to detect (**Fig. 3**).

On MR imaging, islet cell tumors appear hypointense on T1-weighted images with and without fat suppression, and hyperintense on T2-weighted images. Intense enhancement is seen on postcontrast T1-wieghted sequences.[19] Larger tumors are usually malignant and more likely to be associated with metastatic disease. Peptide receptor scintigraphy with the radioactive somatostatin analogue [111]indium-diethylene triamine pentaacetic acid octreotide (^{111}In-DTPA octreotide) is used for identification and localization of intrapancreatic and extrapancreatic gastrinomas and for assessment of metastatic disease.[20]

Nesidioblastomatosis, or persistent hyperinsulimenic hypoglycemia of infancy, is a disorder characterized by proliferation of hyperfunctioning β cells. Two forms have been described, focal and diffuse, with the latter being more common (70%). The diagnosis is based on clinical and biochemical results, because ultrasound, CT, and MR imaging do not provide diagnostic imaging findings.[21]

Pancreatic Cysts

Congenital epithelium-lined cysts of the pancreas are rare and usually found incidentally. Pancreatic cysts may be associated with systemic diseases and syndromes such as von Hippel-Lindau disease, autosomal dominant polycystic kidney disease, and Beckwith-Wiedemann syndrome (**Fig. 4**). Dermoid cysts or mature teratomas of the pancreas are extremely rare; both predominantly cystic and heterogeneous tumors have been described reflecting tumor tissue components (**Fig. 5**).[22,23] Pancreatic pseudocysts, as a consequence of preceding pancreatitis or

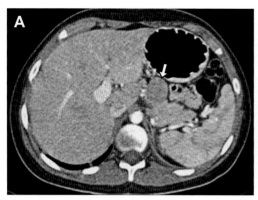
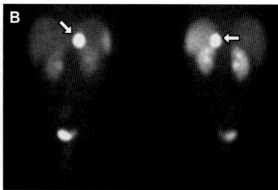

Fig. 3. A 14-year-old boy with gastrinoma. The patient presented with recurrent episodes of abdominal pain associated with hematemesis, weight loss, and fatigue. Endoscopy showed gastritis. (A) Axial contrast-enhanced CT shows a focal mass arising within the body of the pancreas (arrow). (B) Anterior and posterior ^{111}In DTPA-octreotide images show focal uptake of tracer within the mass (arrows). Normal activity is seen within liver, spleen, kidneys, and bladder. No abnormal activity is seen beyond the mass to suggest metastatic disease. (Courtesy of W.H. McAlister, St Louis, MO.)

trauma, are much more common than congenital or neoplastic pancreatic cysts, and therefore are a more likely diagnostic consideration in patients with a cystic pancreatic mass (Fig. 6).

Systemic Malignancy

The pancreas may be encased or displaced by adjacent tumors, such as neuroblastoma or lymphoma. Lymphoma may extend into the pancreas or may involve the pancreas intrinsically. In general, direct pancreatic involvement is rare. Associated disease in other organs and lymph nodes usually suggests the diagnosis. Involvement is most common with large cell lymphoma and is sporadic with Burkitt lymphoma.[4] Focal masses from leukemia (granulocytic sarcoma "chloroma") can rarely affect the pancreas (Fig. 7).[24] Metastatic disease to the pancreas is rare in children but has been reported in rhabdomyosarcoma, neuroblastoma,[25] osteosarcoma,[26,27] and melanoma (Fig. 8).

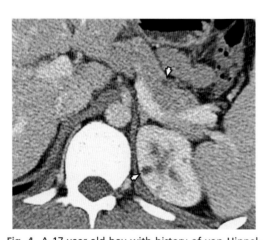

Fig. 4. A 17-year-old boy with history of von Hippel-Lindau syndrome. Axial CT image shows a subcentimeter pancreatic cyst and a small complex cystic lesion in the posterior aspect of the left kidney (arrows). Multiple complex cystic lesions were present in the kidneys (not shown).

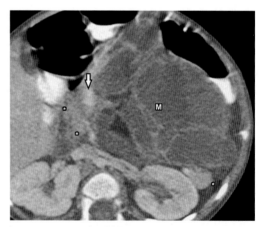

Fig. 5. A 17-month-old boy with palpable abdominal mass and difficulty tolerating feeds. Contrast-enhanced axial CT image shows a predominantly cystic mass with multiple enhancing septations and a few solid enhancing components. Pancreatic head and tail are displaced (asterisk). The mass (M) closely abuts the superior mesenteric artery and vein (arrow), and the portal vein. Pathology showed cystic teratoma composed predominantly of mature elements, with a small component of immature nonneural element.

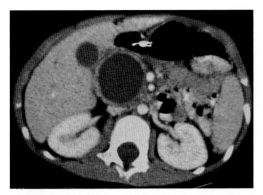

Fig. 6. A 3-year-old boy with a pancreatic cyst. The patient presented with abdominal pain. CT shows a well-defined cystic mass of the pancreatic head. At surgery, the mass was separate from the biliary tree. Although the patient had no history of trauma nor clinical evidence of pancreatitis, pathologic examination showed that the cyst was not lined with epithelium, but rather scar tissue, suggesting a pseudocyst.

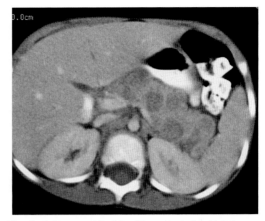

Fig. 8. A 3-year-old girl with metastatic rhabdomyosarcoma to the pancreas at presentation. Multiple low attenuation lesions are seen throughout the pancreas. The primary tumor was in the left infratemporal fossa.

Spleen

Excluding lymphoma, tumors of the spleen are rare in children. Primary vascular neoplasms and congenital epithelial cysts are the most common benign pediatric splenic tumors, and the most common malignant pediatric splenic mass is lymphoma.[28]

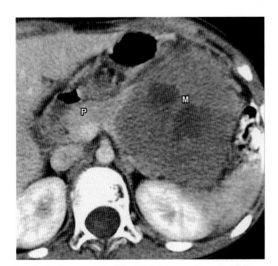

Fig. 7. A 6-year-old girl with history of acute myelogenous leukemia and initial relapse in bone marrow and central nervous system, now presenting with abdominal pain. Contrast-enhanced CT shows a well-defined soft tissue mass (M) arising from the pancreatic body and tail, containing several irregular foci of central low attenuation. Pathologically, the mass proved to be a granulocytic sarcoma (chloroma) of pancreas (P).

Metastatic disease to the spleen is also rare, with neuroblastoma the most frequent.[29–31]

BENIGN VASCULAR TUMORS

Benign vascular tumors of the spleen include hemangioma, lymphangioma and hamartoma.[32,33] These tumors are rare in children; however, hemangioma is the most common benign primary neoplasm of the pediatric spleen. Hemangiomas are usually isolated and asymptomatic but may occur as part of a Klippel-Trénaunay-Weber syndrome or Beckwith-Wiedemann syndrome. Hemangiomas are thought to be congenital in origin, and consist of a proliferation of vascular channels ranging from capillary to cavernous lined by endothelium.[32] Splenic hemangiomas are usually small lesions less than 2 cm; however, size is variable and splenic hemangiomas may be single or multiple. Smaller hemangiomas tend to be solid and larger lesions that demonstrate cystic and solid components with areas of fibrosis. Areas of calcifications may be present. Imaging findings depend on size and internal characteristics. On ultrasound, lesions vary from hypoechoic to hyperechoic relative to the splenic parenchyma, with associated cystic areas and significant blood flow noted on Doppler imaging. If calcification is present, posterior shadowing may be seen. On CT, the solid components show homogeneous or mottled enhancement (**Fig. 9**). On MR imaging, the lesions appear hyperintense or isointense on T1-weighted images and hyperintense on T2-weighted images. Areas of hemorrhage may be present in larger hemangiomas. Contrast-enhancement patterns of

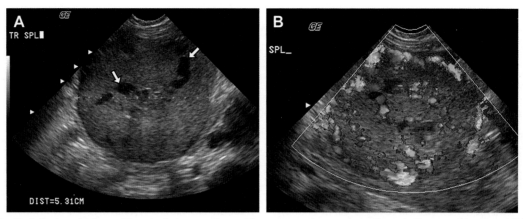

Fig. 9. A 3-year-old boy with splenic hemangioma. The mass was asymptomatic and discovered by the child's pediatrician during a routine physical examination. (*A*) Longitudinal ultrasound showed the mass to be exophytic from the spleen, and solid. Small hypoechoic areas (*arrows*) did not fill with color, and likely represent areas of necrosis, hemorrhage, or stagnant flow. (*B*) On color Doppler imaging, abundant vascular flow is seen within the mass.

splenic hemangiomas vary depending on lesion size. On dynamic post-contrast imaging, small hemangiomas usually show homogenous enhancement. Centripetal enhancement may be seen in larger lesions but is less conspicuous than that of liver hemangiomas. Well-defined enhancing peripheral nodules are not usually present in larger hemangiomas.[33,34]

Splenic lymphangioma, or more correctly "lymphatic malformation of the spleen," is a rare benign tumor that occurs in children, with adult cases being reported less frequently. Lymphangiomas are characterized by endothelium-lined spaces filled with proteinaceous material, and may appear as unilocular or multilocular cystic lesions or may be part of diffuse lymphangiomatosis.[35] The lesions vary in size from a few millimeters to large cystic masses with internal septations and debris. No significant vascularity is present, and therefore enhancement of the septa is minimal on post-contrast imaging. Subtle linear calcifications are better depicted on CT imaging. On MR imaging, these lesions have low signal intensity on T1-weighted images and high signal intensity on T2-weighted images (**Fig. 10**). Isointense to hyperintense signal may sometimes be seen on T1-weighted images because of proteinaceous content.[36]

Splenic hamartoma is a benign lesion composed of disorganized splenic red pulp elements. Some consider this a neoplasm or possibly a posttraumatic lesion, whereas others believe that it might arise as an acquired proliferative process.[32] The lesions have been reported in association with tuberous sclerosis. On ultrasound, splenic hamartomas are usually solid, relatively homogenous masses, and are hyperechoic relative to the spleen parenchyma (**Fig. 11**). A cystic component may be present. Doppler imaging shows hypervascularity likely related to the red pulp component[37]; however, hamartomas do not show hypervascularity to the degree seen with hemangioma. On contrast-enhanced CT, splenic hemangiomas appear isoattenuating to splenic parenchyma. On MR imaging, hamartomas are isointense on T1-weighted images, heterogeneously hyperintense

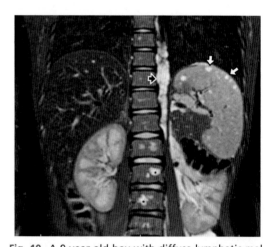

Fig. 10. A 9-year-old boy with diffuse lymphatic malformation involving multiple organs. Coronal short tau inversion recovery image shows multiple small high-signal lesions with the spleen (*white arrows*). Left retrocrural lymphatic malformation (*black arrow*) and vertebral lesions (*asterisk*) are also seen.

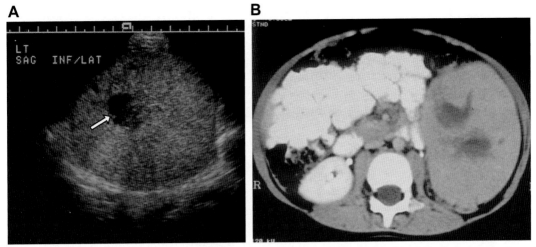

Fig. 11. A 5-year-old boy with a splenic hamartoma. The mass was discovered incidentally during evaluation of abdominal trauma. (*A*) Ultrasound shows a large solid mass. A small area of cystic change is noted (*arrow*). Other images showed the mass to be exophytic from the spleen. (*B*) On CT, the mass appears solid, with small areas of low attenuation corresponding to the ultrasound.

on T2-weighted images, and show heterogeneous enhancement on dynamic post-contrast imaging with more uniform delayed enhancement.[36,38]

Lymphoma

Lymphoma is the most common solid malignancy of the spleen in children. Both Hodgkin disease and non-Hodgkin's lymphoma affect the spleen. Lymphoma may present as a solitary mass, multifocal lesions, or diffuse involvement with splenomegaly. Lesions appear hypoechoic and hypoattenuating relative to the splenic parenchyma. On MR imaging, the lesions are isointense on T1-weighted images and isointense to hyperintense on T2-weighted and short T1 inversion-recovery imaging (**Fig. 12**). Hodgkin disease may present with similar characteristics to those of splenic parenchyma, and diffuse infiltration may not be apparent on imaging studies. Involvement of lymph nodes and other organs often suggests the diagnosis of lymphoma. Imaging with ^{18}F-fluorodeoxiglucose positron emission tomography (^{18}F-FDG PET) is helpful for identifying splenic involvement, particularly in patients with a normal-sized spleen or absent focal lesions.[39]

Other than lymphoma, metastatic disease to the spleen in children is rare. Metastatic neuroblastoma to the spleen has been reported.

Cysts

Congenital cysts of the spleen, also called *true cysts* or *epidermoid cysts*, are epithelial-lined and form because of an infolding of peritoneal mesothelium or a collections of peritoneal mesothelial cells trapped within the splenic sulci.[40] Congenital splenic cysts are usually solitary. On ultrasound, they are anechoic or hypoechoic and may contain thin septations or debris.[41] On CT and MR imaging, splenic cysts follow fluid attenuation or signal intensity. Acquired splenic pseudocysts are much more common than congenital epithelial-lined splenic cysts. Imaging cannot distinguish acquired from congenital cysts; however, patients with acquired cysts usually have a history of trauma.

In addition to acquired pseudocysts, other nonneoplastic differential diagnoses related to the spleen include splenomegaly from nonneoplastic causes, congenital anomalies of the spleen, and infection, including splenic abscess.

Gastrointestinal Tract

Tumors of the gastrointestinal tract are rare in children, and benign tumors are more common than their malignant counterparts. Benign lesions include polyps, hemangiomas, neurofibromas, leiomyomas, gastrointestinal stromal tumors, and lipomas. The most common malignant tumor is lymphoma, and other malignant tumors are exceedingly uncommon. Adenocarcinomas are rare, but may occur isolated or in association with syndromes such as familial adenomatous polyposis syndrome, Peutz-Jeghers syndrome, and Lynch syndrome (hereditary nonpolyposis colorectal cancer syndrome) (**Fig. 13**), and in patients with

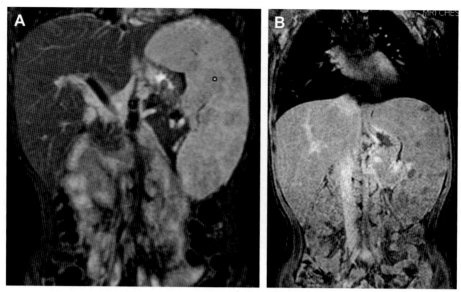

Fig. 12. An 8-year-old boy with history of ataxia telangiectasia and diffuse large B-cell lymphoma. MR imaging was used rather than CT because of the increased sensitivity to radiation in patients with ataxia telangiectasia. (*A*) Coronal T2-weighted image shows splenomegaly with numerous hypointense lesions (*asterisk*) relative to the splenic parenchyma. (*B*) Coronal post-gadolinium T1-weighted with fat-saturation image. The splenic lesions show hypoenhancement relative to adjacent normal parenchyma.

a longstanding diagnoses of ulcerative colitis or Crohn disease.

Carcinoid tumors are neoplasms of neuroendocrine origin, most commonly arising from the appendix but may occur in the small bowel. Fewer than 10% of patients present with carcinoid syndrome, and the tumors are occasionally found incidentally in the appendix without a preoperative diagnosis. Metastatic disease from carcinoid is rare in children.[42]

Lymphoma

Both non-Hodgkin's lymphomas and Hodgkin disease can affect the small bowel and, less frequently, the colon. Burkitt lymphoma is the

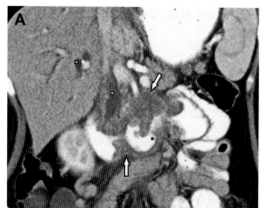

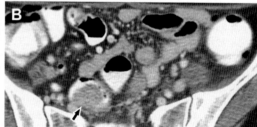

Fig. 13. A 17-year-old girl with subsequent diagnosis of Lynch syndrome and duodenal adenocarcinoma. (*A*) Contrast-enhanced CT coronal reformatted image shows a soft tissue mass in the ampullary region, with irregular circumferential wall thickening of the third and fourth portions of the duodenum (*arrows*). Resultant intrahepatic and extrahepatic biliary ductal dilatation is seen (*asterisk*). The mass abuts the posterior aspect of the pancreatic head. (*B*) A follow-up contrast-enhanced CT axial image in the pelvis performed 3 months later shows a 2-cm lobulated soft tissue mass in the sigmoid colon (*black arrow*). Pathology was consistent with an adenoma.

most frequent subtype of non-Hodgkin's lymphomas in children. In the WHO classification, three clinical variants of Burkitt lymphoma are described: endemic (found in equatorial Africa), sporadic, and immunodeficiency-associated. The sporadic form occurs in North America, and the immunodeficiency-associated type occurs in patients with congenital immunodeficiencies, such as Wiskott-Aldrich syndrome, ataxia-telangiectasia, or X-linked lymphoproliferative disease, and also in allograft recipients.[43] Lymphoma may also occur as a manifestation of posttransplant lymphoproliferative disorder.[44]

Common sites of gastrointestinal tract involvement by lymphoma are the distal small bowel, ileum, cecum, and appendix.[45] Mesenteric and retroperitoneal lymph nodes can also be involved. Patients may present with abdominal pain, a palpable mass, intussusception, or intestinal obstruction (**Fig. 14**). Abdominal radiographs may be unremarkable or may show bowel obstruction or mass effect. On ultrasound, diffuse involvement of the bowel by lymphoma is seen as predominately hypoechoic concentric bowel wall thickening. Enlarged mesenteric or retroperitoneal lymph nodes often suggest the diagnosis. Ultrasound may depict an intussusception, and suggest an underlying lead point. Contrast-enhanced CT at initial diagnosis allows assessment of the bowel, abdominal lymph nodes, and solid organs. Infiltration of the bowel is seen as a concentric bowel wall thickening, frequently associated with dilatation of the bowel lumen and enlarged lymph nodes (**Figs. 15** and **16**). Information on initial CT is used to determine the extent of the disease locally and distantly, which

contributes in the disease staging process once the diagnosis is established. ^{18}F-FDG PET is increasingly used in the initial staging and follow-up of patients with lymphoma.[46]

INTESTINAL POLYPS

The most common type of polyp in the pediatric population is the isolated juvenile polyp. Juvenile polyps are commonly diagnosed in patients younger than 10 years, and clinical presentation is painless rectal bleeding. More frequently, juvenile polyps occur in the rectosigmoid colon and may be single or multiple. Colonoscopy and polypectomy with histologic review is the current management.[47] Juvenile polyposis syndrome is a rare autosomal dominant condition with an increased risk of developing gastrointestinal cancer. This condition may be considered if more than five juvenile polyps are present in the colon, or if juvenile polyps are seen throughout the gastrointestinal tract, or in patients with a family history of juvenile polyposis and any number of polyps.[47]

Peutz-Jeghers syndrome is an uncommon, autosomal dominant syndrome with variable penetrance characterized by hamartomatous polyps and mucocutaneous hyperpigmentation. Polyps most commonly occur in the small bowel, but may also occur in the stomach or colon.[48] Median age of presentation with polyps is 11 to 13 years. Clinical manifestations include anemia, intussusception, and bowel obstruction.[49,50] Patients with this syndrome have a higher risk for intestinal and extraintestinal malignancies, including colon, upper gastrointestinal tract and small bowel, pancreas, breast, ovarian, and testicular cancers. Imaging studies are oriented to screen for polyps and other malignancies. Patients may present acutely with intussusceptions from a polyp lead point (**Fig. 17**).

Familial adenomatous polyposis syndrome is an autosomal dominant disorder related to mutation in the adenomatous polyposis coli gene (*APC* gene).[47] Patients develop hundreds of adenomatous polyps in the colon. Virtually all patients with familial polyposis syndrome will eventually develop adenocarcinoma of the colon or rectum. The average age at presentation is 16 years for adenoma and 39 years for carcinoma. Colon carcinoma rarely occurs in patients younger than 20 years.[47] Patients also develop other gastrointestinal adenocarcinomas and may have extraintestinal manifestations, including desmoid tumor, osteomas, congenital hypertrophy of the retinal pigmented epithelium, nasopharyngeal angiofibromas, lipomas, and fibromas. Patients with familial adenomatous polyposis syndrome have

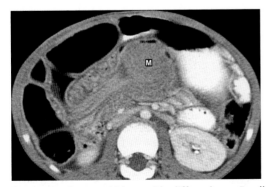

Fig. 14. An 8 year-old boy with diffuse large B-cell lymphoma. He presented with vomiting and abdominal pain. A contrast-enhanced CT axial image shows an ileocolic intussusception with a large soft tissue mass (M) causing incomplete mechanical bowel obstruction.

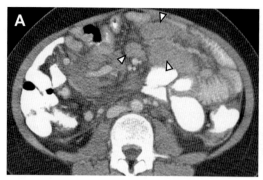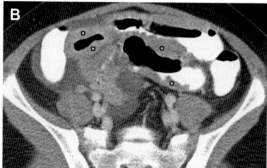

Fig. 15. A 10-year-old girl with Burkitt lymphoma presenting with long-standing abdominal pain and anemia. Axial contrast-enhanced CT images from the lower abdomen (*A*) and upper pelvis (*B*) show multiple enlarged mesenteric lymph nodes (*arrowheads*) and concentric bowel wall thickening and dilatation of the bowel lumen along the distal ileum (*asterisk*).

an increased incidence of hepatoblastoma. Several distinct mutations within the *APC* gene have been associated with other polyposis syndromes, including the attenuated familial adenomatous polyposis, Gardner syndrome, and Turcot syndrome. The attenuated phenotype is characterized by fewer polyps, later onset of polyps, and later onset of cancer. Gardner syndrome is characterized by the development of desmoid tumors. Turcot syndrome is characterized by central nervous system neoplasms, including cerebellar medulloblastoma and glioblastoma multiforme. Colonoscopy and upper endoscopy are used to evaluate patients with familial polyposis and related syndromes. If contrast studies such as double-contrast enema or upper gastrointestinal series are performed, polyps appear as numerous mucosal filling defects of variable size.[51] Imaging evaluation of extraintestinal manifestations includes abdominal ultrasound and/or MR imaging or CT studies.

Isolated leiomyomas, lipomas, hemangiomas, vascular malformations, and neurofibromas may occur within the gastrointestinal tract. Hemangiomas may appear isolated, or as a manifestation of diffuse hemangiomatosis, or in association with Kippel-Trénauney syndrome or Osler-Weber-Rendu disease. Likewise, neurofibromas may appear as isolated masses or in the context of neurofibromatosis.

Fig. 16. A 14-year-old boy with diffuse large B-cell lymphoma. Coronal reformatted image from contrast-enhanced CT shows concentric bowel wall thickening and aneurysmal small bowel involvement with an intussusception (*arrow*). Multiple enlarged retroperitoneal and intra-abdominal lymph nodes are also present (*asterisk*).

GASTROINTESTINAL STROMAL TUMORS

Gastrointestinal stromal tumors (GISTs) are the most common mesenchymal neoplasms of the gastrointestinal tract in adults but rarely occur in children. Histologically, these tumors are characterized by a spindle cell subtype or epithelioid architecture. Tumors may arise as a manifestation of tumor predisposition syndromes, including Carney triad (GIST, pulmonary chondroma, and functioning extra-adrenal paraganglioma),[52] Carney-Stratakis syndrome (paragangliomas and

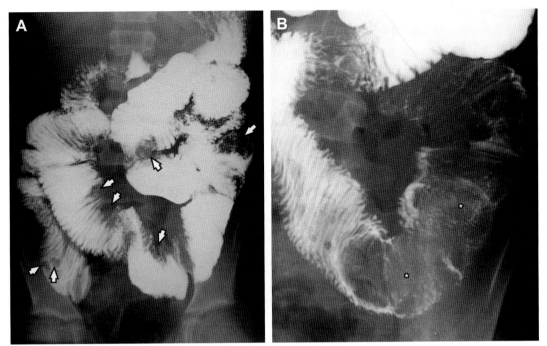

Fig. 17. A 12-year-old boy with Peutz-Jeghers syndrome who presented with recurring abdominal pain and vomiting. (*A*) Overhead image from a barium small bowel follow-through study shows multiple polypoid filling defects scattered within the small bowel (*arrows*). (*B*) Spot image during fluoroscopy shows a transient small bowel intussusception from a polyp *asterisk*.

GIST), or may be associated with neurofibromatosis type I. Pediatric GISTs present during the second decade of life, most commonly affect girls, and are located predominately in the stomach.[53] Tumor size varies in the reported cases from relatively small to large masses up to 35 cm (Fig. 18).[54] Metastatic disease to lymph nodes and liver and multifocality of GIST have been described in pediatric population.[54]

Many nonneoplastic conditions may mimic a tumor of the gastrointestinal tract. Differential considerations may include duplication cyst,

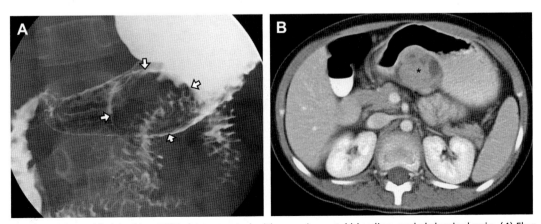

Fig. 18. A 9-year-old girl with a GIST who presented with anemia, rectal bleeding, and abdominal pain. (*A*) Fluoroscopy shows a large mass originating from the distal lesser curve of the stomach (*arrows*). (*B*) On contrast-enhanced CT, the mass is solid (*asterisk*). (*Courtesy of* D.G. Bates, Columbus, OH.)

intussusception, inflammatory bowel disease (Crohn disease, typhlitis, complicated appendicitis), and hematoma.

SUMMARY

Although tumors arising from the spleen, pancreas, and gastrointestinal tract in the pediatric population are relatively uncommon, imaging plays an important role in diagnosis, staging, and treatment planning.

REFERENCES

1. Takano H, Smith WL. Gastrointestinal tumors of childhood. Radiol Clin North Am 1997;35:1367–89.
2. Golden CB, Feusner JH. Malignant abdominal masses in children: quick guide to evaluation and diagnosis. Pediatr Clin North Am 2002;49:1369–92.
3. Milla SS, Lee EY, Buonomo C, et al. Ultrasound evaluation of pediatric abdominal masses. Ultrasound Clin 2007;2:541–59.
4. Chung EM, Travis MD, Conran RM. Pancreatic tumors in children: radiologic-pathologic correlation. Radiographics 2006;26:1211–38.
5. Yu DC, Kozakewich HP, Perez-Atayde AR, et al. Childhood pancreatic tumors: a single institution experience. J Pediatr Surg 2009;44:2267–72.
6. Shorter NA, Glick RD, Klimstra DS, et al. Malignant pancreatic tumors in childhood and adolescence: the Memorial Sloan-Kettering experience, 1967 to present. J Pediatr Surg 2002;37:887–92.
7. Jaksic T, Yaman M, Thorner P, et al. A 20-year review of pediatric pancreatic tumors. J Pediatr Surg 1992; 27:1315–7.
8. Pelizzo G, Conoscenti G, Kalache KD, et al. Antenatal manifestation of congenital pancreatoblastoma in a fetus with Beckwith-Wiedemann syndrome. Prenat Diagn 2003;23:292–4.
9. Solcia E, Capella C, Kloppel G. Tumors of the pancreas. In: Atlas of tumor pathology; 3rd series, fascicle 20. Washington, DC: Armed Forces Institute of Pathology; 1997. p. 103–14.
10. Montemarano H, Lonergan GJ, Bulas DI, et al. Pancreatoblastoma: imaging findings in 10 patients and review of the literature. Radiology 2000;214:476–82.
11. Roebuck DJ, Yuen MK, Wong YC, et al. Imaging features in pancreatoblastoma. Pediatr Radiol 2001;31:501–6.
12. Frantz V. Tumors of the pancreas. In: Atlas of tumor pathology. Section 7, fascicles 27 and 28. Washington, DC: Armed Forces Institute of Pathology; 1959. p. 32–3.
13. Cantisani V, Mortele KJ, Levy A, et al. MR imaging features of solid pseudopapillary tumor of the pancreas in adult and pediatric patients. AJR Am J Roentgenol 2003;181:395–401.
14. Choi JY, Kim MJ, Kim JH, et al. Solid pseudopapillary tumor of the pancreas: typical and atypical manifestations. AJR Am J Roentgenol 2006;187: W178–86.
15. Buetow PC, Buck JL, Pantongrag-Brown L, et al. Solid and papillary epithelial neoplasm of the pancreas: imaging-pathologic correlation in 56 cases. Radiology 1996;199:707–11.
16. Choi BI, Kim KW, Han MC, et al. Solid and papillary epithelial neoplasm of the pancreas: CT findings. Radiology 1988;166:413–6.
17. Khanna G, O'Dorisio SM, Menda Y, et al. Gastroenteropancreatic neuroendocrine tumors in children and young adults. Pediatr Radiol 2008;38:251–9.
18. Service FJ, McMahon MM, O'Brien PC, et al. Functioning insulinoma: incidence, recurrence, and long-term survival of patients a 60 year study. Mayo Clin Proc 1991;66:711–9.
19. Thoeni RF, Mueller-Lise UG, Chan R, et al. Detection of small, functional islet cell tumors in the pancreas: selection of MR imaging sequences for optimal sensibility. Radiology 2000;214:483–90.
20. Kwekkeboom D, Krenning EP, de Jong M. Peptide receptor imaging and therapy. J Nucl Med 2000; 41:1704–13.
21. Berrocal T, Luque AA, Pinilla I, et al. Pancreatic regeneration after near-total pancreatectomy in children with nesidioblastosis. Pediatr Radiol 2005;35: 1066–70.
22. Mester M, Trajber HJ, Compton CC, et al. Cystic teratomas of the pancreas. Arch Surg 1990;125:1215–8.
23. Jacobs JE, Dinsmore BJ. Mature cystic teratoma of the pancreas: sonographic and CT findings. AJR Am J Roentgenol 1993;160:523–4.
24. Guermazi A, Feger C, Rousselot P, et al. Granulocytic sarcoma (chloroma): imaging findings in adults and children. AJR Am J Roentgenol 2002;178:319–25.
25. Kim EY, Yoo SY, Kim JH, et al. Pancreatic metastasis in child suffering with treated stage 4 neuroblastoma. Korean J Radiol 2008;9:84–6.
26. Kim SJ, Choi JA, Lee SH, et al. Imaging findings of extrapulmonary metastases of osteosarcoma. Clin Imaging 2004;28:291–300.
27. Avcu S, Akdeniz H, Arslan H, et al. A case of primary vertebral osteosarcoma metastasizing to pancreas. J Pancreas (Online) 2009;10:438–40.
28. Hilmes MA, Strouse PJ. The pediatric spleen. Semin Ultrasound CT MR 2007;28:3–11.
29. Hickeson MP, Charron M, Maris JM, et al. Biodistribution of post-therapeutic versus diagnostic ^{131}I-MIBG scans in children with neuroblastoma. Pediatr Blood Cancer 2004;42:268–74.
30. Sul HJ, Kang D. Congenital neuroblastoma with multiple metastases: a case report. J Korean Med Sci 2003;18:618–20.
31. Kobrinsky NL, Sjolander DE. Response of metastatic recurrent neuroblastoma to nitisinone: a modulator

of tyrosine metabolism. Pediatr Blood Cancer 2006; 46:517–20.

32. Abbott RM, Levy AD, Aguilera NS, et al. From the archives of the AFIP: primary vascular neoplasms of the spleen: radiologic-pathologic correlation. Radiographics 2004;24:1137–63.

33. Ferrozzi F, Bova D, Draghi F, et al. CT findings in primary vascular tumors of the spleen. AJR Am J Roentgenol 1996;166:1097–101.

34. Ramani M, Reinhold C, Semelka R, et al. Splenic hemangiomas and hamartomas: MR imaging characteristics of 28 lesions. Radiology 1997;202:166–72.

35. Wadsworth DT, Newman B, Abramson SJ, et al. Splenic lymphangiomatosis in children. Radiology 1997;202:173–6.

36. Luna A, Ribes R, Caro P, et al. MRI of focal splenic lesions without and with dynamic gadolinium enhancement. AJR Am J Roentgenol 2006;186: 1533–47.

37. Tang S, Shimizu T, Kikuchi Y, et al. Color Doppler sonographic findings in splenic hamartoma. J Clin Ultrasound 2000;28:249–53.

38. Thompson SE, Walsh EA, Cramer BC, et al. Radiological features of a symptomatic splenic hamartoma. Pediatr Radiol 1996;26:657–60.

39. Rini JN, Leonidas JC, Tomas MB, et al. 18F-FDG versus CT for evaluation of the spleen during initial staging of lymphoma. J Nucl Med 2003;44:1072–4.

40. Urrutia M, Mergo PJ, Ros LH, et al. Cystic masses of the spleen: radiologic-pathologic correlation. Radiographics 1996;16:107–29.

41. Daneman A, Martin DJ. Congenital epithelial cysts in children emphasis on sonographic appearances and some unusual features. Pediatr Radiol 1982; 12:119–25.

42. Iqbal CW, Wahoff DC. Diagnosis and management of pediatric endocrine neoplasms. Curr Opin Pediatr 2009;21:379–85.

43. Ferry JA. Burkitt's lymphoma: clinicopathologic features and differential diagnosis. Oncologist 2006; 11:375–83.

44. Pickhardt PJ, Siegel MJ. Posttransplantation lymphoproliferative disorder of the abdomen: CT evaluation on 51 patients. Radiology 1999;213:73–8.

45. Biko DM, Anupindi SA, Hernandez A, et al. Childhood Burkitt lymphoma: abdominal and pelvic imaging findings. AJR Am J Roentgenol 2009;192: 1304–15.

46. Hernandez-Pampaloni M, Takalkar A, Yu JQ, et al. F-18 FDG-PET imaging and correlation with CT in staging and follow up of pediatric lymphomas. Pediatr Radiol 2006;36:524–31.

47. Durno CA. Colonic polyps in children and adolescents. Can J Gastroenterol 2007;21:233–9.

48. Schreibman IR, Baker M, Amos C, et al. The hamartomatous polyposis syndromes: a clinical and molecular review. Am J Gastroenterol 2005;100: 476–90.

49. Kopacova M, Tacheci I, Rejchrt S, et al. Peutz-Jeghers syndrome: diagnostic and therapeutic approach. World J Gastroenterol 2009;15:5397–408.

50. Rufener SL, Koujok K, McKenna BJ, et al. Small bowel intussusception secondary to Peutz-Jeghers polyp. Radiographics 2008;28:284–8.

51. Schlesinger AE. Colon tumors and tumor-like conditions. In: Slovis TL, editor. Caffeys's pediatric diagnostic imaging, vol. 2. 11th edition. Philadelphia (PA): Mosby Elsevier; 2008. p. 2205–13.

52. Carney JA. Gastric stromal sarcoma, pulmonary chondroma, and extra-adrenal paraganglioma (Carney triad): natural history, adrenocortical component, and possible familial occurrence. Mayo Clin Proc 1999;74:543–52.

53. Miettinen M, Lasota J, Sobin LH. Gastrointestinal stromal tumors of the stomach in children and young adults: a clinicopathologic, immunohistochemical and molecular genetic study of 44 cases with long-term follow-up and review of the literature. Am J Surg Pathol 2005;29:1373–81.

54. Pappo AS, Janeway KA. Pediatric gastrointestinal stromal tumors. Hematol Oncol Clin North Am 2009;23:15–34.

Hepatobiliary Tumors

Ricardo Faingold, MD*, Pedro A.B. Albuquerque, MD,
Lucia Carpineta, MD

KEYWORDS

- Tumor • Ultrasonography • MRI • Liver

Hepatobiliary tumors are uncommon in the pediatric population, representing 5% to 6% of the abdominal tumors. Approximately one-third of hepatic lesions are benign. Metastatic liver tumors are more common than primary disease.[1]

The investigation of hepatobiliary tumors usually begins with an ultrasonographic (US) examination. This technique is readily available without ionizing radiation and does not need sedation. Therefore, US is an outstanding imaging modality for screening and follow-up. Doppler and color Doppler interrogation are part of the examination to assess vascularity of the lesions and vascular anatomy.

The role of computed tomography (CT) is limited, in the pediatric population, because of an increase in the risk of radiation-induced cancer. Therefore, discussion of CT protocols is not the focus of this article.

Magnetic resonance (MR) imaging is a comprehensive imaging modality with multiplanar capability to assess the liver parenchyma, gallbladder, and biliary tree and is free of ionizing radiation. MR imaging provides an assessment of the signal characteristics, vascularity, and pathophysiology of different tumors because of its superior soft tissue contrast resolution that includes the use of gadolinium-enhanced techniques. One has to take into consideration the need for sedation or general anesthesia in infants, toddlers, and young children.

MR imaging protocol consists of T1-weighted and T2-weighted fat-saturated sequences in multiple planes. Breath-hold T2-weighted single-shot fast-spin echo is useful to assess the biliary tree.

Some institutions still use T1 spin echo sequences with and without fat saturation. Two-dimensional dual gradient-echo in-phase and opposed-phase MR images are useful in the evaluation of diffuse and focal fatty infiltrations.

There is a trend toward 3-dimensional T1-weighted gradient-echo breath-hold sequences pregadolinium and postgadolinium administration because of improved spatial resolution. Acquisition as multiphase dynamic gadolinium-enhanced imaging is essential for the assessment of tumor vascularity, vascular anatomy, and segmental anatomy for surgical planning.

BENIGN TUMORS

Infantile Hepatic Hemangioma

Infantile hepatic hemangioma (IHH) has also been referred to, in the literature, as hemangioendothelioma.[2] IHH is the most common benign vascular hepatic tumor in the first year of life and the third most common hepatic tumor in children.[3] This tumor may present with palpable masses, hepatomegaly, or thrombocytopenia. Multifocal lesions may be asymptomatic or may present with a high-output cardiac failure because they demonstrate a variable high-flow shunting. These lesions may be associated with cutaneous hemangiomas.[4]

In 2007, a new classification was proposed.[4] Hepatic hemangiomas are divided into focal (Fig. 1), multifocal (Fig. 2), and diffuse lesions. These hemangiomas have a proliferative phase and then a phase of involution.[5] Alternatively, rapid involuting congenital hemangioma (RICH; Fig. 3) is already developed in the newborn and regresses in the first year of life.[6] RICH also differs from adult hepatic hemangioma, which does not involute.[2]

MR imaging appearance of IHH is usually a low signal on T1-weighted sequences and a very high signal on T2-weighted sequences. The characteristics vary according to the presence of high-flow vessels, thrombosis, and large vascular spaces. Following intravenous gadolinium

Department of Medical Imaging, Montreal Children's Hospital, McGill University, Montreal, Quebec, Canada
* Corresponding author. Room C-309, 2300 Tupper Street, Montreal, Quebec, H3H 1P3, Canada.
E-mail address: Ricardo.Faingold@muhc.mcgill.ca

Radiol Clin N Am 49 (2011) 679–687
doi:10.1016/j.rcl.2011.05.002

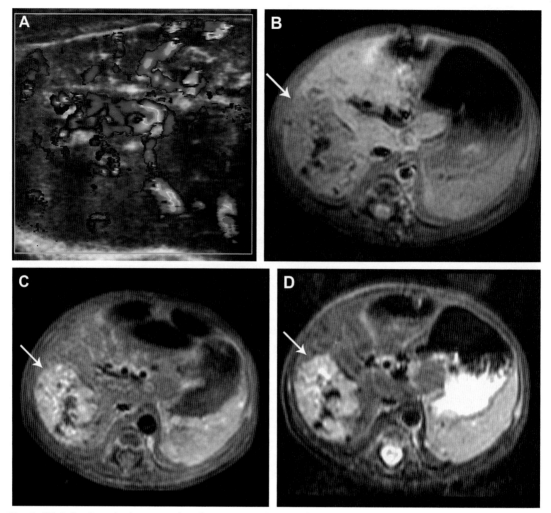

Fig. 1. (*A*) Color Doppler interrogation demonstrates increased vascularity within a heterogeneous lesion in the right hepatic lobe. (*B*) T1-weighted image shows hypointense lesion (*arrow*) with high-flow vessels. (*C*) Fat-saturated T1-weighted image demonstrates avid enhancement of the lesion (*arrow*) with areas of signal void. (*D*) The same lesion (*arrow*) is hyperintense on T2-weighted sequence.

administration, they may enhance from the periphery to the center or homogenously.[2]

US usually demonstrates hypoechoic lesions. Some lesions may be hyperechoic or with calcifications. Doppler interrogation shows abnormal vessels and may show evidence of shunting.[2]

Most lesions resolve spontaneously and can be followed-up with MR imaging and US.

In case of cardiac failure or severe thrombocytopenia, one may consider medical therapy. Embolization following angiography is the next step, in case medical therapy fails.

Mesenchymal Hamartoma

Mesenchymal hamartoma is usually seen in children up to 2 years of age and is considered the second most common benign hepatic tumor.

Mesenchymal hamartoma can be cystic/multicystic or can have a more predominant stromal component with a Swiss cheese appearance. It is considered a developmental lesion containing mesenchymal tissue with bile ducts.

Mesenchymal hamartoma is usually cystic and septated with US and may contain a solid component.

The MR imaging appearance is of low signal on T1-weighted sequences and of very high signal on T2-weighted sequences.[1] The solid component may show some degree of enhancement after intravenous gadolinium administration and may have a low T2 signal.

Hepatic Adenoma

Hepatic adenoma (HA) is an uncommon benign hepatic tumor in the pediatric population,

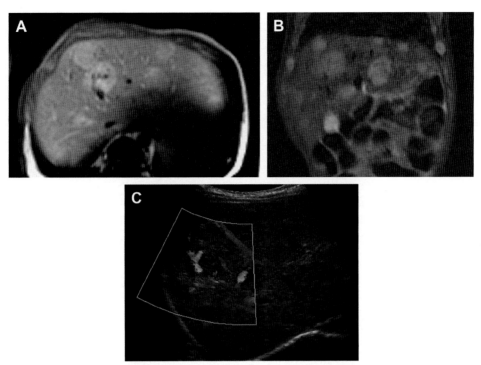

Fig. 2. (A) Axial T1-weighted postgadolinium image showing multiple enhancing lesions of different sizes throughout the liver. (B) Coronal T2-weighted image demonstrates hyperintense lesions. (C) Color Doppler US shows one of the hypoechoic lesions with increased flow.

predominantly associated with certain predisposing conditions, such as glycogen storage disease type 1 and Fanconi anemia, and those patients using oral contraceptives or anabolic steroids.[7] HAs can be single or multiple (**Fig. 4**), and the presence of 4 or more lesions is referred to as hepatic adenomatosis. HA is more commonly asymptomatic; however, patients may present with hepatomegaly and abdominal pain secondary to tumoral necrosis/hemorrhage. In rare cases, HA may also rupture, causing hemoperitoneum. On US, the HA is of variable echogenicity and may be hypoechoic, isoechoic, or hyperechoic to the liver.[8] CT without intravenous contrast shows these

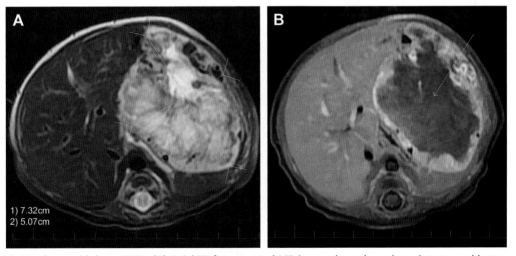

Fig. 3. Newborn with large RICH. (A) Axial T2 fat-saturated MR image shows large hyperintense and heterogeneous mass with flow voids within the left hepatic lobe. The indicator represents measurement of the lesion. (B) Fat-saturated T1-weighted image demonstrates peripheral enhancement with no significant vascularity of the center of the lesion (arrow).

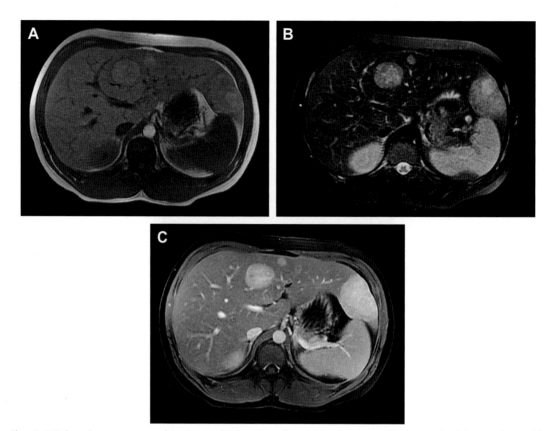

Fig. 4. MR imaging sequences showing multiples HAs of variable sizes in a 15-years-old adolescent boy with a history of glycogen storage disease type 1. (*A*) Axial, breath-hold, spoiled gradient recalled (SPGR) image shows 3 well-delineated lesions that are slightly heterogeneous but with predominantly high signal intensity, involving the segments 4 and 2. (*B*) Axial, fat-suppressed, breath-hold, T2-weighted, fast-relaxation fast-spin echo sequence demonstrates the lesions to have heterogeneous but predominantly high signal intensity. (*C*) Postcontrast, axial, fat-suppressed, breath-hold, SPGR image shows significant enhancement of the adenomas.

lesions to be predominantly hypodense. Both CT and MR imaging show most HAs to have a peak enhancement during the arterial phase, with a rapid washout that may become isodense or isointense to the liver on the delayed phase. HA may present variable signal intensity characteristics on MR imaging, depending on the presence of internal hemorrhage, necrosis, or fat. T1-weighted MR sequences may show a signal intensity varying from hypointense to hyperintense. The out-of-phase T1-weighted sequences are useful to assess for the presence of a signal drop of the tumoral fatty component. On T2-weighted sequences, HA is predominantly hyperintense, but some may also be isointense to the liver.[9,10] Large adenomas may show areas of heterogeneous enhancement secondary to internal necrotic/hemorrhagic changes.

Focal Nodular Hyperplasia

Focal nodular hyperplasia (FNH) accounts for 2% to 6% of the hepatic tumors in childhood; usually these are tumors with less than 5 cm in diameter. Most cases occur in women. FNH usually presents as a single lesion; however, it can be multifocal in up to 20% of cases. FNH is surrounded by dense fibrous septa with a central prominent scar.[1] On US, it appears as a well-delineated mass, isoechoic to the liver with a more-hyperechoic central scar.[11] Color Doppler evaluation shows the increased vascularity of the fibrous septa and the central portion of the tumor, resulting in the spoke wheel pattern. The nonenhanced CT shows the lesion to be predominantly isodense to the liver. On MR imaging, FNH is usually isointense to the liver on both T1- and T2-weighted sequences; sometimes it may also be mildly hypointense on T1-weighted or mildly hyperintense on T2-weighted sequences. The central scar appears hyperintense on T2-weighted sequences. Contrast-enhanced CT and MR imaging show an intense arterial enhancement that becomes isointense to the liver on the delayed sequences and also on delayed enhancement of the central scar (**Fig. 5**).[10,12]

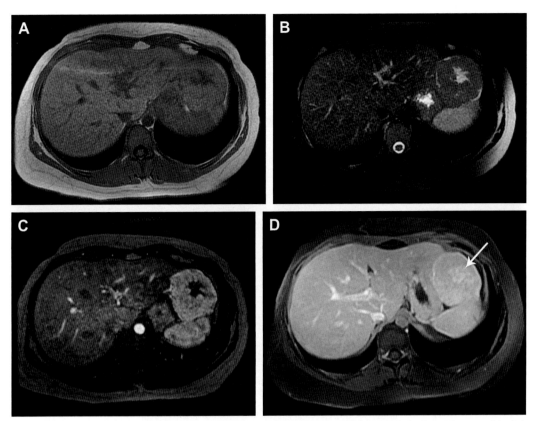

Fig. 5. MR imaging showing the presence of a large FNH involving the left hepatic lobe in a 15-years-old adolescent girl. (*A*) Axial, breath-hold, spoiled gradient recalled (SPGR) image shows the lesion to be isointense to the hepatic parenchyma, with the central scar showing low signal intensity. (*B*) Axial, fat-suppressed, breath-hold, T2-weighted, fast-relaxation fast-spin echo image demonstrates the lesion to have a slightly higher signal to the liver and the central scar to have a hyperintense signal intensity. (*C*) Postcontrast, axial, fat-suppressed, breath-hold, 3-dimensional, SPGR image shows significant enhancement of the lesion in the arterial phase. (*D*) Delayed, postcontrast, axial, fat-suppressed, breath-hold, T1-weighted image shows the lesion to be almost isointense to the liver and the delayed enhancement of central scar (*arrow*).

MALIGNANT TUMORS
Hepatoblastoma

Hepatoblastoma is the most common primary hepatic neoplasm of childhood and accounts for 79% of all liver tumors in children.[13] The typical presentation is that of an asymptomatic abdominal mass in a young child, usually younger than 3 years,[14] with a peak incidence seen between the ages of 18 and 24 months. Rarely, the patient may present with an acute abdomen at instances of tumor rupture. An increased incidence has been noted in patients with Beckwith-Wiedemann syndrome, hemihypertrophy syndromes, and familial adenomatous polyposis coli.[15] Low–birth weight infants have also been found to have an increased incidence of this tumor.[16,17]

The tumor is usually a well-circumscribed solitary lesion (**Fig. 6**) with a nodular surface and usually involves the right hepatic lobe, but it can be multifocal (**Fig. 7**) in up to 15% of cases.[18] The average size at the time of diagnosis is 10 to 12 cm. Metastases, when they occur, are usually encountered in the lungs and local lymph nodes and only rarely in the brain and bony skeleton. Approximately 10% to 20% of cases are found to have metastatic disease at the time of diagnosis.[18] Elevated α-fetoprotein (α-FP) levels are present in as many as 90% of patients.[19] On US, the lesion is usually hyperechoic, and, occasionally, intravascular tumor thrombus is seen, which can extend as far as the right atrium. On CT, calcifications can be seen in about half the cases. With intravenous contrast, the lesions show slight enhancement compared with nearby liver parenchyma in the early phase of imaging, only to become isodense to hypodense with respect to liver parenchyma on delayed imaging.[8] The appearance of hepatoblastoma on

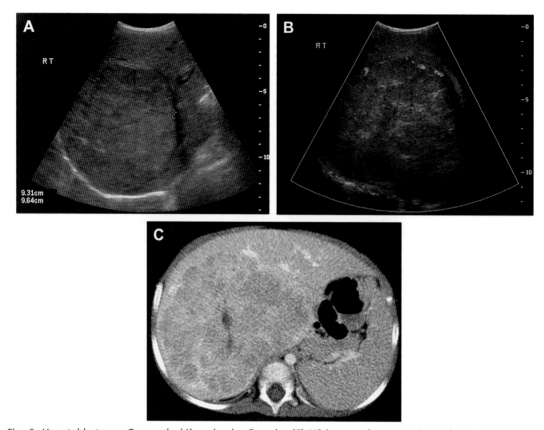

Fig. 6. Hepatoblastoma. Gray-scale (*A*) and color Doppler (*B*) US images demonstrating a large circumscribed heterogeneously slightly hyperechoic mass in the right lobe of liver with some internal flow, associated with splaying of intrahepatic vessels. (*C*) Enhanced CT image in portal venous phase imaging depicting the heterogeneous nature of the mass with central necrosis.

MR imaging varies with the histologic type. The epithelial type has a more homogeneous internal nature and appearance, whereas the mixed epithelial/mesenchymal type is more heterogeneous, containing fibrotic bands. On MR imaging, conventional spin echo sequences, the lesions show a hypointense signal relative to adjacent liver parenchyma on T1-weighted images. Occasionally, however, small hemorrhages can be seen as foci of increased signal intensity. On T2-weighted

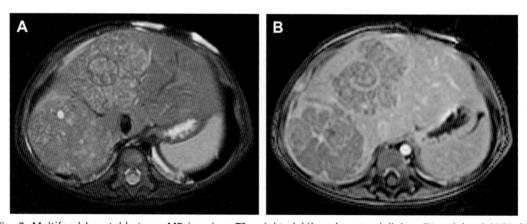

Fig. 7. Multifocal hepatoblastoma MR imaging. T2-weighted (*A*) and postgadolinium T1-weighted SPGR (*B*) images show heterogeneous lesions in the liver that are slightly hyperintense on T2-weighted image and hypointense with poor enhancement on T1-weighted postgadolinium image.

images, the tumors appear heterogeneously hyperintense in signal. Areas of fibrosis appear as bands of hypointense signal on both T1- and T2-weighted sequences. Spoiled gradient recalled pulse sequences or MR angiography (MRA) can help delineate the effect of the tumor on vessels, such as displacement or encasement, and also help determine whether there is vascular invasion.

Hepatocellular Carcinoma

Hepatocellular carcinoma (HCC) is the second most common malignant liver tumor, accounting for 35% of all primary hepatic malignancies. There are 2 age peaks in the pediatric population: one peak at 12 to 14 years of age and a second less-frequent peak at 2 to 4 years of age.[8] The typical presentation is that of a palpable abdominal mass. Conditions predisposing to cirrhosis, such as biliary atresia, infantile cholestasis, hepatitis, glycogen storage disorders, hemochromatosis, hereditary tyrosinemia, α_1-antitrypsin deficiency, porphyria cutanea tarda, and Wilson disease, are associated with an increased risk for developing HCC.[1,8] Elevation of serum α-FP levels is seen in up to 80% of pediatric patients with HCC.[20] Up to 50% of patients present with metastases at the time of diagnosis.[21]

Both focal and diffuse forms of HCC can be encountered. In the focal form, smaller lesions, generally not exceeding 3 cm in diameter, appear on US as hypoechoic circumscribed foci, whereas the larger lesions appear either hyperechoic or heterogeneous. Up to 40% of these lesions show internal calcifications with posterior shadowing. On color Doppler interrogation, flow is seen at the periphery of the lesion but without distortion of the hepatic vasculature. On multiphase CT, HCC appears as a mass showing precocious enhancement in the arterial phase with rapid subsequent washout on delayed imaging with capsular enhancement.[22] Invasion of hepatic vessels can also be seen. On MR imaging, HCC usually appears hypointense to isointense with respect to liver parenchyma on T1-weighted images and isointense to hyperintense on T2-weighted images. On postgadolinium images, the behavior of the lesions is as on CT, with early arterial phase enhancement of the mass with rapid washout and capsular enhancement on delayed imaging.[10] MRA is an excellent tool for depicting neovascularity, tortuous feeding vessels, tumor blush, and even signs of arteriovenous shunt.[23]

Fibrolamellar Carcinoma

This histologic variant of HCC is generally seen in adolescents and young women. The appearance on US is that of a well-circumscribed lobulated mass of variable echogenicity containing a central more-hyperechoic scar.[24] On CT, calcifications can be seen within these lesions. On multiphase imaging, the arterial phase shows the central scar, which can be hypervascular. Delayed portal venous phase images can show the lesion as isoattenuating, hypoattenuating, or hyperattenuating. On MR imaging spin echo sequences, fibrolamellar HCC appears hypointense on T1-weighted images and hyperintense on T2-weighted images. The internal scar appears as a central stellate region that retains contrast on portal venous phase images because of the slow washout.[25] Because this central scar is fibrous, the signal is low on both T1- and T2-sequences, and this feature is a key to distinguishing between this entity and FNH.

Undifferentiated Embryonal Sarcoma

Undifferentiated embryonal sarcoma (UES) is the third most common hepatic malignancy, comprising 6% of all pediatric liver tumors. This tumor typically presents as a rapidly growing abdominal mass, sometimes associated with pain, in an older child, usually 6 to 10 years.[26] Metastatic disease, when present, usually involves the lungs and bones. A clinically important feature is that serum α-FP levels remain in the normal range. According to some investigators, UES is believed to be the malignant counterpart of mesenchymal hamartoma.[27]

The key imaging finding with this entity is that there is discordance between the appearance on US and on CT, with the former clearly solid with iso-echoic or hyperechoic appearance and the latter more as a well-delineated, multiseptated, fluid-appearing structure with enhancing solid septations and a pseudocapsule. On MR imaging, UES has a heterogeneous multiseptated cystic appearance, with hypointense signal on T1-weighted images and hyperintense signal on T2-weighted images.[28] A pseudocapsule with peripheral enhancement, because of compressed adjacent hepatic parenchyma, can also be seen in the early arterial phase of imaging, whereas delayed images best reveal any enhancing tumor nodules.[8]

Liver Metastases

Metastases to the liver (**Figs. 8** and **9**) are most commonly from tumors arising from other intra-abdominal organs. In children, the most common tumors metastasizing to the liver are neuroblastoma and Wilm tumor.[29]

The main role of imaging is detection, characterization, and staging. The lesions tend to be multiple. The US appearance can be variable but

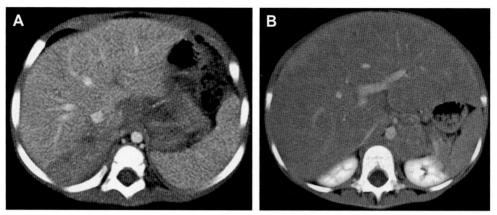

Fig. 8. Metastases from neuroblastoma in 2 different patients. (*A*) CT image shows hypodense lesion in the right hepatic lobe with significant associated retroperitoneal tumor. (*B*) Enhanced CT demonstrates large liver with heterogeneous and hypodense parenchyma in keeping with diffuse metastatic disease from left adrenal neuroblastoma.

is more often hypoechoic. On CT, the appearance is also protean but tends to be hypodense as compared with adjacent liver parenchyma and shows variable degrees of enhancement,[8] all depending on the primary tumor. The contrast-enhanced appearance can vary from targetlike to fairly intense and homogeneous enhancements. MR imaging is a highly sensitive modality for the detection of liver metastases, and it has been shown to be more sensitive and more specific than other modalities. The MR imaging characteristics depend to a large extent on the tumor of origin. On MR imaging, most liver metastases display moderately hypointense signal on T1-weighted images and moderately hyperintense signal on T2-weighted images. Even tiny metastases are often clearly depicted on nonenhanced fat-saturated T2-weighted images because liver metastases have extracellular matrices containing abundant free water. Occasionally, metastases with intratumoral hemorrhage or necrosis or those containing mucin may show mixed signal intensity on T1-weighted images, and those metastases with intratumoral fibrosis or necrosis may exhibit decreased signal intensity on T2-weighted images.[30]

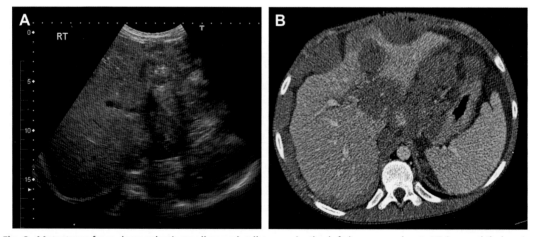

Fig. 9. Metastases from desmoplastic small round cell tumor in the left lower quadrant. US image (*A*) showing numerous vaguely hypoechoic mass lesions around the periphery of the liver and within the liver along the main portal vein and left branch portal vein. On CT image (*B*), the peripheral lesions appear extracapsular. Nodular masses in the region of the gastrohepatic ligament and along the anteromedial stomach are consistent with peritoneal implants.

REFERENCES

1. Das CJ, Dhingra S, Gupta AK, et al. Imaging of paediatric liver tumors with pathological correlation. Clin Radiol 2009;64:1015–25.

2. Kassarjian A, Zurakowski D, Dubois J. Infantile hepatic hemangiomas: clinical and imaging findings and their correlation with therapy. AJR Am J Roentgenol 2004;182:785–95.

3. Van der Meijs BB, Merks JH, de Haan TR, et al. Neonatal hepatic haemangioendotheliomas: treatment options and dilemmas. Pediatr Radiol 2009; 39:277–81.

4. Christison-Lagay ER, Burrow PE, Alomari A, et al. Hepatic hemangiomas: subtype classification and development of a clinical practice algorithm and registry. J Pediatr Surg 2007;42:62–8.

5. Kassarjian A, Dubois J, Burrows PE. Angiographic classification of hepatic hemangiomas in infants. Radiology 2002;222:693–8.

6. Zenzen W, Perez-Atayde AR, Elisofon SA, et al. Hepatic failure in a rapidly involuting congenital hemangioma of the liver: failure of embolotherapy. Pediatr Radiol 2009;39:1118–23.

7. Choi BY, Nguyen MH. The diagnosis and management of benign hepatic tumors. J Clin Gastroenterol 2005;39:401–12.

8. Jha P, Chawla SC, Tavri S, et al. Pediatric liver tumors—a pictorial review. Eur Radiol 2009;19:209–19.

9. Siegel M, Hoffer FA. Pediatric body applications of MRI. In: Edelman RR, Hesselink JR, Zlatkin MB, et al, editors. Clinical magnetic resonance imaging. Philadelphia: Saunders; 2006. p. 3086–116.

10. Martin DR, Semelka RC. Imaging of benign and malignant focal liver lesions. Magn Reson Imaging Clin N Am 2001;9(4):785–802.

11. Caseiro-Alves F, Zins M, Mahfouz AE, et al. Calcification in focal nodular hyperplasia: a new problem for differentiation from fibrolamellar hepatocellular carcinoma. Radiology 1996;198:889–92.

12. Mergo PJ, Ros PR. Benign lesions of the liver. Radiol Clin North Am 1998;36:319–31.

13. Willert JR, Dahl G. Hepatoblastoma. Available at: http://emedicine.medscape.com/article/986802-overview. Accessed April 15, 2010.

14. Schlesinger AE, Parker BR. Tumors and tumor-like conditions. In: Kuhn JP, Slovis TL, Haller JO, editors. Caffey's pediatric diagnostic imaging. Philadelphia: Mosby; 2004. p. 1500–2.

15. Hughes LJ, Michels VV. Risk of hepatoblastoma in familial adenomatous polyposis. Am J Med Genet 1992;43:1023–5.

16. Ikeda H, Matsuyama S, Tanimura M. Association between hepatoblastoma and very low birth weight: a trend or a chance? J Pediatr 1997;130:557–60.

17. Tanimura M, Matsui I, Abe J, et al. Increased risk of hepatoblastoma among immature children with a lower birth weight. Cancer Res 1998;33:585–6.

18. Herzog CE, Andrassy RJ, Eftekhari F. Childhood cancers: hepatoblastoma. Oncologist 2000;5:445–53.

19. Han SJ, Yoo S, Choi SH, et al. Actual half life of alpha feto-protein as a prognostic tool in pediatric malignant tumors. Pediatr Surg Int 1997;12:599–602.

20. Donnelly LF, Bisset GS 3rd. Pediatric hepatic imaging. Radiol Clin North Am 1998;36:413–27.

21. Ni YH, Chang MH, Hsu HY, et al. Hepatocellular carcinoma in childhood. Clinical manifestations and prognosis. Cancer 1994;68:1737–41.

22. Oto A, Tamm EP, Szklaruk J. Multidetector row CT of the liver. Radiol Clin North Am 2005;43:827–48.

23. Buetow PC, Midkiff RB. MRI imaging of the liver. Primary malignant neoplasms in the adult. Magn Reson Imaging Clin N Am 1997;5:289–318.

24. Ichikawa T, Federle MP, Grazioli L, et al. Fibrolamellar hepatocellular carcinoma: imaging and pathologic findings in 31 recent cases. Radiology 1999; 213:352–61.

25. Stocker JT, Ishak KG. Undifferentiated (embryonal) sarcoma of the liver: report of 31 cases. Cancer 1978;42:336–48.

26. Lauwers GY, Grant LD, Donnelly WH, et al. Hepatic undifferentiated (embryonal) sarcoma arising in a mesenchymal hamartoma. Am J Surg Pathol 1997;21:1248–54.

27. Moon WK, Kim WS, Kim IO, et al. Undifferentiated embryonal sarcoma of the liver: US and CT findings. Pediatr Radiol 1994;24:500–3.

28. Yoon W, Kim JK, Kang HK. Hepatic undifferentiated embryonal sarcoma: MRI findings. J Comput Assist Tomogr 1997;21:100–2.

29. Bader TR, Salamah AB, Semelka RC. Focal liver lesions. In: Edelman RR, Hesselink JR, Zlatkin MB, et al, editors. Clinical magnetic resonance imaging. Philadelphia: Saunders; 2006. p. 2554–88.

30. Albuquerque PA, Morales Ramos A, Faingold R. Magnetic resonance imaging of the liver and biliary tree in children. Curr Probl Diagn Radiol 2009;38: 126–34.

Renal Neoplasms of Childhood

Evan Geller, MD[a,b],*, Polly S. Kochan, MD[a,b]

KEYWORDS

• Renal • Neoplasm • Childhood • Abdominal mass

An abdominal mass in a child in the first year of life is usually of renal origin. The most common renal masses in the perinatal period are nonneoplastic and include hydronephrosis and multicystic dysplastic kidney. Only 20% of renal masses in the first year of life are true neoplasms.[1] The most common solid neoplasm in this age group is the mesoblastic nephroma. Other neoplasms occur, but these are far less common; these include Wilms tumor, rhabdoid tumor of the kidney (RTK), and ossifying renal tumor of infancy (ORTI). Beyond the first year of life and during the first decade, primary tumors of the kidney become more common. With the development of new therapeutic regimens and standardization of treatment protocols, the cure rate for the most common renal neoplasm, Wilms tumor, has risen from 10% in 1920 to more than 90% today.[2] This article reviews the role of imaging in the diagnosis, staging, and follow-up of children with renal neoplasms. Pertinent epidemiologic, clinical, and histopathologic considerations are reviewed, and current recommendations for management are presented.

WILMS TUMOR
Epidemiology

Wilms tumor is a malignant neoplasm that arises from persistent embryonal tissue. It is the most common abdominal malignancy in children.[3] It occurs with an annual incidence of 7.8 cases per million children less than the age of 15 years.[4] This is equivalent to approximately 400 to 500 newly diagnosed cases per year. There is no racial or gender predilection. Approximately 80% of children with this tumor present between 1 and 5 years of age, with a peak incidence between 3 and 4 years of age.[5] In a large, multicenter, international retrospective data review of 750 children diagnosed with a renal tumor in the first 7 months of life, Wilms tumor was identified in 58%, making this the most common tumor in this age group (however, congenital mesoblastic nephroma was more commonly seen in the first 2 months of life).[6] The most common presentation is an incidentally discovered abdominal mass. Approximately 5% to 7% of patients with Wilms tumor have bilateral disease.[7] Most bilateral tumors occur synchronously[8]; metachronous tumors do occur, although these are less frequently diagnosed. One explanation is that metachronous tumors are treated and cured with chemotherapy before they can be diagnosed.[9] Bilateral tumors have been correlated with an earlier presentation, a high incidence of associated congenital anomalies, and a higher incidence of nephroblastomatosis than seen in unilateral Wilms tumor.[8,10] Children with Wilms tumor and associated congenital anomalies tend to present at an earlier age. Up to 12% of children with Wilms tumors have associated congenital anomalies.[10] The incidence of coexistent genitourinary anomalies is highest (5%), followed by hemihypertrophy (2.5%) and aniridia (1%).[10,11] Of those with genitourinary anomalies, children with cryptorchidism or hypospadias have the strongest association with Wilms tumor (2.8% and 1.8% respectively).[11] Wilms tumor is 1.96 times more common in horseshoe kidney than in the general population (**Fig. 1**).[12] Wilms tumor has been reported to arise in multicystic dysplastic kidneys; it has been suggested that these kidneys should be monitored

[a] Department of Radiology, St Christopher's Hospital for Children, 3601 A Street, Philadelphia, PA 19134, USA
[b] Departments of Radiology and Pediatrics, Drexel University College of Medicine, Philadelphia, PA, USA
* Corresponding author. Department of Radiology, St Christopher's Hospital for Children, 3601 A Street, Philadelphia, PA 19134.
E-mail address: evan.geller@tenethealth.com

Radiol Clin N Am 49 (2011) 689–709
doi:10.1016/j.rcl.2011.05.003

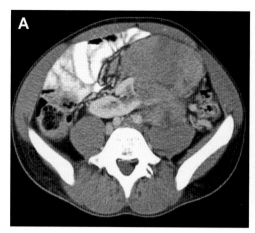
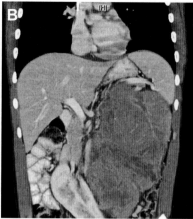
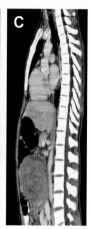

Fig. 1. (*A–C*) Contrast-enhanced transaxial abdominal CT with coronal and sagittal reformats in a 9-year-old boy with Wilms tumor of the left moiety of a horseshoe kidney.

for any deviation from the normally expected course of progressive involution.[13,14]

Children with hemihypertrophy have a 3% incidence of Wilms tumor. These tumors may develop ipsilateral or contralateral to the hypertrophy.[8] Wilms tumor is the most common abdominal neoplasm in children with Beckwith-Wiedemann syndrome. The combined incidence of this and other abdominal tumors (hepatoblastoma and adrenal cortical carcinoma) in this syndrome is approximately 10%.[15] Thirty-three percent of children with sporadic aniridia develop Wilms tumor, and these tumors are often bilateral.[8] Other congenital anomalies associated with Wilms tumor include the WAGR syndrome (Wilms, aniridia, genitourinary abnormalities, and retardation), Drash syndrome[16] (male pseudohermaphroditism, glomerular disease, and Wilms tumor), Bloom syndrome[17] (diminished growth and immunity, facial telangiectasia), trisomy,[17,18] and imperforate anus with rectourethral fistula.[19] There is a 3% incidence of musculoskeletal malformations (club foot, rib fusion, hip dysplasia) in children with Wilms tumor.[20]

Histopathology

The gross appearance of a Wilms tumor is that of a large, bulky, solid mass surrounded by a pseudo-capsule of compressed renal parenchyma. Foci of hemorrhage, necrosis, and cyst formation are commonly found, especially if the tumor is large or has previously been treated with radiation or chemotherapy. Tumors tend to arise in the periphery of the kidney, sparing the central collecting system. This location may account for the large size (approximately 500 g) these tumors attain before diagnosis, because findings of gross hematuria and compromised renal function are usually

lacking. Wilms tumor uncommonly may arise from the renal pelvis or calyces as a polypoid lesion. The incidence of hematuria in these children is stated to be much greater than in those with the more typical parenchymal origin of Wilms (87% vs 25%) and, in contrast with classic Wilms tumor, only 37.5% present with an abdominal mass.[21] Most Wilms tumors arise in a single location within the kidney, although they may occasionally be multicentric in origin. If 2 or more masses are discovered within the same kidney, there is a greater likelihood of nephroblastomatosis in the contralateral kidney.[22]

Extrarenal Wilms tumors are rare. They are believed to arise from extrarenal displacement of metanephric or mesonephric rests.[23] The most common extrarenal locations are within the retroperitoneum, inguinal region, pelvis, and thorax. Their behavior and histology are identical to an intrarenal tumor location. The mean age at diagnosis is 3.6 years.[24]

The classic Wilms tumor shows triphasic histology, containing epithelial (tubular, glomerular), blastemal (small round cells), and stromal (spindle, myxoid) cell lines. However, not all tumors contain all cell lines, and the proportion as well as the degree of differentiation of cell lines is highly variable from one tumor to the next.[25] The prognosis of children with Wilms tumor is heavily dependent on the presence of anaplasia. A Wilms tumor with favorable histology lacks anaplastic changes, whereas one with unfavorable histology shows extreme nuclear and mitotic atypia characteristic of anaplasia. Approximately 90% of Wilms tumors are of favorable histology. The distribution of anaplasia (focal vs diffuse), rather than absolute quantity, has been found to be a more sensitive indicator of clinical outcome in Wilms tumor; it has been found to be more significant than tumor staging in assigning a prognosis.[26] Anaplastic histology generally predicts a poor response to chemotherapy and is associated with an increased risk of recurrent disease.[27]

Anaplastic changes are found in 4% of Wilms tumors. Anaplastic Wilms tumor occurs in an older age group and is associated with a higher incidence of lymph node metastases at diagnosis.[28]

Box 1
National Wilms Tumor Study Group staging system for Wilms tumor

Stage I (43% of patients)

- In stage I tumor, all of the following criteria must be met:
  - Tumor is limited to the kidney and is completely resected.
  - The renal capsule is intact.
  - The tumor is not ruptured or biopsied before removal.
  - No involvement of renal sinus vessels.
  - No evidence of tumor at or beyond the margins of resection.

Stage II (20% of patients)

- In stage II Wilms tumor, the tumor is completely resected, and there is no evidence of tumor at or beyond the margins of resection. The tumor extends beyond the kidney as shown by any 1 of the following criteria:
  - There is regional extension of tumor (ie, penetration of the renal sinus capsule or extensive invasion of the soft tissues of the renal sinus).
  - Blood vessels within the nephrectomy specimen outside the renal parenchyma, including those of the renal sinus, contain tumor.

(Note: rupture or spillage confined to the flank, including biopsy of the tumor, is no longer included in stage II and is now included in stage III.)

Stage III (21% of patients)

- In stage III Wilms tumor, there is residual nonhematogenous tumor present following surgery that is confined to the abdomen. Any 1 of the following may occur:
  - Lymph nodes within the abdomen or pelvis are involved by tumor. (Lymph node involvement in the thorax or other extra-abdominal sites is a criterion for stage IV.)
  - The tumor has penetrated through the peritoneal surface.
  - Tumor implants are found on the peritoneal surface.
  - Gross or microscopic tumor remains after surgery (eg, tumor cells are found at the margin of surgical resection on microscopic examination).
  - The tumor is not completely resectable because of local infiltration into vital structures.
  - Tumor spillage occurs either before or during surgery.
  - The tumor is treated with preoperative chemotherapy and was biopsied (using Tru-cut biopsy, open biopsy, or fine needle aspiration) before removal.
  - The tumor is removed in more than 1 piece (eg, tumor cells are found in a separately excised adrenal gland; a tumor thrombus within the renal vein is removed separately from the nephrectomy specimen). Extension of the primary tumor within vena cava into thoracic vena cava and heart is considered stage III, even though outside the abdomen.

Stage IV (11% of patients)

- In stage IV Wilms tumor, hematogenous metastases (lung, liver, bone, brain), or lymph node metastases outside the abdominopelvic region are present. (The presence of tumor within the adrenal gland is not interpreted as metastases and staging depends on all other staging parameters present.)

Stage V (5% of patients)

- In stage V Wilms tumor, bilateral involvement by tumor is present at diagnosis. An attempt should be made to stage each side according to the criteria listed earlier according to the extent of disease. The 4-year survival is 94% for those patients whose most advanced lesion is stage I or stage II, and 76% for those whose most advanced lesion is stage III.

Reprinted from National Cancer Institute: PDQ Wilms tumor and other childhood kidney tumors treatment. Bethesda, MD: National Cancer Institute. Date last modified February 8, 2011. Available at: http://cancer.gov/cancertopics/pdq/treatments/Wilms/HealthProfessional. Accessed August 7, 2009.

Staging of Wilms tumor incorporates issues of surgical resectability and local and distant spread as determined by imaging and microscopic evaluation (**Box 1**).[29] Wilms tumor may extend into contiguous vascular structures. Extension into the ipsilateral or contralateral renal vein is common. Propagation of tumor thrombus into the inferior vena cava or right atrium has been reported to occur in 4.1% of patients with Wilms tumor; of these, 21% show atrial extension.[30] Caval thrombus may extend into its tributaries, including the gonadal, adrenal, and hepatic veins. Extension into the hepatic veins may result in the Budd-Chiari syndrome.[31] Imaging plays a major role in the documentation of intravascular propagation of tumor thrombus and may alter surgical management considerably. Despite having to undergo a surgically difficult procedure, those children with atrial tumor thrombus tend to have a good prognosis.[32] Wilms tumor often metastasizes to regional lymph nodes within the renal hilum and periaortic chain. Hematogenous dissemination typically is to the lungs and, less often, to the liver. Bone metastases are rare. Most tumors with skeletal metastases previously classified as clear cell and rhabdoid variants of Wilms tumor are now classified as distinct neoplasms manifesting different biologic behaviors.[33,34]

Clinical Features

Most children with Wilms tumor appear to be in good health. Constitutional symptoms usually are lacking, although occasionally these children present with weight loss, diminished appetite, and malaise. Children with Wilms tumor most often present with a palpable abdominal mass. This presentation occurs with an incidence of between 75% and 95%.[29] Approximately 25% of children with Wilms tumor present with microscopic hematuria.[21] Gross hematuria is uncommon; when present it may signify invasion of the collecting system from a primary parenchymal lesion or, less commonly, tumor arising from the renal pelvis proper.[21] Hypertension is present in 25% of patients with Wilms tumor and has been shown to be directly related to increased rennin production by tumor cells.[35]

Diagnostic Imaging

Typical radiographic findings in patients with Wilms tumor are nonspecific and include a large flank mass with obliteration of the psoas shadow and displacement of gas-distended bowel loops. Calcifications may be identified in approximately 9% of tumors.[36]

Sonographic evaluation of Wilms tumor shows a large mass of homogeneous echogenicity interrupted by hypoechoic (or frankly cystic) regions as well as regions of increased echogenicity. These regions correspond with foci of tumor necrosis and calcium or fat deposition, respectively. The periphery of the tumor is typically well demarcated (**Fig. 2**). The tumor-kidney interface may be sharply defined by an echogenic rim corresponding with the tumor pseudocapsule or by a hypoechoic band of compressed renal parenchyma.[37] The ipsilateral renal vein and inferior vena cava should be examined for tumor thrombus; its presence may alter the clinical staging and surgical approach, especially if there is involvement of the supradiaphragmatic vena cava or right atrium. Such patients may benefit from chemotherapy before nephrectomy to

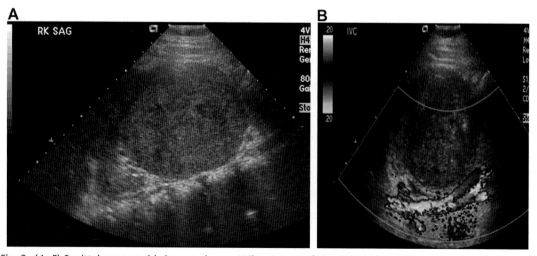

Fig. 2. (*A, B*) Sagittal sonographic images show a Wilms tumor of the right kidney. The tumor shows heterogenous echotexture and is well defined. Note the claw sign of compressed renal parenchyma superiorly, and vascular displacement.

promote shrinkage of the intravascular tumor and facilitate subsequent surgical removal. The contralateral kidney must be carefully inspected for synchronous tumor or congenital anomalies; unilateral agenesis or ureteropelvic junction obstruction may alter operative management.

Abdominal computed tomography (CT) scan is more sensitive than ultrasound in identifying tumor extent and nodal and liver involvement.[38] However, its specificity for Wilms tumor is low because imaging features may show considerable overlap with those of non-Wilms tumor.[39] Wilms tumor is seen as a large, well-defined mass of heterogeneous attenuation. Areas of low attenuation coincide with tumor necrosis and/or fat deposition. Calcifications may be identified on precontrast studies. There is minimal enhancement of tumor tissue relative to the adjacent rind of compressed renal parenchyma (**Fig. 3**). Capsular invasion may be suggested by a pattern of exophytic growth and contour irregularity.[10] CT scan may identify regional adenopathy, although it cannot differentiate tumor replacement from reactive adenopathy. Acute hemorrhage within a Wilms tumor may be seen as a fluid-fluid level. As with ultrasound, contrast-enhanced CT scan allows evaluation of the renal veins and inferior vena cava for tumor thrombus. It has been reported to be slightly less sensitive than ultrasound, although data from the National Wilms Tumor Study (NWTS)-III reveal that neither modality is sensitive in showing tumor thrombus.[30]

Chest CT scan has been shown to be superior to plain films in the detection of lung metastases from Wilms tumor. CT scan can identify lesions not visible on chest radiography and is more sensitive in the detection of calcifications within a nodule (**Fig. 4**).[10,40] However, the role of chest CT in the initial staging of Wilms tumor has historically been widely debated.[41,42] It was designated as an elective study in the NWTS-IV. It was required in the NWTS-V protocol, although all discordant lesions (eg, those that are visible only on CT scan) were ignored and were not considered in staging and management decisions.[40] Current Central Oncology Group (COG) protocols call for the use of chest CT for documentation and follow-up of pulmonary metastases.[43]

MR imaging has been shown to be a valuable tool in Wilms tumor imaging. As with CT scan, it can accurately identify the primary tumor and its renal origin, although it cannot distinguish between Wilms tumor and other primary intrarenal neoplasms found in a similar age group. MR imaging can accurately assess tumor size, gross composition, and regional spread, although, as with all other imaging modalities, it cannot define subtle capsular invasion.[44,45] Wilms tumor shows signal intensities consistent with prolonged T1 and T2 relaxation times. The tumor typically appears of heterogeneous signal intensity because of the presence of blood, tissue necrosis, fat, and cystic change. Gadolinium-enhanced T1-weighted images show inhomogeneous enhancement of tumor tissue with an overall diminished enhancement pattern relative to the brightly enhancing normal renal tissue. Tumor borders are more accurately defined following contrast administration.

MR imaging cannot differentiate tumor-replaced regional lymph nodes from those that are enlarged because of reactive hyperplasia; in either case, they show the same signal intensity as the primary tumor.[44] MR imaging can accurately identify the presence of liver metastases and caval thrombus. Weese and colleagues[46] compared MR imaging, CT, and ultrasound in the detection of tumor thrombus and found MR imaging to be superior to other modalities. Advantages compared with US and CT scan include the use of specific flow sequences in the search for tumor thrombus and

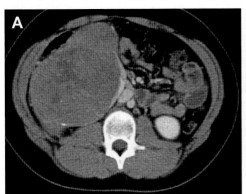
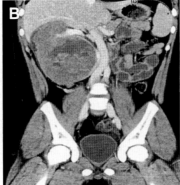
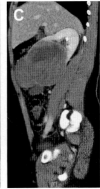

Fig. 3. (A–C) The same patient as in **Fig. 2**. Contrast-enhanced abdominal CT with coronal and sagittal reformation showing a large Wilms tumor of the right kidney with a characteristic claw sign of compressed renal parenchyma indicating slowly progressive growth. Note heterogeneous internal architecture and caval displacement.

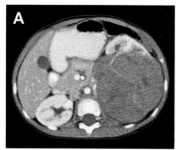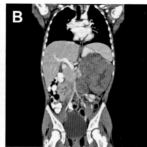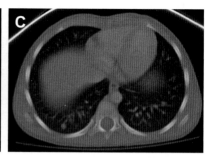

Fig. 4. (*A–C*) Contrast-enhanced abdominal CT showing a large heterogeneous mass of the left kidney with pulmonary metastases consistent with a stage IV Wilms tumor.

multiplanar imaging in evaluating caval displacement by tumor; vessel examination is not hampered by overlying bowel gas as may be the case with US.[44]

Screening is recommended for those children at high risk for developing Wilms tumor. These children include those with sporadic aniridia, hemihypertrophy, Beckwith-Wiedemann syndrome, Drash syndrome, WAGR, and nephroblastomatosis. US is the modality of choice and should be performed every 3 to 6 months until the child is between 6 and 10 years of age.[10] CT scan is the modality of choice for surveillance of children with resected Wilms tumors. Most relapses occur within the chest and abdomen,[47] and 94% of relapses occur within the first 2 years following diagnosis.[48] It is therefore recommended that CT scan of the chest and abdomen be performed 3 times per year for 2 years following initial diagnosis.[10]

Management

Nephrectomy followed by postoperative adjuvant chemotherapy remains the mainstay of treatment of unilateral Wilms tumor in North America. Because recent treatment methods have produced consistently high levels of disease-free survival, current COG protocols are intended to refine chemotherapeutic regimens to reduce overall morbidity.

The type of chemotherapy and the need for additional abdominal or whole lung irradiation varies according to histologic grade, stage at presentation, biologic markers such as loss of heterozygosity at chromosomes 1p and 16q, and response to initial treatment.[49] Chemotherapy may be administered before surgery to facilitate resection of tumor associated with caval and/or atrial tumor thrombus.[50] By promoting tumor shrinkage, preoperative chemotherapy has also allowed resection of tumors initially considered unresectable from imaging findings. Radiation to the tumor bed and across the midline may be used in certain circumstances, and whole-abdominal radiation is used in the setting of gross tumor spillage at surgery and/or peritoneal tumor

implants. Treatment of bilateral Wilms tumors is conservative; rather than unilateral nephrectomy (the kidney with the largest tumor burden) and parenchyma-sparing resection of the other kidney, the current surgical approach is to attempt bilateral kidney salvage through directed, imaging-guided excision.[51] This approach has resulted in a 4-year survival, which is comparable with the previous surgical approach, and provides the additional benefit of a lower incidence of complicating renal failure.[50]

It is noteworthy that, in Europe, staging and initial management of patients with Wilms tumor is according to the Single Integrated Operational Plan (SIOP) protocol, which involves neoadjuvant chemotherapy for presumed Wilms tumor based on characteristic imaging findings, followed by nephrectomy. In a review of Wilms tumor management, Sonn and Shortliffe[49] describe several advantages of the SIOP protocol including the reduction of tumor volume and diminished risk of intraoperative rupture. Furthermore, these investigators comment on reported tumor downstaging that may occur with preoperative chemotherapy.

Criticisms of this approach include the potential for an incorrect initial imaging diagnosis of Wilms tumor and the institution of inappropriate therapy, as well as the potential for undertreatment owing to incorrect tumor staging following chemotherapy.[50]

NEPHROBLASTOMATOSIS
Epidemiology

Nephrogenic rests represent islands of primitive blastemal elements that persist in the kidneys beyond 36 weeks' gestation and have the potential of malignant transformation into Wilms tumor. Nephroblastomatosis is defined as the presence of multifocal or diffuse nephrogenic rests.[22] It has been identified in 41% of patients with unilateral Wilms tumor and in 94% and 99% of metachronous and synchronous bilateral tumors, respectively.[22] Perilobar nephrogenic rests (PLNR) are associated with such entities as Beckwith-Wiedemann syndrome, Perlman syndrome, trisomy 18, and hemihypertrophy. Intralobar nephrogenic rests are less common than the perilobar type, although there is a higher association with Wilms tumor. These rests are found in association with sporadic aniridia, WAGR syndrome, and Denys-Drash syndrome.[52] Nephrogenic rests have been noted in fewer than 1% of normal perinatal autopsies.[53]

Histopathology

Nephrogenic rests may be classified as perilobar or intralobar from their location. Perilobar rests lie within the peripheral cortex or columns of Bertin. They may be unifocal, multifocal, or diffuse in distribution and are further subdivided into dormant, sclerosing, hyperplastic, or neoplastic types. Dormant and sclerosing rests are not considered premalignant. The finding of perilobar nephrogenic rests is associated with a 1% to 2% incidence of Wilms tumor; the incidence of Wilms tumor in kidneys with intralobar nephrogenic rests is 4% to 5%.[54] Nephrogenic rests may become grossly visible with hyperplastic or neoplastic transformation. Histologically, hyperplastic nephrogenic rests may be identical to Wilms tumor. The absence of a fibrous pseudocapsule may help to distinguish these from a small Wilms tumor.[55]

Imaging

Sonographic evaluation of the kidneys for nephroblastomatosis lacks the sensitivity of CT scan and MR imaging.[52] The affected kidney(s) may be enlarged and have an indistinct corticomedullary junction. It may contain focal areas of diminished echogenicity or may be diffusely hypoechoic, corresponding with focal or diffuse nephroblastomatosis.[56] Differential diagnosis of diffuse nephroblastomatosis on ultrasound includes Wilms tumor, renal lymphoma, leukemia, and polycystic kidneys.

CT scan with contrast enhancement shows a pattern of poorly enhancing peripherally based lesions in cases of focal perilobar nephroblastomatosis. In cases of diffuse hyperplastic perilobar nephroblastomatosis (DHPLN), CT scan show diffuse rindlike proliferation and therefore enlargement of the kidney(s) with homogeneously poor enhancement compared with the attenuated but otherwise normal renal tissue (Fig. 5).[57] MR imaging of nephroblastomatosis reveals diminished signal intensity relative to normal renal cortex on all imaging sequences. There is variability of signal intensity within the histologic subtypes, and the higher signal intensity of the highly cellular, hyperplastic, and neoplastic subtypes (isointense to Wilms tumor) contrasts with the hypointense foci of sclerotic nephroblastomatosis.[54] MR short-tau inversion recovery sequences therefore show the bright signal intensity of DHPLN and Wilms tumor as contrasted with the low signal intensity of sclerotic PLNR. Gadolinium enhancement adds to the conspicuity of these lesions. Foci of nephroblastomatosis show a uniformly nonenhancing pattern following gadolinium administration; this contrasts with the heterogeneous pattern of enhancement seen with Wilms tumor and may serve to differentiate the two.[54,57] In a study of 12 patients with nephroblastomatosis, the overall sensitivity of gadolinium-enhanced MR imaging in lesion detection was 57%.[54] Wilms tumors tend to take on a rounded contour; this may further help to distinguish these from the lenticular shape of nephrogenic rests.[57]

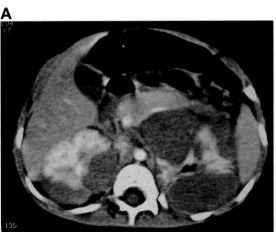 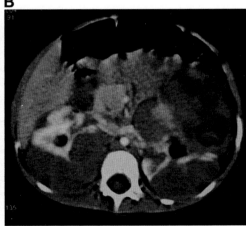

Fig. 5. (A, B) A 3-year-old with bilateral DHPLN. Both kidneys are enlarged by a thick peripheral rind of nonenhancing/poorly enhancing nephrogenic rests. Note normal enhancement of compressed renal parenchyma.

Management

Imaging plays an important role in the management of children with nephrogenic rests because many cannot be reliably identified at surgery. Patients are followed by imaging for a minimum of 7 years, at a maximal interval of 3 months.[43] A biopsy may not be able to distinguish these from Wilms tumor. Nephroblastomatosis in conjunction with Wilms tumor is treated according to the stage of the tumor, as per the NWTS protocol.

Although nephrogenic rests may spontaneously involute, current recommendations for treatment of nephrogenic rests call for chemotherapy with vincristine and dactinomycin. Even with treatment, Wilms tumor develops in approximately 50% of these children within an average of 36 months following diagnosis. Of these, approximately 33% are of anaplastic histology, perhaps because of selection of chemotherapy-resistant tumors.[43] These patients, therefore require close follow-up for lesion transformation. Bilateral nephrogenic rests that attain a larger size on follow-up examinations are excised surgically with sparing of normal renal tissue.

CLEAR CELL SARCOMA OF THE KIDNEY
Epidemiology

Formerly considered a highly aggressive variant of Wilms tumor, clear cell sarcoma of the kidney (CCSK) is now recognized as a distinct tumor from a histologic and clinical standpoint. This tumor was first described in 1970 by Kidd, who noted its tendency to metastasize to bone.[58,59] Clear cell sarcoma represents approximately 4% of all childhood renal neoplasms and has a marked male predilection.[60] It has been reported in children as young as 3 days of age and in adults as old as 57 years; however, its peak incidence is similar to that of Wilms tumor and lies between 3 and 5 years, or slightly younger.[61] As distinct from Wilms tumor, CCSK has not been reported in association with sporadic aniridia, hemihypertrophy, or nephroblastomatosis. There have been no reports of bilateral tumors.[25]

Histopathology

The classic histologic pattern (90%) consists of nests/cords of ovoid, epithelioid, or spindled cells with bland nuclei separated by a distinctive, evenly spaced fibrovascular network that has been likened to a chicken-wire appearance.[55] On gross inspection, these tumors are solid, but may contain cystic areas and may mimic multilocular cystic nephroma. They do not have a pseudocapsule and tend to infiltrate the normal adjacent renal parenchyma.[62]

Recently, a translocation t(10;17) and deletion 14q have been described in CCSK, suggesting that they may play a role in its pathogenesis.[63]

Metastatic disease at presentation is uncommon, in contrast with Wilms tumor. Another differentiating feature, historically, has been its propensity to metastasize to bone, in addition to local nodal spread and pulmonary metastases. Metastases to the brain have also been reported and may have exceeded bone metastases as the most common site of recurrence in recently released reports from the NWTS-5 and SIOP93-01/GPOH.[64]

Imaging

There are no specific imaging features of CCSK to help distinguish it from Wilms tumor. Both tumors are seen as heterogeneous masses of renal origin on US, CT scan, and MR imaging. They may enhance and contain foci of cystic necrosis.[65] Extracapsular tumor spread occurs in approximately 70% of patients. In contrast with Wilms tumor, extension into the renal vein is rare and occurs in less than 5% of cases.[66] Skeletal metastases have been variably described as having an osteolytic or osteoblastic appearance.[67]

Management

The approach to treatment of children with CCSK differs considerably from treatment of Wilms tumor with favorable histology. Current standard of care following nephrectomy and lymph node dissection is based on results from the NWTS-5. For stages I to IV, this includes a 4-drug regimen of vincristine, doxorubicin, cyclophosphamide, and etoposide. Overall survival is 100% for stage I tumor, 97% for stage II, 87% for stage III, and 45% for stage IV tumor.[58] In previous years, long-term relapses (up to 10 years) were commonplace but, with current chemotherapeutic regimens, relapses after 3 years are uncommon.[68]

RHABDOID TUMOR OF THE KIDNEY
Epidemiology

RTK is the most aggressive malignant neoplasm of the kidney in children, and accounts for 2% to 3% of all renal neoplasms in the NWTS.[69] Its name is derived from a histologic similarity to skeletal muscle. Along with anaplastic Wilms and CCSK, it is included in the unfavorable histology category of the NWTS. It is seen only in childhood, with most cases diagnosed during the first year of life. There is a slight male preponderance.[69] Fever and gross hematuria are presenting symptoms in approximately 50% to 60% of these patients, respectively.[70] Hypercalcemia secondary to increased parathormone levels has also been reported as an unusual clinical finding; this usually resolves spontaneously following tumor resection.[71]

Histopathology

Unlike Wilms tumor, RTK usually arises from the central medullary portion of the kidney and involves the renal hilum.[33] These tumors often are large at presentation (>9 cm) and spread throughout the renal parenchyma. Invasion of the renal vein is common. Metastatic spread to the lungs and liver is common, as with Wilms tumor, and metastases to the brain and skeleton also have been reported.[69] An association of RTK with synchronous or metachronous embryonal tumors of the central nervous system is distinctive to this type of renal tumor.[52] These tumors are mostly of posterior fossa origin and include medulloblastoma and primitive neuroectodermal tumor.[72]

Imaging

These tumors have a similar appearance to Wilms tumor and, in most instances, they are indistinguishable from each other. Several distinguishing features are suggested: the presence of subcapsular fluid (44%), tumor lobules separated by areas of low-density hemorrhage or necrosis (44%), and calcifications outlining tumor lobules may suggest the diagnosis of RTK (**Fig. 6**).[33] Subcapsular fluid collections, representing tumor necrosis or hemorrhage, are noted in 50% to 70% of cases. Although these collections are characteristic, they may also be found in those with Wilms tumor and CCK.[59] The finding of a centrally located tumor with involvement of the hilum is characteristic.[33,69] Local or distant dissemination and/or vascular invasion may be detected on cross-sectional imaging, although this does not serve to distinguish RTK from other primary renal neoplasms of children.

Management and Prognosis

Of all primary pediatric renal tumors, the prognosis of children with RTK is the poorest. Most patients present with advanced stage disease (stage III–IV). A young age at presentation has been correlated with a poorer outcome.[70] There is a high rate of local tumor recurrence following surgical resection. An 80% mortality was reported in a series of 111 children with RTK.[69] Of 31 patients with RTK reported by the NWTS-III, there was a 4-year survival rate of only 25%.[48]

PRIMITIVE NEUROECTODERMAL TUMOR OF THE KIDNEY
Epidemiology

Primitive neuroectodermal tumor (PNET) of the kidney is a rare, small, round cell tumor belonging to the Ewing family of tumors. The mean age at diagnosis is 24 years. Clinical presentation includes flank pain, hematuria and a palpable mass, in declining order.[73] Metastases are most often to the regional lymph nodes, lung, liver, and bone.

Histopathology

PNET of the kidney usually presents as a large mass with the cut surface showing foci of hemorrhage and necrosis. The tumor may be surrounded by a fibrous capsule and may contain calcifications. The histologic hallmarks of PNET are small, round to ovoid hyperchromatic cells often arranged in nests, with the formation of rosettes or pseudorosettes.[73] Ewing sarcoma and PNET share a common and unique t(11;22) chromosomal translocation that produces the EWS-FLI1 fusion gene, which acts as a transcription factor to drive cellular proliferation.[74]

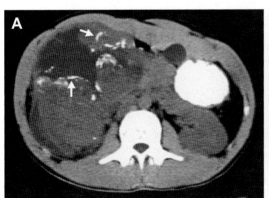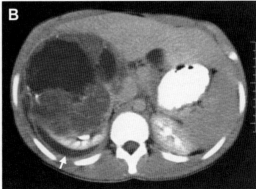

Fig. 6. (*A, B*) Rhabdoid tumor of the right kidney. Note curvilinear calcifications and subcapsular fluid (*arrows*). (*Courtesy of* Archana Malik, MD.)

Imaging

There are no specific imaging findings for PNET of the kidney. The tumor may be isoechoic/hypoechoic to normal renal parenchyma on sonography. CT shows large mixed-density lesions with mild to moderate enhancement. On MR imaging, these tumors appear isointense or hypointense on T1-weighting imaging, and heterogeneous on T2-weighted imaging, owing to foci of necrosis and hemorrhage (**Fig. 7**).[73] Calcifications may occur, but are uncommon. Tumor tissue may extend to the renal vein and inferior vena cava. There may be invasion of the liver and psoas muscle. Regional lymphadenopathy is noted. These tumors do not cross the midline.[75]

Management and Prognosis

Treatment of renal PNET is by a combination of radical nephrectomy, multidrug chemotherapy, and radiation. Despite this, prognosis is poor, with 25% to 50% of patients presenting with metastatic disease and a 5-year disease-free survival of 45% to 55%.[74]

OSSIFYING RENAL TUMOR OF INFANCY
Epidemiology

ORTI is a rare, benign renal tumor that, along with congenital mesoblastic nephroma and Wilms tumor, comprises most of the tumors occurring in infancy. It was first described by Chatten and colleagues[76] and, since then, only 11 cases have been reported.[77] Age at presentation is from 9 days to 6 months. Gross hematuria has been reported to be a characteristic presentation. Boys are more commonly affected than girls and the left kidney has been found to be involved more commonly than the right (9 of 11 cases).[52]

Histopathology

This tumor is believed to arise from the urothelium within the papillary region of the renal pyramids. It then extends into the collecting system of the kidney in a polypoid fashion. It is usually less than 2 to 3 cm in diameter. Microscopic analysis shows 3 components: osteoblasts and spindle cells surrounding an osteoid core.[77] Mature osteoid elements are said to be more characteristic of older patients.

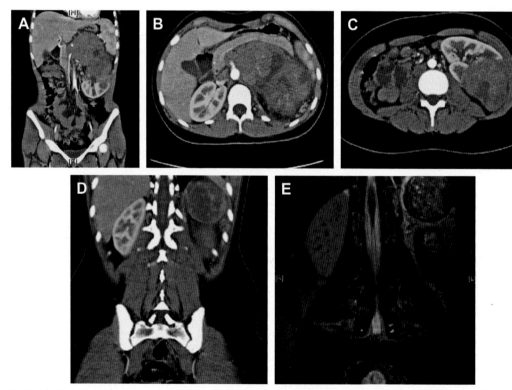

Fig. 7. (*A–C*) A 15-year-old girl with PNET of left kidney. Note heterogeneous attenuation, anterior displacement of residual functioning kidney, and extension across midline to encase aorta. (*D, E*) Coronal CT and MR imaging depicting the posterior and superior extent of this tumor. Note the heterogeneous signal intensity on MR T1-weighted imaging.

Speculation regarding the origin and natural course of these lesions include the ossifying potential of urothelial cells, and a similarity of the spindle cell component to intralobar nephrogenic rests.[52] It is hypothesized that these lesions may therefore lie within the pathologic spectrum of Wilms tumor, although no cases of this transition have been reported to date.[52]

Imaging

Abdominal ultrasound may show an echogenic, shadowing mass with or without associated hydronephrosis.

On contrast-enhanced CT imaging, ORTI most often appears as a calcified (ossified) renal mass within the collecting system, having the appearance of a staghorn calculus (**Fig. 8**).[52] Filling defects may be seen within the outline of the contrast-filled collecting system in lieu of, or in combination with, these calcifications. There may be partial obstruction of the collecting system. This tumor typically does not distort the renal outline and shows poor contrast enhancement.

Management and Prognosis

ORTI is considered a benign tumor and has been historically treated with nephrectomy or partial nephrectomy without chemotherapy or radiation.[78] There have been no incidences of metachronous or contralateral Wilms tumor to date.

RENAL MEDULLARY CARCINOMA
Epidemiology

Renal medullary carcinoma (RMC) is a recently described, highly aggressive tumor seen almost exclusively in patients with sickle cell trait or sickle SC disease. The age range at presentation is 10 to 39 years. It presents with a triad of clinical symptoms including hematuria, flank pain, and a palpable mass. In children, male/female ratio is 3:1. Gender predilection disappears beyond 25 years. Recent reports have postulated a relationship between chronic hypoxia and tumor development.[79]

Histopathology

These tumors arise at the renal pelvic-mucosal interface and rapidly proliferate to fill the renal pelvis and invade adjacent vessel and lymphatics. Intrarenal satellite lesions have been found in many resected specimens.[80] These tumors are variable in architecture, containing drepanocytes (sickle cells), foci of hemorrhage and necrosis, and prominent stromal desmoplasia with inflammation.

Imaging

A review of the CT and MR imaging findings of RMC describes features that are considered to be characteristic, including a centrally located lesion with invasion of the renal sinus, peripheral caliectasis, and retroperitoneal lymphadenopathy.[81] In this series of 6 patients with RMC, Blitman and colleagues[81] reported on the similarity in radiographic appearance of these lesions. All were right sided and showed an infiltrative pattern with obstructive caliectasis. Most lesions exhibited regional lymphadenopathy, hemorrhage, and necrosis. A reniform outline was usually maintained.

MR imaging is felt to be slightly superior to CT scan because of its multiplanar capability in the assessment of parenchymal extent and nodal invasion. MR imaging is also felt to be superior in showing intratumoral hemorrhage and liver metastases.[81] Evaluation with ultrasound exclusively is cautioned because of alterations in renal echogenicity that may be attributed to other, nonneoplastic lesions.[81,82]

Management and Prognosis

The overall survival in patients with RMC is dismal. In a review of 28 published cases from 1995 to 2003, survival averaged 32 weeks (range 2–68 weeks) from diagnosis.[83] In a more recent series of 9 patients, overall survival ranged from 4 to 16 months using a variety of chemotherapeutic regimens.[80]

CONGENITAL MESOBLASTIC NEPHROMA

Congenital mesoblastic nephroma (CMN) is the most common solid renal tumor in the newborn period. This tumor is now recognized as a distinct

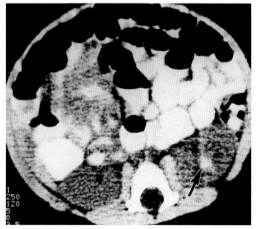

Fig. 8. ORTI, left kidney. Note the central ossified density (*arrow*). (*Courtesy of* Archana Malik, MD.)

entity from Wilms tumor, characterized by a more benign clinical behavior and lack of the malignant epithelial components typical of Wilms tumor.[25] It is considered a predominantly benign lesion, but one with some malignant potential.

Epidemiology

The tumor usually presents as a palpable abdominal mass in young infants, with a mean age at presentation of approximately 3 months. Hematuria is occasionally noted.[84] There is a male predominance. Unusual presenting findings include hypercalcemia[85] and hemorrhagic cyst.[86] Hypertension caused by hyperreninism has been reported in 9 cases, 6 of whom were neonates.[87] The tumor often is congenital and may be associated with maternal polyhydramnios (10%), believed to be related to impaired gastrointestinal function, increased renal blood flow, or impaired renal concentrating ability, with or without hypercalcemia.[88]

Histopathology

The tumors may be large (8–30 cm) and may replace much of the normal kidney. They tend to infiltrate locally, have poorly defined margins, and lack a capsule.[89,90] Microscopically, the tumors are composed of benign connective tissue and mature spindle cells that infiltrate between, and tend to entrap, intact nephrons.[89] A more aggressive variant of this tumor is more densely cellular, with a high number of active mitoses; this variant occurs primarily in infants older than 3 months and carries a less favorable prognosis with greater potential for local recurrence and metastasis.[10] Necrosis is uncommon except with this more aggressive variant.

Imaging

Ultrasound characteristically shows a well-defined, solid renal mass, which is usually homogeneous in echotexture, unless there is associated hemorrhage or necrosis (Fig. 9). CT scan is important to show the mass and nodal metastases, foci of calcification, and fat. MR imaging shows low signal intensity on T1-weighted images and high signal intensity on T2 weighting. These findings may be indistinguishable from those of Wilms tumor. Because of entrapment of renal tissue or urine within the mass, there is occasional contrast excretion within the mass on cross-sectional imaging.[10] Following resection, imaging plays a role in evaluation for local recurrence or distant metastases, particularly in children with the more aggressive, cellular subtype of tumor.

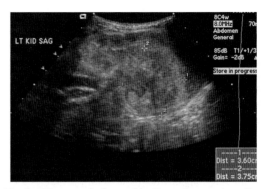

Fig. 9. Ultrasound of mesoblastic nephroma. Longitudinal image of the left kidney shows a well-circumscribed solid mass of mixed echogenicity within the inferior pole.

Management and Prognosis

Therapy consists of nephrectomy, with wide margins to ensure adequate resection of the infiltrative tumor. With the conventional, benign type of histology, prognosis is excellent and generally no further therapy is required.[84] In patients with the cellular subtype of mesoblastic nephroma, there is the potential for metastasis or local recurrence, which is greater when diagnosis and resection have occurred after the age of 3 months.[25] In such patients, chemotherapy may be indicated, particularly when there is extensive local invasion or recurrence following resection. Multimodal treatment (surgery, radiation, and chemotherapy) may rarely be necessary in patients with distant metastases.[84]

MULTILOCULAR CYSTIC RENAL TUMOR

The term multilocular cystic renal tumor refers to 2 types of generally benign renal tumors: cystic nephroma (CN) and cystic poorly differentiated nephroblastoma (CPDN).[91] These are well-circumscribed, discrete lesions consisting entirely of cysts and septae, without solid tumor components except for the septae. These lesions are at one end of a spectrum of nephroblastoma, but behave in a benign fashion.[92] These tumors follow a generally benign course; nephrectomy alone usually is curative, and no adjunctive chemotherapy is recommended.

Epidemiology and Clinical Features

The lesion presents as an abdominal mass in a young child between the ages of 3 months and 4 years. Most children present in the first 2 years of life, with a male predominance; boys are almost always less than 4 years of age. Girls usually are more than 4 years old and show a biphasic age distribution: 4 to 20 years of age and fifth to sixth decades. The most common symptom in children is a painless abdominal mass. The mass may increase in size slowly and progressively, or may show rapid growth. Systemic symptoms are uncommon in children.[93]

Histopathology

CN and CPDN are indistinguishable on gross examination. The masses are often large, averaging 8 to 10 cm in diameter; they are single, unilateral, and involve only part of a kidney.[10] Individual cysts may vary in size from microscopic to 2 to 4 cm.[94] There is no communication between cysts or with the collecting system. Two histologic subtypes are seen: cellular CPDN (potentially malignant) and classic CN (benign).[92] CPDN resembles CN in every feature except that the septae contain blastemal cells, with or without other embryonal stromal cells. There are no solid elements (other than septae) in this lesion, differentiating this entity from Wilms tumor and other renal neoplasms, which may contain cystic spaces caused by hemorrhage and necrosis.[94]

Imaging

Just as CN and CPDN cannot be distinguished on gross examination, they are also indistinguishable radiographically. Plain film findings may show a soft tissue mass with displacement of bowel. Small curvilinear calcifications occasionally may be visible.[92] Ultrasound shows a complex intrarenal mass with acoustic enhancement. Septations, dividing the mass into discrete anechoic locules, may be seen if the cysts are of sufficient size (**Fig. 10**). However, when individual cysts are small, sonography may show numerous internal echoes but no distinct loculations.[93] The finding of a peripheral crescentic rim of renal tissue

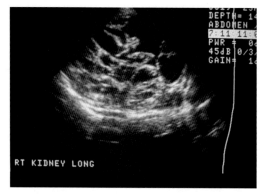

Fig. 10. Multilocular CN. Longitudinal ultrasound of the right kidney shows multiple septations within a cystic mass.

surrounding a well-defined mass, as well as splaying or displacement of the renal collecting system, is helpful to confirm the renal origin of the tumor.[94] On CT scan, a sharply circumscribed, multiseptated mass is shown, with cystic spaces between the septae (**Fig. 11**). The contents of the cysts may be similar to, or slightly greater than, water attenuation. In some tumors, the cystic spaces are very small, resulting in the appearance of a solid soft tissue mass. Enhancement of septae may be seen following intravenous contrast; however, no filling of cystic spaces with contrast occurs.[93] MR imaging shows an encapsulated multilocular renal mass, with the capsule showing low signal intensity on all pulse sequences, variable signal intensity of cyst contents on T1-weighted images, and high signal intensity of cyst contents on T2-weighted images.[95]

Management and Prognosis

All cases of CN follow a benign course. However, CPDN may show more aggressive behavior with a potential for recurrence following resection. Because these 2 entities cannot be distinguished by imaging or by gross appearance, the treatment is complete surgical resection, with careful noninvasive imaging for follow-up. If the tumor proves to be renal cellular CMN with gross residual disease or after recurrence, these patients receive adjuvant chemotherapy.[92] In most series, the prognosis is excellent, with metastases being rare.[10]

RENAL CELL CARCINOMA

Renal cell carcinoma (RCC) is primarily a tumor of adulthood; although it can be seen in children more than 5 years of age, only 0.3% to 1.3% of all cases of RCC present in childhood. RCC represents a small percentage (2.3%–6.6%) of all renal neoplasms in childhood. Wilms tumor is more common than RCC in the first decade of life, whereas Wilms tumor and RCC are equally uncommon in the second decade of life.[96] RCC has been reported in a child as young as 3 months of age. Histologically, RCC in children is identical to that seen in adults. The tumor probably originates in the epithelium of renal tubules. It forms a solid mass that may contain hemorrhage, necrosis, cystic degeneration, calcification, or fibrosis. It invades the kidney parenchyma, forms a pseudocapsule, distorts renal architecture, and spreads to contiguous nodes and to the adjacent retroperitoneum. Metastases to lungs, liver, brain, or skeleton are present in 20% of patients at diagnosis. Compared with Wilms tumor, RCC in children is more likely to metastasize to bone and more likely to be bilateral.[96] The classic triad of

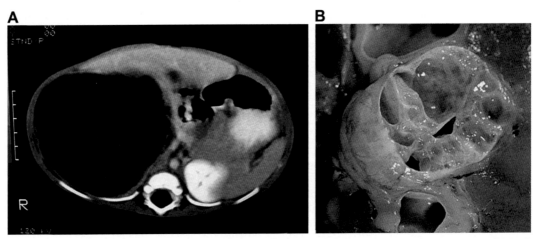

Fig. 11. (*A, B*) Multilocular CN. (*A*) Transaxial contrast-enhanced CT shows a large cystic mass arising from the right kidney, with multiple septations. (*B*) Gross specimen.

flank pain, hematuria, and palpable mass seen in adults usually is not present in children. Presenting symptoms include a palpable mass and hematuria (40%).[97]

The clinical course of RCC presenting in childhood is similar to that seen in adults. There is some controversy as to whether radical surgery, including nephrectomy and lymphadenectomy, is warranted. This approach has been advocated in pediatric patients because those with isolated lymph node metastasis have better survival rates than adults with disease at similar stages.[98] RCC is more likely to metastasize to bone and more likely to be bilateral in the adolescent age group than is Wilms tumor; however, RCC cannot be distinguished from Wilms tumor from imaging.[96] The tumor is a solid intrarenal mass on sonographic imaging (**Fig. 12**).

The 2 most important prognostic factors are stage of disease and age of presentation.[99] Management remains primarily surgical. In select patients, partial nephrectomy is effective in providing local control. The current trend is toward nephron-sparing techniques.[100]

The association of RCC with von Hippel-Lindau syndrome has been described, with the youngest reported case being a 16-year-old boy. Keeler and Klauber[101] found malignant cells in the lining of several renal cysts in a 16-year-old boy with von Hippel-Lindau disease and RCC; the investigators proposed that the presence of cysts in von Hippel-Lindau may indicate risk for progression to solid mass. Any teenager with a renal mass should be examined for other signs of von Hippel-Lindau disease.[96] Screening with ultrasound in early adolescence is advocated for patients with von

Hippel-Lindau, and kidney-sparing surgery is recommended if masses develop.[101]

Several cases of RCC associated with tuberous sclerosis have been reported.[102] In contrast with adults, RCC in children with tuberous sclerosis seems to behave in a more benign fashion, and the cases reported had no recurrences at a median 3.5-year follow-up. Isolated cases of RCC also have been reported in very young patients with other risk factors. RCC has been reported in a 3-year-old child with Beckwith-Wiedemann syndrome, appearing as a hyperechoic mass on US and having high attenuation on CT scan.[103] RCC has also been reported in a 2-year-old child following chemotherapy for neuroblastoma.[104]

ANGIOMYOLIPOMA

Angiomyolipomas (AMLs) are benign hamartomatous masses in the kidney that contain fat, smooth muscle, and abnormal blood vessels in varying proportions.

AML is uncommon in the general population (1%–2%); when found in children, they are almost exclusively associated with tuberous sclerosis. Up to 80% of all patients with tuberous sclerosis, including adults and children, have AMLs. AMLs are the most common renal lesion in tuberous sclerosis (50%–75%), far outnumbering cystic lesions (17%) and RCC (1%–2%).[97] AML is seen at a younger age and is more often symptomatic in patients with tuberous sclerosis; these tumors are more likely to be multifocal, bilateral, and of greater size than in patients without tuberous sclerosis. The tumors can expand and compress surrounding renal tissue. Between 20% and 27%

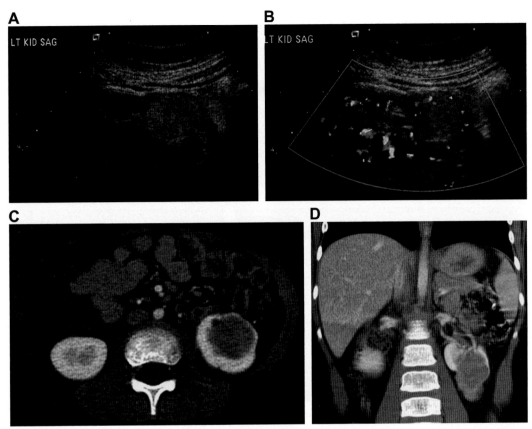

Fig. 12. (A, B) RCC. Longitudinal ultrasound of the left kidney in a 5-year-old child shows a solid, poorly vascularized echogenic mass arising from the lower pole. (C, D) Corresponding contrast-enhanced abdominal CT in axial and coronal reformatted plane shows a well-defined, low-attenuation mass extending from the interpolar region through the inferior pole, terminating as an exophytic, nonenhancing mass.

of AMLs smaller than 4 cm, and 46% of those larger than 4 cm, can be expected to grow if followed for as long as 5 years.[105]

The vessels in the tumor have deficient elastic walls and tend to be tortuous and to develop small and large aneurysms prone to spontaneous bleeding. The appearance of symptoms is correlated with the size of the tumor. Masses less than 4 cm in diameter usually are asymptomatic, but those larger than 3.5 or 4 cm often cause flank pain, hematuria, and anemia, and carry a significant risk for catastrophic hemorrhage. AMLs increase in size during adolescence, most notably in girls, suggesting possible hormonal modulation of tumor growth.[106] Hemorrhage is rare in patients less than 10 years of age, but, in the second and third decades of life, bleeding may be severe enough to produce hypovolemic shock in up to 10% of patients.[107]

Imaging studies can be diagnostic if a characteristic fatty component is identified. Ultrasound shows brightly echogenic fatty foci, which are

easily identifiable in the renal cortex (**Fig. 13**). However, small masses lying near the renal sinus may be missed. In small lesions, CT scan with thin sections and single-voxel measurements may be helpful to confirm the diagnosis.[108] MR imaging provides superior soft tissue contrast of renal and extrarenal abnormalities (hemorrhage, perinephric collections, renal cysts, hepatic AMLs) and is the best alternative to ultrasound in children with tuberous sclerosis (**Fig. 14**).[109]

Conservative management is recommended for patients with known masses smaller than 4 cm, with serial US examination every 6 months to 1 year. Partial nephrectomy or selective catheter embolization is advocated for masses larger than 4 cm.[110] Selective arterial embolization is the treatment of choice, because it has been shown to shrink most tumors and control symptoms in 83% to 90% of renal tumors.[111] In addition, selective embolization can be directed to a site of acute hemorrhage and can be repeated as necessary with maximum sparing of functional renal tissue.

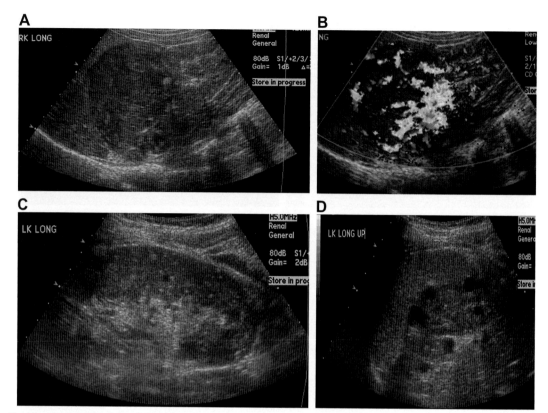

Fig. 13. Large AML of the right kidney in a patient with tuberous sclerosis. There is a large, well-defined, hyper-vascular lesion of mixed echogenicity within the superior pole of the right kidney (*A, B*). Longitudinal images of the left kidney show multiple tiny echogenic foci and fewer, larger anechoic lesions consistent with angiolipomas and cysts, respectively (*C, D*).

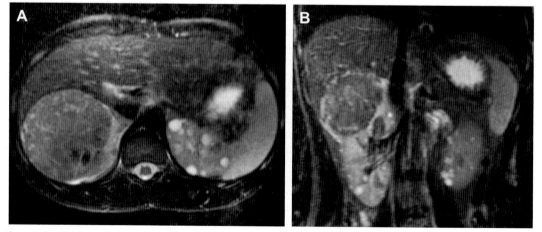

Fig. 14. (*A, B*) The same patient as **Fig. 13**. Corresponding T2-weighted MR images. Note low signal intensity of large AML containing bright internal septations. Also note cysts with high signal intensity and small angiolipomas with low signal intensity.

It has been suggested that postprocedural imaging at 1 to 3 months and again at 6 to 12 months should be used to evaluate for regression or regrowth. Ultrasound evaluation is recommended in patients with tuberous sclerosis every 2 to 3 years before puberty and yearly after that.[112]

LYMPHOMA AND LEUKEMIA

There is still debate about the existence of primary lymphoma of the kidney.[113] Although the kidneys contain no lymph tissue, rare cases of lymphoma confined to the kidney have been reported, usually showing multinodular renal enlargement on ultrasound or CT imaging.[114] Diagnostic criteria are unclear, and the possibility of metastasis from another site lingers when there is extrarenal involvement. Nevertheless, Arranz Arija and colleagues[113] reported 3 cases, including 2 in children, and proposed that renal biopsy and abdominal imaging findings should be sufficient to guide therapy without the need for staging laparotomy.

Lymphoma commonly involves the kidney secondarily from direct retroperitoneal extension or hematogenous metastases. In children, non-Hodgkin lymphoma, especially Burkitt, is more likely to involve the kidney.[115] Between 24% and 40% of cases of non-Hodgkin lymphoma occur primarily at extranodal sites; however, primary renal lymphoma is a rare condition.

Lymphoma usually presents with an abdominal or chest mass with adenopathy. When the kidney is involved, the most common radiologic pattern is multiple parenchymal masses or nodules that occasionally distort the renal contour and collecting system (**Fig. 15**).[52]

The patient may present with renal failure, or renal failure may be induced on initiation of chemotherapy because of breakdown of malignant cells and massive excretion of uric acid. Leukemic

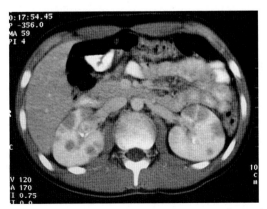

Fig. 15. Large cell lymphoma. Contrast-enhanced axial CT image showing multiple hypodense nodules throughout both kidneys.

infiltration of the kidneys may cause bilateral, diffuse renal enlargement. Renal symptoms such as hypertension or renal failure are rare.

MISCELLANEOUS RENAL TUMORS

Renal invasion by extrarenal neuroblastoma can be diagnosed accurately by CT examination of the abdomen. A 20% incidence of extension of abdominal neuroblastoma into the kidney is reported.[116] It is more common in patients with higher stage (III or IV) tumor and with undifferentiated histology. Extension may occur by tumor spread along vessels or by direct infiltration of the renal capsule, especially the upper pole contiguous with the adrenal gland.[116] Neuroblastoma arising within the kidney is rare. The lesion may resemble Wilms tumor on imaging examination, although, in 50% of cases, the mass is not completely surrounded by renal parenchyma. The appearance at surgery may resemble Wilms tumor and, in some cases, the lesion initially has been confused with undifferentiated Wilms tumor. The histologic finding is invariably highly anaplastic, and there is rapidly progressive clinical deterioration.[117]

Nephrogenic adenofibroma is a rare renal neoplasm first characterized in 1992.[118] The mean age at presentation is 13 years, although the tumor has been reported in patients as young as 15 months and as old as 83 years.[52] Patients present with a mass, hypercalcemia, polycythemia, hypertension, or hematuria. The mass has been confused with Wilms tumor, but the histology is a distinctive proliferation of spindled mesenchymal cells, with nodules of embryonal epithelium. Unlike Wilms tumor, nephrogenic adenofibroma is not encapsulated. The active proliferation of Wilms tumor is absent. In addition, nephrogenic adenofibroma lacks immunoreactivity for muscle-specific actin and fails to immunostain for desmin, findings that separate it from similar-appearing mesoblastic nephroma. Clinical symptoms resolve following nephrectomy.

Nephrogenic adenofibroma may be indistinguishable from Wilms tumor by imaging. Ultrasound may show a well-defined solid mass that is hypoechoic or hyperechoic or even cystic with a mural nodule. It is hypovascular by Doppler imaging. Noncontrast CT shows an isoattenuating or hyperattenuating mass with small flecks of calcification.[119]

REFERENCES

1. McVee JJ, Grosfeld JL, Smith JP. Abdominal masses in the newborn: 63 cases. J Urol 1971; 106:770–5.

2. Paulino AC, Coppes MJ. Wilms tumor. emedicine pediatrics. 2009. Available at: emedicine.medscape. com. Updated May 4, 2011.

3. Feinstein KF. Renal neoplasms. In: Kuhn JP, Slovis TL, Haller JO, editors. Caffey's pediatric diagnostic imaging. 10th edition. St Louis (MO): CV Mosby; 2004. p. 1788.

4. Mesrobian HG. Wilms tumor: past, present, future. J Urol 1988;140:231–8.

5. Breslow NE, Beckwith JB, Ciol M, et al. Age distribution of Wilms' tumor: report from the National Wilms Tumor Study. Cancer Res 1988; 48:1653–7.

6. Van den Heuvel-Eibrink MM, Grundy P, Graf N, et al. Characteristics and survival of 750 children diagnosed with a renal tumor in the first seven months of life: a collaborative study by the SIOP/GPOH/NWTSG/and UKCCSG Wilms tumor study groups. Pediatr Blood Cancer 2008;50: 1130–4.

7. Davidoff AM, Giel DW, Jones DP, et al. The feasibility and outcome of nephron-sparing surgery for children with bilateral Wilms tumor. The St. Jude Children's Hospital Experience: 1999–2006. Cancer 2008;112(9):2060–70.

8. Bond JV. Bilateral Wilms' tumour: age at diagnosis, associated congenital anomalies, and possible patterns of inheritance. Lancet 1975;2:482–4.

9. Casale AI, Flanigan RC, Moore PJ, et al. Survival in bilateral metachronous (asynchronous) Wilms tumors. J Urol 1982;128:766–9.

10. Cohen MD. Genitourinary tumors (imaging of the primary tumor). In: Cohen MD, editor. Imaging of children with cancer. 1st edition. St Louis: Mosby-Year Book; 1992. p. 60–74.

11. Breslow NE, Beckwith JB. Epidemiological features of Wilms' tumor: results of the National Wilms' Tumor Study. J Natl Cancer Inst 1982;68:429–36.

12. Neville H, Ritchey ML, Shamberger RC, et al. The occurrence of Wilms tumor in horseshoe kidneys: a report of the National Wilms Tumor Study Group (NWTSG). J Pediatr Surg 2002;37(8):1134–7.

13. Hartman GE, Smolik LM, Shochat SJ. The dilemma of the multicystic dysplastic kidney. Am J Dis Child 1986;140:925.

14. Oddone M, Marino C, Sergi C, et al. Wilms' tumor arising in a multicystic kidney. Pediatr Radiol 1994;24:236–8.

15. Tank ES, Kay R. Neoplasms associated with hemihypertrophy, Beckwith-Wiedemann syndrome and aniridia. J Urol 1980;124:266–8.

16. Goldman SM, Garfinkel DJ, Oh KS, et al. The Drash syndrome: male pseudohermaphroditism, nephritis, and Wilms' tumor. Radiology 1981;141:87–91.

17. Cairney AEL, Andrews M, Greenberg M, et al. Wilms tumor in three patients with Bloom syndrome. J Pediatr 1987;111:414–6.

18. Karayalcin J, Shanske A, Honigman R. Wilms' tumor in a 13-year-old girl with trisomy 18. Am J Dis Child 1981;135:665–6.

19. Early CK, Rosen D, Mirza M. The coexistence of Wilms' tumor and imperforate anus with rectourethral fistula. J Pediatr Surg 1981;16:756–7.

20. Pendergrass TW. Congenital anomalies in children with Wilms' tumor; a new survey. Cancer 1976;37: 403–9.

21. Niu CK, Chen WF, Chuang JH, et al. Intrapelvic Wilms tumor: report of two cases and review of the literature. J Urol 1993;150:936–9.

22. Beckwith JB, Kiviat NB, Bonadio JF. Nephrogenic rests, nephroblastomatosis and the pathogenesis of Wilms' tumor. Pediatr Pathol 1990;10:1–36.

23. Coppes M, Wilson P, Weitzman S. Extrarenal Wilms' tumor: staging, management and prognosis. J Clin Oncol 1991;9:167–74.

24. Suzuki K, Tashiro M, Mori H, et al. Extrarenal Wilms' tumor. Pediatr Radiol 1993;23:149–50.

25. White KS, Grossman H. Wilms' and associated renal tumors of childhood. Pediatr Radiol 1990; 21:81–8.

26. Faria P, Beckwith JB, Mishra K. Focal versus diffuse anaplasia in Wilms' tumor: new definitions with prognostic significance-a report from the National Wilms Tumor Study Group. Am J Surg Pathol 1996;20:909–20.

27. Kim S, Chung DH. Pediatric solid malignancies: neuroblastoma and Wilms tumor. Surg Clin North Am 2006;86:469–87.

28. Bonadio JF, Storer B, Norkool P, et al. Anaplastic Wilms' tumor: clinical and pathologic studies. J Clin Oncol 1985;3:513–20.

29. Exelby PR. Retroperitoneal malignant tumors: Wilms' tumor and neuroblastoma. Surg Clin North Am 1981;61:1219–27.

30. Ritchey ML, Kelalis PP, Breslow NE, et al. Intracaval and atrial involvement with nephroblastoma: review of National Wilms' Tumor Study-3. J Urol 1988;140: 1113.

31. Schraut WH, Chilcote RR. Metastatic Wilms' tumor causing acute hepatic vein occlusion (Budd-Chiari syndrome). Gastroenterology 1985;88:576–9.

32. Nakayama DK, deLorimier AA, O'Neill JA, et al. Intracardiac extension of Wilms' tumor. Ann Surg 1986;204:693.

33. Chung CJ, Lorenzo R, Rayder S, et al. Rhabdoid tumors of the kidney in children: CT findings. Am J Roentgenol 1995;164:697–700.

34. Khalil RM, Aubel S. Clear cell sarcoma of the kidney: a case report. Pediatr Radiol 1993;23: 407–8.

35. Yokomori K, Hori T, Takemura T, et al. Demonstration of both primary and secondary reninism in renal tumors in children. J Pediatr Surg 1988;23: 403–9.

36. Kaufman RA, Holt JP, Heidelberger KP. Calcification in primary and metastatic Wilms' tumor. Am J Roentgenol 1978;130:783.

37. Hartman DS, Sanders RC. Wilms' tumor versus neuroblastoma: usefulness of ultrasound in differentiation. J Ultrasound Med 1982;1:117–22.

38. Reiman TAH, Siegel MJ, Shackelford GD. Wilms' tumor in children: abdominal CT and US evaluation. Radiology 1986;160:501–5.

39. Miniati D, Gay AN, Parks KV, et al. Imaging accuracy and incidence of Wilms' and non-Wilms' renal tumors in children. J Pediatr Surg 2008;43:1301–7.

40. Cohen MD. Commentary: imaging and staging of Wilms' tumors: problems and controversies. Pediatr Radiol 1996;26:307–11.

41. Green DM, Fernbach DI, Norkool P, et al. The treatment of Wilms' tumor patients with pulmonary metastases detected only with computed tomography: a report from the National Wilms' Tumor Study. J Clin Oncol 1991;9:1776–81.

42. Wilmas JA, Douglass EC, Magill HL, et al. Significance of pulmonary computed tomography at diagnosis in Wilms tumor. J Clin Oncol 1988;6:1144–6.

43. National Cancer Institute: PDQ Wilms tumor and other childhood kidney tumors treatment. Bethesda, MD: National Cancer Institute. Date last modified February 8, 2011. Available at: http://cancer.gov/cancertopics/pdq/treatments/Wilms/HealthProfessional. Accessed August 7, 2009.

44. Belt TG, Cohen MD, Smith JA, et al. MRI of Wilms' tumor: promise as the primary imaging modality. Am J Roentgenol 1986;146:955–61.

45. Schenk JP, Graf N, Gunther P, et al. Role of MRI in the management of patients with nephroblastoma. Eur Radiol 2008;18:683–91.

46. Weese DL, Applebaum H, Taber P. Mapping intravascular extension of Wilms' tumour with magnetic resonance imaging. J Pediatr Surg 1991;26:64–7.

47. Breslow NE, Churchill G, Beckwith JB, et al. Prognosis for Wilms' tumor patients with nonmetastatic disease at diagnosis-Results of the second National Wilms' Tumor Study. J Clin Oncol 1985;3:521–31.

48. D'Angio GI, Breslow N, Beckwith JB, et al. Treatment of Wilms' tumor: results of the third National Wilms' Tumor Study. Cancer 1989;64:349–60.

49. Sonn G, Shortliffe LM. Management of Wilms tumor: current standard of care. Nat Clin Pract Urol 2008;5(10):551–60.

50. Habib F, McLorie GA, Mckenna PH, et al. Effectiveness of preoperative chemotherapy in the treatment of Wilms tumor with vena caval and intracardiac extension. J Urol 1993;150:933–5.

51. Longaker MT, Harrison MR, Adzick NS, et al. Nephron-sparing approach to bilateral Wilms' tumor: in situ or ex vivo surgery and radiation therapy. J Pediatr Surg 1990;25:411–4.

52. Lowe LH, Isuani BH, Heller RM, et al. Pediatric renal masses: Wilms tumor and beyond. Radiographics 2000;20:1585–603.

53. Beckwith JB. Wilms' tumor and other renal tumors of childhood: an update. J Urol 1986;136:320–4.

54. Gylys-Morin V, Hoffer FA, Kozakewich H, et al. Wilms' tumor and nephroblastomatosis: imaging characteristics at gadolinium-enhanced MR imaging. Radiology 1993;188:517–21.

55. Sebire NJ, Vujanic GM. Pediatric renal tumors: recent developments, new entities and pathologic features. Histopathology 2009;54:516–28.

56. Fernbach SK, Feinstein KA. Renal tumors in children. Semin Roentgenol 1995;30(2):200–17.

57. Perlman EJ, Faria P, Soares A, et al. Hyperplastic perilobar nephroblastomatosis: long-term survival of 52 patients. Pediatr Blood Cancer 2006;46:203–21.

58. Kidd JM. Exclusion of certain renal neoplasms from the category of Wilms tumor [abstract]. Am J Pathol 1970;58:16a.

59. Prasad SR, Humphrey PA, Menias CO, et al. Neoplasms of the renal medulla: radiologic-pathologic correlation. Radiographics 2005;25:369–80.

60. Haas JE, Bonadio JF, Beckwith JB. Clear cell sarcoma of the kidney with emphasis on ultrastructural studies. Cancer 1984;54:2978.

61. Kagan RA, Steckel RJ. Clear cell sarcoma of the kidney: a renal tumor of childhood that metastasizes to bone. AJR Am J Roentgenol 1986;146:64–6.

62. Beckwith JB. Wilms' tumor and other renal tumors of childhood: a selective review from the National Wilms' Tumor Study Pathology Center. Hum Pathol 1983;14:481–92.

63. Brownlee NA, Perkins LA, Stewart W, et al. Recurring translocation (10:17) and deletion (14q) in clear cell sarcoma of the kidney. Arch Pathol Lab Med 2007;131:446–51.

64. Radulescu VC, Gerrard M, Moertel C, et al. Treatment of recurrent clear cell sarcoma of the kidney with brain metastasis. Pediatr Blood Cancer 2008;50(2):246–9.

65. Glass RB, Davidson AI, Fernbach SK. Clear cell sarcoma of the kidney: CT, sonographic and pathologic correlation. Radiology 1991;180:715–7.

66. Argani P, Perlman EJ, Breslow NE, et al. Clear cell sarcoma of the kidney: a review of 351 cases from the National Wilms Tumor Study Group Pathology Center. Am J Surg Pathol 2000;24:4–18.

67. Eklöf O, Mortensson W, Sandstedt B, et al. Bone metastases in Wilms' tumor: occurrence and radiological appearance. Ann Radiol (Paris) 1984;27:97–103.

68. Seibel NL, Li S, Breslow NE, et al. Effect of duration of treatment on treatment outcome for patients with clear cell sarcoma of the kidney: a report from the

National Wilms Tumor Study Group. J Clin Oncol 2004;22(3):468–73.

69. Weeks DA, Beckwith JB, Mierau GW, et al. Rhabdoid tumor of kidney. A report of 111 cases from the National Wilms' Tumor Study Pathology Center. Am J Surg Pathol 1989;13:439.

70. Geller JI, Leslie ND, Yin H. Malignant rhabdoid tumor. In: Coppes MJ, editor. Available at: emedicine. medscape.com/article993084-overview. Updated December 18, 2009.

71. Jafri SZ, Freeman JL, Rosenberg BF, et al. Clinical and imaging features of rhabdoid tumor of the kidney. Urol Radiol 1991;13:94–7.

72. Bonnin JM, Rubinstein LI, Palmer NF, et al. The association of embryonal tumors originating in the kidney and in the brain. A report of seven cases. Cancer 1984;54:2137–46.

73. Ellinger J, Bastian PJ, Hauser S, et al. Primitive neuroectodermal tumor: rare, highly aggressive differential diagnosis in urologic malignancies. Urology 2006;68(2):257–62.

74. Ishii H, Ogaki K. Primitive neuroectodermal tumor of the kidney. Med Mol Morphol 2009;42:175–9.

75. Hari S, Jain TP, Thulkar S, et al. Imaging features of peripheral neuroectodermal tumours. Br J Radiol 2008;81:975–83.

76. Chatten J, Cromie WJ, Duckett JW. Ossifying tumor of infantile kidney: report of two cases. Cancer 1980;45:609–12.

77. Glick RD, Hicks MJ, Nuchtern JG, et al. Renal tumors in infants less than 6 months of age. J Pediatr Surg 2004;39(4):522–5.

78. Vazquez JL, Barnewolt CE, Shamberger RC, et al. Ossifying renal tumor of infancy presenting as a palpable abdominal mass. Pediatr Radiol 1998; 28:454–7.

79. Swartz MA, Karth J, Schneider DT, et al. Renal medullary carcinoma: clinical, pathologic, immuno-histochemical and genetic analysis with pathogenetic implications. Urology 2002;60:1083–9.

80. Hakimi AA, Kol PT, Milhoua PM, et al. Renal medullary carcinoma: the Bronx experience. Urology 2007;70(5):878–82.

81. Blitman NM, Berkenblit RG, Rozenblit AM, et al. Renal medullary carcinoma: CT and MRI features. Am J Roentgenol 2005;185:268–72.

82. Wesche WA, Wilimas J, Khare V, et al. Renal medullary carcinoma: a potential sickle cell nephropathy of children and adolescents. Pediatr Pathol Lab Med 1998;18:97–113.

83. Simpson L, He X, Pins M, et al. Renal medullary carcinoma and ABL gene amplification. J Urol 2005;173:1883–8.

84. Howell C, Othersen H, Kiviat N. Therapy and outcome in 51 children with mesoblastic nephroma: a report of the national Wilms' tumor study. J Pediatr Surg 1982;17:826–31.

85. Ferraro E, Klein S, Fakhry M, et al. Hypercalcemia in association with mesoblastic nephroma: report of a case and review of the literature. Pediatr Radiol 1986;16:516–7.

86. Christmann D, Becmeur F, Marcellin L, et al. Mesoblastic nephroma presenting as a hemorrhagic cyst. Pediatr Radiol 1990;20:553.

87. Khashu M, Osiovich H, Sargent M. Congenital mesoblastic nephroma presenting with neonatal hypertension. J Perinatol 2005;25:433–5.

88. Chaudry G, Perez-Atayde A, Ngan B, et al. Imaging of congenital mesoblastic nephroma with pathological correlation. Pediatr Radiol 2009;39:1080–6.

89. Hartman D, Lesar M, Madewell J. Mesoblastic nephroma: radiologic-pathologic correlation of 20 cases. Am J Roentgenol 1981;136:69–74.

90. Loeb DM, Hill DA, Dome JS. Complete response of recurrent cellular congenital mesoblastic nephroma to chemotherapy. J Pediatr Hematol Oncol 2002;24(6):478–81.

91. Joshi V, Beckwith J. Multilocular cyst of the kidney (cystic nephroma) and cystic, partially differentiated nephroblastoma. Cancer 1989;64:466–79.

92. Perlman E. Pediatric renal tumors: practical updates for the pathologist. Pediatr Dev Pathol 2005;8:320–38.

93. Madewell J, Goldman S, Davis C, et al. Multilocular cystic nephroma: a radiographic-pathologic correlation of 58 patients. Radiology 1983;146:309–21.

94. Agrons G, Wagner B, Davidson A, et al. Multilocular cystic renal tumor in children: radiologic-pathologic correlation. Radiographics 1995;15:653–69.

95. Abara O, Liu P, Churchill B, et al. Magnetic resonance imaging of cystic, partially differentiated nephroblastoma. Urology 1990;36:424–7.

96. Hartman DS, Davis CJ Jr, Madewell IE, et al. Primary malignant renal tumors in the second decade of life: Wilms' tumor versus renal cell carcinoma. J Urol 1982;127:888–91.

97. Hicks J. Review of pediatric renal neoplasms: from USCAP Annual Symposium. Boston (MA), March 1, 1998.

98. Freedman AL, Yates TS, Stewart T, et al. Renal cell carcinoma in children: the Detroit experience. J Urol 1996;155:1708–10.

99. Manion S, Hayani A, Husain A, et al. Partial nephrectomy for pediatric renal cell carcinoma: an unusual case presentation. Urology 1997;49(3).

100. Cook A, Lorenzo A, Salle J, et al. Pediatric renal cell carcinoma: single institution 25-year case series and initial experience with partial nephrectomy. J Urol 2006;175:1456–60.

101. Keeler LL 3rd, Klauber GT. von Hippel-Lindau disease and renal cell carcinoma in a 16-year old boy. J Urol 1992;147:1588–91.

102. Washeka R, Hanna M. Malignant renal tumors in tuberous sclerosis. Urology 1991;37:340–3.

103. Yamaguchi T, Fukuda T, Uetani M, et al. Renal cell carcinoma in a patient with Beckwith-Wiedemann syndrome. Pediatr Radiol 1996;26:312–4.

104. Fenton DS, Taub JW, Amundson GM, et al. Renal cell carcinoma occurring in a child 2 years after chemotherapy for neuroblastoma. Am J Roentgenol 1993;161:165–6.

105. Steiner MS, Goldman SM, Fishman EK, et al. The natural history of renal angiomyolipoma. J Urol 1993;150:1782–6.

106. Ewalt DH, Sheffield E, Sparagana SP, et al. Renal lesion growth in children with tuberous sclerosis complex. J Urol 1988;160:140–5.

107. Van Baal JG, Smits NJ, Keeman IN, et al. The evolution of renal angiomyolipomas in patients with tuberous sclerosis. J Urol 1994;152:35–8.

108. Kurosaki Y, Tanaka Y, Kuramoto K, et al. Improved CT fat detection in small kidney angiomyolipomas using thin sections and single voxel measurements. J Comput Assist Tomogr 1993;17:745–8.

109. Winterkorn E, Daouk G, Anupindi S, et al. Tuberous sclerosis complex and renal angiomyolipoma: case report and review of the literature. Pediatr Nephrol 2006;21:1189–93.

110. Kennelly MJ, Grossman HB, Cho KJ. Outcome analysis of 42 cases of renal angiomyolipoma. J Urol 1994;152:1988–91.

111. Harabayashi T, Shinohara N, Katano H, et al. Management of renal angiomyolipomas associated with tuberous sclerosis complex. J Urol 2004;171:102–5.

112. Kothary N, Soulen MC, Clark TW, et al. Renal angiomyolipoma: long term results after arterial embolization. J Vasc Interv Radiol 2005;16:45–50.

113. Arranz Arija JA, Carrion JR, Garcia FR, et al. Primary renal lymphoma: report of 3 cases and review of the literature. Am J Nephrol 1994;14:148–53.

114. Kandel LB, McCullough DL, Harrison LH, et al. Primary renal lymphoma: does it exist? Cancer 1987;60:386–91.

115. Sheth S, Ali S, Fishman E. Imaging of renal lymphoma: patterns of disease with pathologic correlation. Radiographics 2006;26(4):1151–68.

116. Albregts AE, Cohen MD, Galliani CA. Neuroblastoma invading the kidney. J Pediatr Surg 1994;29:930–3.

117. Rosenfield NS, Leonidas JC, Barwick KW. Aggressive neuroblastoma simulating Wilms' tumor. Radiology 1988;166:165–7.

118. Henninger RA, Beckwith JB. Nephrogenic adenofibroma. A novel kidney tumor of young people. Am J Surg Pathol 1992;16:325–34.

119. Navarro O, Conolly B, Taylor G, et al. Metanephric adenoma of the kidney: a case report. Pediatr Radiol 1999;29:100–3.

Adrenal Masses in Children

Csilla Balassy, MD[a,b,c], Oscar M. Navarro, MD[a,b],
Alan Daneman, MD[a,b],*

KEYWORDS

• Adrenal gland • Mass lesions • Pediatric

The adrenal glands are small organs that are located in the retroperitoneal space, within the fascia of Gerota, superior and medial to the upper pole of the kidneys. During fetal life, because of the presence of the prominent fetal cortex, they are proportionately much larger than in adults, being approximately one-half to one-third the size of the kidneys. Normal adrenal glands can already be visualized prenatally, both with ultrasound (US) and with magnetic resonance (MR) imaging. Their prominent fetal size remains evident in early neonatal life (**Fig. 1**). With the physiologic atrophy of the fetal adrenal cortex, the glands lose one-third of their weight by the end of the second week of life. Beyond this age, usually from late infancy, the adrenal limbs are normally thinner than the adjacent crura of the diaphragm. Therefore, they are much more difficult to detect with US, but can be easily visualized on computed tomography (CT) or MR imaging.

US is the primary modality for imaging the abdomen in children, including those with known or suspected abnormalities of the adrenal glands. Conventional plain radiographs have become obsolete for this purpose; however, subtle, often incidental findings on abdominal radiographs can be suggestive for the presence of adrenal tumors. CT and MR imaging are required for lesion characterization, more accurate assessment of tumor size, to determine relationship to adjacent tissues and anatomic structures, and to differentiate benign from malignant masses.

Functional imaging modalities, such as positron emission tomography (PET) and single-photon emission CT (SPECT) can be used for the primary diagnosis, and for the evaluation of recurrent and metastatic disease. In recent years, the combination of nuclear medicine modalities and anatomic imaging in PET-CT has been shown to have a large impact on the management of the pediatric oncologic population as well.[1–4] PET-CT has been shown to have significantly higher sensitivity than PET alone in the detection of distant metastasis in several malignant diseases, including neoplasms of the adrenal gland.[5]

ADRENAL MASSES

Adrenal masses may occur as a result of neoplasms, hemorrhage, infection, or cysts. Such lesions are often discovered incidentally; therefore, the evaluation and management of these incidentally detected adrenal masses are discussed briefly later in this article.

Primary adrenal neoplasms can be categorized by their origin and function. They may arise from the medulla or cortex, and they can be hyperfunctioning or nonfunctioning. Primary medullary neoplasms originate from the neural crest, and, in addition to the adrenal gland itself, may occur anywhere along the sympathetic neural chain. This group of neoplasms includes neuroblastoma, ganglioneuroblastoma, ganglioneuroma, and

The authors have nothing to disclose.

a Department of Diagnostic Imaging, The Hospital for Sick Children, 555 University Avenue, Toronto, ON M5G 1X8, Canada

b Department of Medical Imaging, University of Toronto, 555 University Avenue, Toronto, ON M5G 1X8, Canada

c Department of Radiology, Vienna General Hospital, Medical University of Vienna, Waehringer Guertel 18-20, 1090 Vienna, Austria

* Corresponding author. Department of Diagnostic Imaging, The Hospital for Sick Children, 555 University Avenue, Toronto, ON M5G 1X8, Canada.

E-mail address: alan.daneman@utoronto.ca

Radiol Clin N Am 49 (2011) 711–727

doi:10.1016/j.rcl.2011.05.001

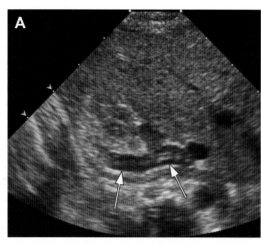
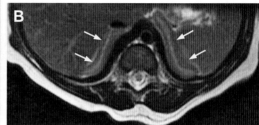

Fig. 1. Normal neonatal adrenal gland. (*A*) Transverse US scan shows the Y-shaped right adrenal gland (*arrows*) with characteristic hypoechoic peripheral component and a thin central hyperechoic band. (*B*) Axial T2-weighted MR image shows both adrenal glands (*arrows*) with a peripheral hypointense component and a central hyperintense band. These peripheral and central components of different echogenicity on US and of different signal intensity on MR imaging do not correlate with the cortex and medulla. At this age, most of the adrenal gland is formed by fetal cortex, whereas the microscopic medulla is not definable. The central echoes seen on US are related to vessels and connective tissue.

pheochromocytoma. Neoplasms that arise from the adrenal cortex include adrenocortical carcinoma and adenoma. Other, much rarer, neoplasms that may occur in children include smooth muscle tumor in patients with acquired immune deficiency syndrome (AIDS), and teratoid rhabdoid tumor.

In addition to masses of adrenal origin, there are extra-adrenal masses in the suprarenal fossa, which, because of their location, may be difficult to differentiate from masses arising primary from the adrenal glands. The most common of these extra-adrenal suprarenal masses in the pediatric age group include intra-abdominal extralobar pulmonary sequestration and retroperitoneal lymphatic malformations.

MEDULLARY NEOPLASMS

Neuroblastoma, ganglioneuroblastoma, and ganglioneuroma are histologically related entities that arise from the primordial neural crest cells of the sympathetic nervous system, and are referred to collectively as neuroblastic tumors.[6] However, they are distinct entities with different degrees of cell maturation and differentiation, and thus are associated with different biologic behavior.

Neuroblastoma is the most frequent and most malignant of the 3 tumor types. It contains the least differentiated malignant small round cells. Ganglioneuroma is the most mature, and is a benign entity, whereas ganglioneuroblastoma shows mixed histology, and is considered to be borderline malignant.

NEUROBLASTOMA

Neuroblastoma is the most common extracranial solid neoplasm in children, accounting for 10% of all pediatric neoplasms, and 15% of all childhood mortality from neoplasms.[7] In three-quarters of pediatric cases, neuroblastomas arise in the abdomen, with one-third of these in the adrenal glands. The remainder of the neuroblastomas may occur anywhere along the sympathetic nerve chain from the neck to the pelvis.[8] Considering its incidence, neuroblastoma represents the second most common intra-abdominal neoplasm after Wilms tumor and the third most common pediatric tumor after leukemia and tumors of the central nervous system.

The typical age of presentation for neuroblastoma is between 1 and 5 years (90% of cases), with a median just less than 2 years of age. Up to 50% of cases occur in the first months of life, and can occur during the antenatal period, in which case it may be detected on fetal US and MR imaging (**Fig. 2**). Perinatal neuroblastoma has some particular features and its diagnosis is usually challenging because of specific entities seen at this age, particularly adrenal hemorrhage and extralobar pulmonary sequestration that may mimic its appearance. For these reasons, it is briefly discussed separately later in this article.

Neuroblastoma has no sex predominance. Rarely, the disease may be familial, or may be associated with neurofibromatosis, aganglionosis

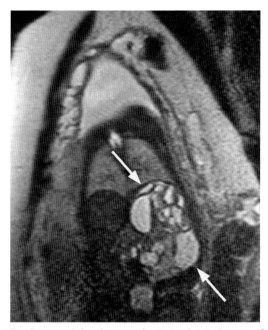

Fig. 2. T2-weighted coronal prenatal MR image of a fetus (gestational age 31+4 weeks), in whom US screening detected a large cystic mass in the left adrenal region. MR imaging confirms the finding of a predominantly cystic mass, with multiple septations and fluid-fluid levels (*arrows*). The lesion was operated after birth and the diagnosis of cystic neuroblastoma with intracystic hemorrhages was established.

of the colon (Hirschprung disease), Beckwith-Wiedemann syndrome, and central hypoventilation syndrome.[9]

Clinically, neuroblastoma most commonly presents as a palpable mass, but may be detected incidentally on abdominal US or radiographs or in association with minor abdominal trauma. Abdominal radiographs can be entirely unremarkable; however, they may show subtle findings, such as broadening of the paravertebral line (**Fig. 3**), or some mass effect with or without calcifications. When symptomatic, children typically present with signs related to direct tumor growth or invasion into the neighboring structures, or with symptoms secondary to metastatic disease. In addition, symptoms in association with hormone production, such as catecholamines and vasoactive intestine polypeptides (VIP), may be observed. The increased serum catecholamine levels can lead to high blood pressure, whereas the increased level of VIP may manifest in diarrhea. Urinary catecholamines are increased in 90% of the cases beyond infancy,[10] so their measurement is helpful when neuroblastoma is suspected. A less common, but typical and specific, paraneoplastic syndrome is opsoclonus-myoclonus with nystagmus and ataxia (Kinsbourne syndrome), which is the result of a distant, nonmetastatic effect on the cerebellum.

Local invasion can occur into the liver, kidneys, and through the neural foramina into the spinal canal, causing cord compression symptoms, depending on the level of invasion (**Fig. 4**). Neuroblastomas typically show encasement and displacement of the vascular structures (see **Fig. 3**; **Fig. 5**), and only rarely invasion of the vasculature (**Fig. 6**) or ureter.

Distant metastases are present in half the cases at the time of the diagnosis, the pattern of which is age related. The most common sites of metastatic disease are lymph nodes, bone marrow, liver, and skin (blueberry muffin skin) (see **Figs. 3** and **5**; **Fig. 7**). Metastasis to skin, bone marrow, and liver are more common in infants. Symptoms caused by metastatic disease also include skeletal pain that can mimic arthritis. Proptosis and periorbital ecchymosis (raccoon eye) may be present in cases with metastasis in the orbits (see **Fig. 3**).

At present, there are 2 systems used for the staging of neuroblastoma. The original International Neuroblastoma Staging System (INSS) was first established in 1988 and revised in 1993.[11] It is a surgically based staging system based on tumor resectability, lymph node metastasis, and metastatic sites. However, patients with locoregional disease can have different INSS stages, based on the degree of surgical resection. In addition, nonoperated patients cannot be staged accurately. Therefore, the International Neuroblastoma Risk Group (INRG) Task Force developed new guidelines for a preoperative staging system, which are based on clinical criteria and a detailed list of imaging-defined risk factors (IDRF), according to the location of the tumor.[12] The main difference between the 2 systems is that INSS is based on surgical resection, the INRG staging system (INRGSS) is based on the preoperative imaging characteristics of the tumor, and that lymph node involvement and midline involvement are not included in the staging criteria in the latter. Currently, these IDRF and INRGSS should be used at the time of the diagnosis.

According to the INRGSS criteria, stage L1 applies to localized tumor not involving vital structures, as defined by the list of IDRF, and confined to 1 body compartment. Stage L1 corresponds to stage 1 in the INSS. Stage L2 refers to locoregional tumor with presence of 1 or more IDRF, and corresponds to stages 2A, 2B, and 3 in the INSS. Stage M and MS of the INRGSS correspond to stage 4 and 4S in the INSS respectively, with a difference in the age limit (infants younger than 12 months in stage 4, and younger than 18 months in 4S). Imaging modalities required for staging include either CT or MR imaging, and [123]I-*meta*-iodobenzylguanidine

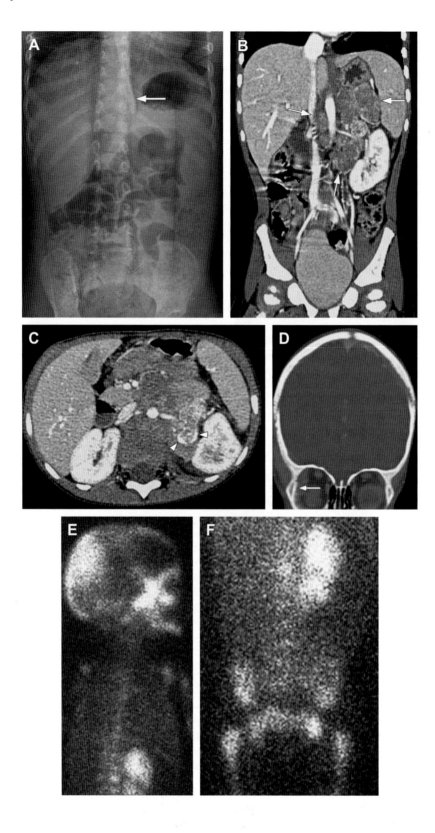

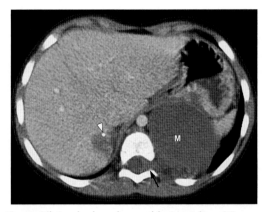

Fig. 4. Bilateral adrenal neuroblastoma in a 4.5-year-old boy. Axial contrast-enhanced CT image shows a large left adrenal mass (M) that extends into the spinal canal through a widened neural foramen (*arrow*). The spinal cord is slightly displaced to the right. The most cranial aspect of the right-sided mass is also seen containing a tiny intralesional calcification (*arrowhead*).

(MIBG) scintigraphy. The prognosis is highly dependent on the stage of the tumor. According to the INRGSS, patients with an L1 stage have a significantly higher overall survival rate than patients with an L2 stage.[13] However, the patient's age and the location of the tumor are also important determining factors.[14] The best prognostic factors are younger age (<1 year, especially those diagnosed in fetal life), lower stage, and extra-abdominal tumor origin. In these cases, the survival rate is approximately 80%, as opposed to 5% in those patients with distant metastasis. Genetic markers, such as the presence of a high amplification of N-myc oncogenes, allelic host chromosomes, and a diploic karyotype, are also associated with a poor prognosis.[15] A more favorable prognosis is seen with an aneuploic N-myc oncogene, well-differentiated tumor stroma, a normal short arm of chromosome 1, and triploid karyotypes. Based on these parameters, tumors are categorized by the INRG as high, intermediate, or low risk.

Therapy options depend on the stage at the time of the initial diagnosis and on tumor size. Patients less than 18 months of age at the time of the diagnosis, with favorable tumor biology and no distant metastasis, are often curable with surgery alone.[16] Surgery, chemotherapy, radiotherapy, and bone marrow transplantation, or a combination of these, play a role, especially in cases initially not amenable to surgery, to achieve tumor size reduction for potential operation.

The initial diagnosis of neuroblastoma arising from the adrenal gland or retroperitoneum is usually performed by US, or by cross-sectional imaging. Multidetector CT and MR imaging are the standard imaging modalities for more accurate measurement and delineation of the primary tumor and its relationship to adjacent organs and anatomic structures, and for showing metastatic disease; thus, these modalities are suited for the assessment of IDRF according to the new INRGSS. CT and MR imaging are helpful in cases with a considerable tumor size, where US may underestimate the true extent of the lesion, and in cases with very small masses, where the detection with US may be difficult. MR imaging is preferred for staging and follow-up in very young children, because of the lack of radiation exposure.

On US, the neuroblastoma usually appears as a heterogeneous mass, with hyperechoic areas caused by calcifications, which, when small, do not cause typical acoustic shadowing. Hypoechoic and anechoic areas correspond to cystic, hemorrhagic, or necrotic changes (see **Fig. 5**), and are typically less common than in Wilms tumor. Larger cystic areas are more often present in neonates, in whom bilateral cystic neuroblastoma with acute intracystic hemorrhage may occur (see **Fig. 2**; **Fig. 8**).[17] US is also helpful in the diagnosis of metastatic disease, especially liver involvement (see **Fig. 7**).

On CT, neuroblastomas present as isodense or hypodense masses compared with the musculature, with areas of calcification in most cases

Fig. 3. Left adrenal neuroblastoma in a 2-month-old girl, who presented with a 2-week history of vomiting. (*A*) Upright plain radiograph of the abdomen shows subtle broadening of the left paravertebral line (*arrow*). This finding should always raise suspicion for the presence of a retroperitoneal mass. (*B*, *C*) Contrast-enhanced CT in coronal (*B*) and axial (*C*) planes shows a large left-sided adrenal neuroblastoma (*arrows*). The mass is hypodense with multiple calcifications (*arrowheads*) (*C*) that were not apparent on the plain radiograph. A typical feature of neuroblastoma is the encasement of the vessels, the renal arteries on these particular images. (*D*) Contrast-enhanced coronal CT scan of the head shows osteolytic changes of the right orbit (*arrow*), a typical location for metastasis of neuroblastoma. There is also metastatic disease involving the right parietal bone and left parietal bone. (*E*, *F*) *meta*-Iodobenzylguanidine (MIBG) scan shows increased metabolite activity at the site of the primary lesion in the left adrenal gland, as well as in the periorbital region, skull, spine, pelvis, and proximal femurs, indicating metastatic disease. Multiple foci in the spine and pelvis were not evident on CT.

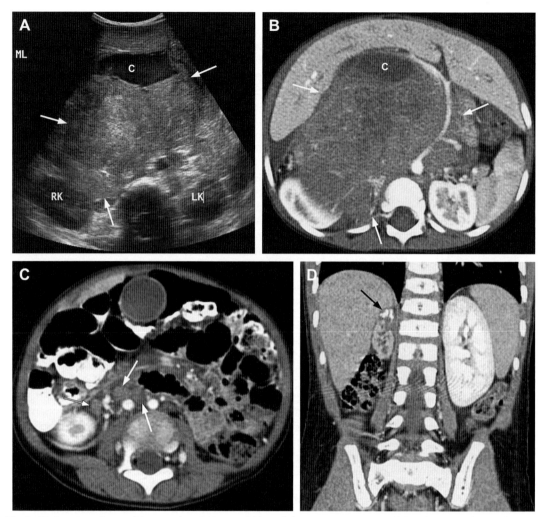

Fig. 5. Right adrenal neuroblastoma in a 2.5-year-old boy. (*A*) Transverse US scan of the abdomen shows the presence of a large, heterogeneous, right adrenal mass (*arrows*) that crosses to the left of the midline. The mass contains a cystic hypoechoic component anteriorly (C). RK, right kidney; LK, left kidney; ML, midline. (*B*) Axial contrast-enhanced CT image of the upper abdomen shows the large right-sided heterogeneous neuroblastoma (*arrows*) with the anterior cystic component (C) as shown on (*A*). The mass is crossing to the left of the midline with characteristic encasement and displacement of the vessels. Significant compression and displacement of the liver and right kidney are also noted. (*C*) Axial contrast-enhanced CT image of the midabdomen shows multiple enlarged retroperitoneal lymph nodes (*arrows*), compatible with metastatic disease. (*D*) Coronal contrast-enhanced CT performed 8 months after the initial diagnosis and 3 months after completing chemotherapy shows a small, calcified residual soft tissue mass in the right adrenal region (*arrow*). The right kidney has undergone interval atrophy and the left kidney shows compensatory hypertrophy.

(approximately 85%) (see **Fig. 3**).[18] Calcifications may be coarse, punctate, or linear. Intravenous contrast material, ideally administered with a power injector, must always be used, because it greatly facilitates the delineation of the exact size and extent of the tumor, as well as its relation to surrounding vessels. Contrast enhancement also shows the vascularity of the lesion, and helps to depict hemorrhagic, cystic, or necrotic areas within it. Multiplanar reformations facilitate better delineation of the tumor from adjacent organs to determine invasion. CT also shows the typical encasement and displacement of the mesenteric, renal, and retroperitoneal vessels, the presence of lymphadenopathy (see **Figs. 3** and **5**), as well as liver or pulmonary metastasis. Compression of the renal vessels may lead to renal infarction and organ atrophy (see **Fig. 5**). Less commonly than

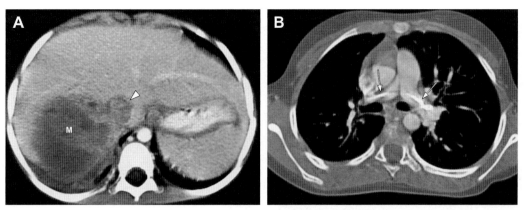

Fig. 6. A 7-year-old boy with right adrenal neuroblastoma. (*A*) Axial contrast-enhanced CT image of the upper abdomen at the time of diagnosis shows large, heterogeneous, predominantly hypodense right adrenal mass (M) with invasion into the inferior vena cava (*arrowhead*). (*B*) Follow-up axial contrast-enhanced CT image of the chest 2 years after the diagnosis shows bilateral calcified emboli in the main pulmonary arteries (*arrows*). This patient already had these tumoral pulmonary emboli at the time of diagnosis and, with the chemotherapy, they underwent calcification similar to the primary tumor.

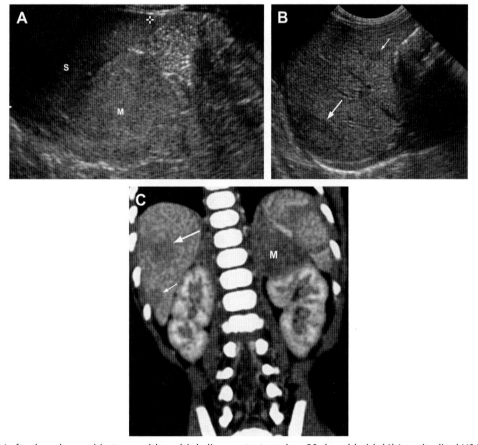

Fig. 7. Left adrenal neuroblastoma with multiple liver metastases in a 29-day-old girl. (*A*) Longitudinal US image of the left upper quadrant shows a large, homogeneous mass (M) of intermediate echogenicity in the suprarenal region. Note the spleen (S) between electronic cursors. (*B*) Longitudinal US image of the liver shows several hypoechoic intraparenchymal nodules that indicate metastatic disease (*arrows*). (*C*) Coronal contrast-enhanced CT image shows the left adrenal mass (M) and multiple metastatic nodules in the liver (*arrows*).

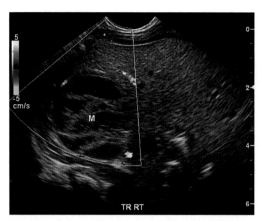

Fig. 8. Congenital cystic neuroblastoma in an 8-day-old girl with antenatal diagnosis of suprarenal mass in the third trimester. Color Doppler US scan in the transverse plane shows a heterogeneous right suprarenal mass (M) with cystic-appearing hypoechoic components, as well as more echogenic areas. The absence of internal flow may suggest the diagnosis of hemorrhage; however, cystic or hemorrhagic neuroblastomas may mimic this appearance, as illustrated in this case. Therefore, the differentiation between neuroblastoma and adrenal hemorrhage is not possible with a single US, and these cases require follow-up as well as correlation with urine catecholamines.

in Wilms tumor, neuroblastomas may also invade the inferior vena cava and extend up to the heart (see **Fig. 6**).

On MR imaging, neuroblastomas show low signal intensity on T1-weighted images and high signal intensity on T2-weighted images, as well as heterogeneous enhancement after the administration of intravenous contrast material. MR imaging is the modality of choice to show spinal invasion with leptomeningeal or epidural extension and bone marrow disease. Intraspinal extension occurs more often in neuroblastomas that arise in the chest, and less commonly in those of retroperitoneal origin, and is seldom seen in cases with an adrenal origin. However, a significant degree of invasion may be present with a lack of obvious clinical symptoms; thus, the evaluation of possible intraspinal components is essential in all cases. Intraspinal invasion may be limited to 1 vertebral level (see **Fig. 4**), or it may grow more extensively and cause multilevel involvement with widening of the neural foramina, even distant from the primary tumor site.

Nuclear medicine studies, preferably ^{123}I-MIBG examination, are essential during the initial phase to establish diagnosis and to search for distant metastasis, particularly bone metastasis (see **Fig. 3**). Alternatively, ^{131}I-MIBG or technetium 99m (TC) methyldiphosphonate scintigraphy may be used

for the same purpose. Nuclear medicine studies are also used to follow response to therapy.

Imaging diagnosis is more accurate when anatomic images, provided by CT, and metabolic images, provided by PET, are fused, compared with PET alone, or in a side-by-side comparison of PET and CT images.[19,20] In recent years, several papers have shown the high impact of PET and PET-CT in the oncologic management of the pediatric patient population as well.[2,3,5] Furthermore, in addition to the use of CT, MIBG scintigraphy and fludeoxyglucose (FDG) PET-CT have been found to play an important role in the follow-up after surgery and/or chemotherapy. In cases of relapsed neuroblastomas, FDG-PET-CT was found to be more sensitive than MIBG, because the initial MIBG-positive tumor may became MIBG-negative when it recurs.[21,22]

Follow-up imaging is required to assess for residual tumor after surgery, response to chemotherapy, to decide possible operability, to assess tumor recurrence, and to search for distant metastasis. Follow-up is performed with CT, MR imaging, MIBG, or PET-CT. Lesions that respond to chemotherapy typically decrease in size significantly and become more calcified (see **Fig. 5**). However, the differentiation between residual scar and viable tumor may be difficult with all imaging modalities, and may require biopsy.

Perinatal neuroblastoma deserves special mention because of its challenging diagnosis. The antenatal diagnosis of neuroblastoma has increased with the routine use of prenatal US, and one-fifth of all neuroblastomas are diagnosed either antenatally or in the first 3 months of life (see **Fig. 2**).[23] Most of these neuroblastomas are localized tumors with favorable biologic features, showing a 4-year survival of greater than 95%, and are associated with a high rate of spontaneous regression. Increase of urinary catecholamines is less common than in older children, being seen only in 50% of cases,[24] and the sensitivity of the otherwise very sensitive ^{123}I-MIBG examination is not known in infancy. The main differential diagnoses for perinatal neuroblastoma include adrenal hemorrhage and extralobar pulmonary sequestration, as well as primary renal tumors, such as mesoblastic nephroma.

In newborns, adrenal hemorrhage occurs almost 4 times more frequently than neuroblastoma.[25] It may occur in large infants or after difficult delivery. It is also more frequent in infants of diabetic mothers, and in those with breech delivery, perinatal asphyxia, or neonatal sepsis. Almost 70% of adrenal hemorrhages present on the right side, 30% on the left side, and up to 10% may occur bilaterally.[26] US differentiation of adrenal hemorrhage from

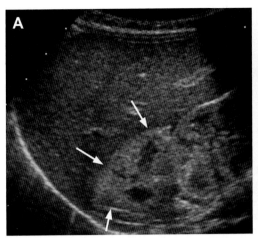 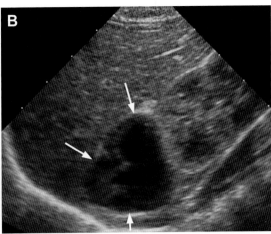

Fig. 9. Incidentally discovered adrenal hemorrhage in a term neonate, who had an abdominal US because of increased serum creatinine level. (*A*) Longitudinal US scan of the right suprarenal region at 1 day of age shows a right suprarenal mass (*arrows*), which is predominantly hyperechoic, although with central hypoechoic areas. No flow was shown on color Doppler evaluation (not shown). At this age and with this appearance, the differential diagnosis includes adrenal hemorrhage and neuroblastoma. (*B*) Follow-up US 8 days after (*A*) shows enlargement of hypoechoic areas within the right suprarenal mass (*arrows*) suggestive of further liquefaction of the hemorrhage. The lesion remained avascular on color Doppler interrogation (not shown). This pattern of rapid change in the echogenicity of the lesion associated with lack of vascularity strongly favors the diagnosis of hemorrhage rather than neuroblastoma.

neuroblastoma is difficult, because both entities are usually echogenic and may appear cystic (see **Fig. 8**; **Fig. 9**).[27,28] Furthermore, adrenal hemorrhage may occur within a congenital neuroblastoma, which makes evaluation even more complicated.[29] Because of the favorable biology of neuroblastoma in neonates, an expectant approach with serial short-term follow-up US is recommended. This follow-up typically shows progressive cystic transformation, gradual decrease in size, and appearance of calcifications in infants with adrenal hemorrhage (see **Fig. 9**). Another helpful tool is color and/or power Doppler US, which shows absent flow in hemorrhages.[30] However, if the mass does not decrease in size or shows interval growth, and/or shows increasing echogenicity, a neuroblastoma should be considered.[30]

Intra-abdominal extralobar pulmonary sequestrations are usually located in the left suprarenal region, and appear as well-defined, hyperechoic masses (**Fig. 10**), and, in some cases, with 1 or more well-defined feeding arteries. Calcification is usually not present; however, small cysts are often seen, which represent components of congenital pulmonary airway malformation.[31] Extralobar sequestrations are usually first identified in the second trimester US, and in follow-up US are either stable in size or show gradual shrinking with advancing gestational age, or in the postnatal period.[32] In contrast, antenatal neuroblastomas are more frequently right sided, and are almost always

first detected in the third trimester of the pregnancy, with normal US in the second trimester. The reason for this is likely that neural tissue in the adrenal gland only appears in the third trimester of pregnancy.[32] In addition, neuroblastomas are

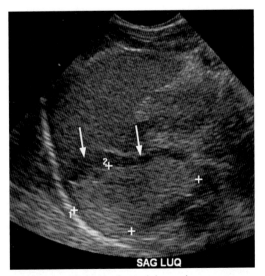

Fig. 10. Intra-abdominal extralobar pulmonary sequestration in a 5-day-old girl with antenatal diagnosis of left suprarenal mass in the second trimester. The sequestration (between electronic cursors) appears as a diffusely hyperechoic mass in the left suprarenal region. The normal hypoechoic left adrenal (*arrows*) can be seen anterior to the sequestration.

more heterogeneous on US, with predominantly cystic and/or complex appearance.[32]

On prenatal US, it is often difficult to localize the exact origin of a mass in the suprarenal region. However, on postnatal US it is usually possible to distinguish between lesions arising from the adrenal gland and extra-adrenal lesions in the suprarenal fossa, which usually displace the otherwise normal adrenal gland.[33]

GANGLIONEUROBLASTOMA

Ganglioneuroblastomas are composed of mature ganglion cells and of immature cells similar to those found in neuroblastomas, resulting in a potentially malignant behavior. One-third of the cases arise in the adrenal gland, one-third in the retroperitoneum, and the remaining one-third mainly in the posterior mediastinum, or, rarely, in the neck or pelvis.

Symptoms and imaging characteristics resemble those of neuroblastoma more than the benign ganglioneuroma. Abdominal pain and distension are frequent symptoms caused by the primary lesion or its metastasis.[34] On CT, they may be mainly solid or predominantly cystic, and heterogeneous (**Fig. 11**). Heterogeneous appearance is typical on precontrast and postcontrast MR imaging. As with neuroblastomas, ganglioneuroblastomas may also have irregular margins and may cause invasion into neighboring organs and vessels.

GANGLIONEUROMA

Ganglioneuroma is the most mature form of the tumors of neural crest origin and are histologically benign. These tumors consist of mature ganglion cells and encapsulated nerve fibers. They occur less frequently than neuroblastomas and can arise de novo, or may transform from previous malignant neuroblastomas. The most common site of occurrence for ganglioneuroma is the posterior mediastinum. One-third of the cases arise in the retroperitoneum and, rarely, in the adrenal gland. An association with neurofibromatosis type I has been reported.

Ganglioneuromas occur in older children, often without clinical symptoms; therefore, they are often incidental findings on US or chest radiographs. When they invade the spine, neurologic symptoms may appear caused by cord compression. Occasionally, myoclonic encephalopathy, diarrhea, or hypertonia can be seen at presentation. As opposed to neuroblastoma, urinary catecholamine levels are usually not increased.

On CT, ganglioneuromas present as well-defined, ovoid or crescent shaped masses, with homogeneous low attenuation on images obtained before intravenous contrast material administration, and mild to moderate enhancement on images obtained after contrast material injection. Calcification is seen in approximately half of the cases.[35] On MR imaging, ganglioneuromas show low signal intensity on T1-weighted images, and often heterogeneous high signal intensity on T2-weighted images, because of the combination of myxoid stroma and mature ganglion cells.[35] The content of the tumor may also have a whirl-like appearance, as a result of the collagen fibers and Schwann cells mixed in the stroma.[34] Occasionally, a fibrous pseudocapsule can be identified, which shows low signal intensity on both T1-weighted and T2-weighted sequences.

Ganglioneuromas cannot be distinguished from neuroblastoma with imaging alone. The definite diagnosis must be established based on histology. Total resection of large tumors may be difficult, especially when they are in close anatomic relation to adjacent organs, or invade into the neural foramina. Patients with such tumor presentation are monitored by imaging alone, particularly when these patients are clinically asymptomatic. A change in the appearance, or an increase in size, is a signal for malignant transformation and should prompt biopsy. Currently, no standard imaging protocol exists that describes how often and how long patients with ganglioneuromas that are managed nonoperatively should be followed up with imaging.

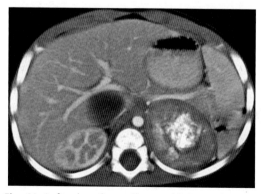

Fig. 11. Left adrenal ganglioneuroblastoma in a 16-month-old boy. Axial contrast-enhanced CT image shows coarse heterogeneous calcification within a large mass arising from the left adrenal gland. The imaging findings alone do not allow differentiation from neuroblastoma.

PHEOCHROMOCYTOMA

According to the World Health Organization classification of endocrine tumors, pheochromocytoma is defined as an intra-adrenal paraganglioma, whereas the term extra-axial paraganglioma is applied for paragangliomas with an extra-adrenal location.[36]

Pheochromocytoma is an uncommon pediatric neoplasm, with an incidence of only 5% in childhood and, thus, it accounts for less than 1% of all tumors seen in large pediatric centers. It is a potentially curable, hormonally functioning tumor that arises from the chromaffin cells in the adrenal gland. In the pediatric age group, 80% of pheochromocytomas occur in the adrenal gland,[37] and, in 25% of these, both adrenal glands are involved (**Fig. 12**).[38] In the remaining 20%, the most frequent site is the upper abdomen.[18] Less common extra-adrenal sites include the sympathetic chain in a cervical (formerly referred to as glomus tumor), thoracic, or pelvic location, and, in rare cases, they may occur in the urinary bladder, spinal cord, and vagina. Multiple tumors are present in 30% to 70% of the patients, especially in those with a positive family history for pheochromocytoma. Malignant pheochromocytoma is less frequent than in adults, and is proved by the presence of metastasis rather than by histology.

Pheochromocytoma usually presents in older children, with a mean age of 11 years,[38] but has been reported in infancy as well. Often, it is familial and is inherited as an autosomal dominant trait. Familial pheochromocytoma may be part of the multiple endocrine neoplasia (MEN) type II, in association with medullary thyroid carcinoma and hyperplasia of the parathyroid gland. Pheochromocytoma may also occur in association with neurofibromatosis type I, von Hippel-Lindau disease, and hemihyperplasia.

The clinical presentation is typically determined by tumor function, which is usually caused by the production of epinephrine and norepinephrine, but may also be caused by the overproduction of VIP. Symptoms include hypertension, tachycardia, hypertensive encephalopathy, sweating, headaches, visual blurring, papilla edema, flushing, diarrhea, weight loss, or chronic diarrhea. In the rare cases with metastatic disease, symptoms may be caused by the metastasis.

The usual size of the tumor at the time of the presentation ranges between 2 and 5 cm; however,

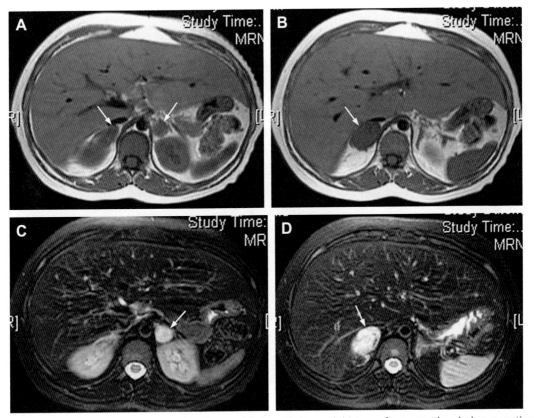

Fig. 12. Bilateral pheochromocytomas in a 9-year-old girl with 6-month history of recurrent headaches, sweating episodes, and increased urine homovanillic acid. (*A–D*) Axial MR images of the upper abdomen show bilateral homogeneous adrenal masses (*arrows*), larger on the right, which are hypointense on T1-weighted (*A, B*) and hyperintense on fat-suppressed T2-weighted images (*C, D*).

they may exceed 10 cm. They appear as well-defined, rounded tumors with high vascularization, and may contain hemorrhage and necrosis. Surgical resection is the treatment of choice and is curative when the disease is benign; therefore, accurate localization is mandatory before operation.

The first-line imaging modality is US, on which pheochromocytoma may present as a homogeneous soft tissue mass (**Fig. 13**), but it may also contain heterogeneous areas, caused by hemorrhage, necrosis, or calcifications. MIBG scanning must be performed, because it is more sensitive than US, and can be positive, even when US shows no abnormalities. Furthermore, MIBG is essential in evaluating the whole body to determine multifocal disease before surgery.[17] CT and MR imaging are useful for precise surgical planning.

On CT, pheochromocytomas have soft tissue attenuation and typically intense contrast enhancement, the pattern of which may be diffuse, mottled, or rimlike. Adrenergic blockade is not required to prevent hypertensive crisis when using nonionic intravenous contrast agent.[17] Chest CT is useful to detect paragangliomas in the posterior mediastinum, and in those patients with suspected metastasis in the lung parenchyma.

On MR imaging, pheochromocytomas have low signal intensity on T1-weighted images, markedly high signal intensity on T2-weighted images, and avid enhancement of contrast material, with prolonged washout phase.[17] After successful surgical removal, clinical and laboratory (urinary catecholamine levels) follow-up is needed to detect recurrence or de novo lesions.

ADRENOCORTICAL MASSES

Primary tumors of the adrenal cortex are rare in children, with a worldwide incidence of 0.3/1 million/y before the age of 15 years.[39] They are significantly less common than neuroblastoma, but more common than pheochromocytoma, and are the most common tumors in the pediatric adrenal cortex.[40] Because reliable histologic differentiation of cortical adenomas and cortical carcinomas in children is not possible, the term adrenocortical neoplasm is used to designate benign and malignant neoplasms of the adrenal cortex in the pediatric age group.[41] Most tumors occur before the age of 5 years, with a female predominance, although the sex ratio is equal in adolescents.

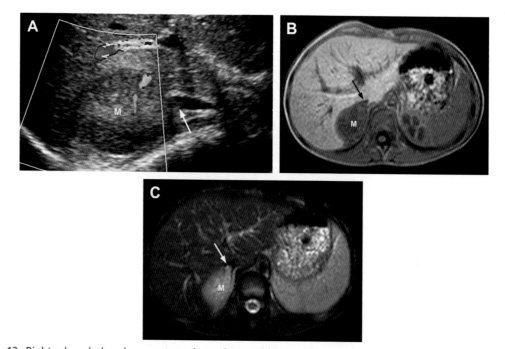

Fig. 13. Right adrenal pheochromocytoma in an 8-year-old boy who presented with arterial hypertension. (*A*) Transverse color Doppler US image of the right suprarenal region shows a rounded, solid right adrenal mass (M) with some internal vascularity. The mass invades the inferior vena cava (*arrow*). (*B, C*) Axial MR images of the upper abdomen show that the right adrenal mass (M) is of fairly homogeneous signal intensity, hypointense on T1-weighted (*B*) and hyperintense on fat-suppressed T2-weighted images (*C*). The mass extends into the inferior vena cava medially (*arrow*).

As opposed to adults, where adrenocortical neoplasms are usually nonfunctioning, most pediatric cases are hormonally active and manifest with endocrine abnormalities. The overproduction of androgens leads to the clinical symptoms of virilization in girls and precocious puberty in boys. Overproduction of glucocorticoids is less common in young children than in adolescents or adults, but more pediatric adrenocortical tumors cause overproduction of mineralocorticoids, compared with adults. The detection of increased hormone levels is not only useful for the initial diagnosis but also for the detection of tumor recurrence during follow-up.

Most children with adrenocortical neoplasm have no underlying disorder; however, an association with Beckwith-Wiedemann syndrome, Li-Fraumeni syndrome (mutation of p53 tumor suppressor gene), and developmental abnormalities of the urinary tract have been reported.[41]

At presentation, the tumors are usually small, and may not be apparent at physical examination, but they can also be sizable, and, in such instances, the tumors are more often carcinomas. US is the first-line imaging method, and is particularly useful in the detection of tumor invasion into the inferior vena cava. For more detailed evaluation of focal tumor invasion or tumor spread, MR imaging or, when it is not available, CT should be used, especially when the lesion is very large (**Fig. 14**). The lung is the most common site for distant metastasis; therefore, chest CT should be performed at the time of initial diagnosis. On all modalities, smaller lesions are generally more homogeneous than larger ones, which more often contain areas of hemorrhage, necrosis, or calcification. In such large lesions, a characteristic central scar with linear bands may be visible, caused by the presence of foci of necrosis and calcification.

The histologic distinction between benign and malignant adrenocortical lesions is not clearly defined in childhood; however, there are findings that favor malignancy, when present. These findings include a size greater than 5 to 10 cm, weight more than 200 g, and aggressive growth features, such as local spread and invasion into the periadrenal soft tissues, kidneys, or inferior vena cava,[17] or evidence of distant metastasis, most commonly in the lung, liver, and bone.[18]

Surgical resection of the tumor is essential for survival, combined with chemotherapy and radical lymph node resection in malignant cases. The role of chemotherapy and radiotherapy is limited. Completely removed noninfiltrative, nonmetastatic disease in the younger age group carries a good prognosis. However, even clinical, laboratory, and imaging follow-up is necessary in such cases,

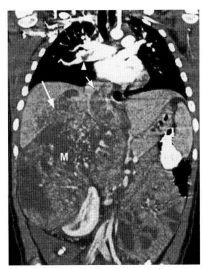

Fig. 14. Adrenocortical carcinoma in a 2-year-old girl with precocious puberty. Contrast-enhanced CT image reformatted in the coronal plane shows a large, heterogeneous right adrenal solid mass (M) with areas of necrosis and calcification. There is evidence of tumor invasion into the right lobe of the liver (*long arrow*), inferior vena cava (*short arrow*), and into the right atrium with embolus in the right main pulmonary artery (*arrowhead*).

because of the lack of clear histologic differentiation between adenoma and carcinoma.

OTHER ADRENAL NEOPLASMS

Malignant rhabdoid tumor (MRT) is a rare pediatric malignancy that accounts for 1.8% of malignant renal tumors, but can also occur in the adrenal gland.[42] This is a highly aggressive neoplasm with poor prognosis and, despite the presence of rhabdoid features, it lacks evidence of rhabdomyoblastic differentiation.[43] Renal and extrarenal MRT show similar clinical and histopathologic features; however, extrarenal MRT has no association with brain tumors as renal MRTs do.[44] The imaging features are similar to those of neuroblastoma, and differentiation between these 2 entities is not possible based on imaging alone (**Fig. 15**).

Smooth muscle tumors have been reported in the adrenal glands of children infected by human immunodeficiency virus (HIV). These lesions are leiomyomas histologically, and arise in the walls of adrenal vessels. They may be unilateral or bilateral, and their presentation may be linked to Epstein-Barr virus infection.

Teratoma occurring in the retroperitoneum is rare in childhood, and is extremely uncommon in the adrenal glands,[45] but it may be detected prenatally.[46] Neonates usually present with a palpable mass

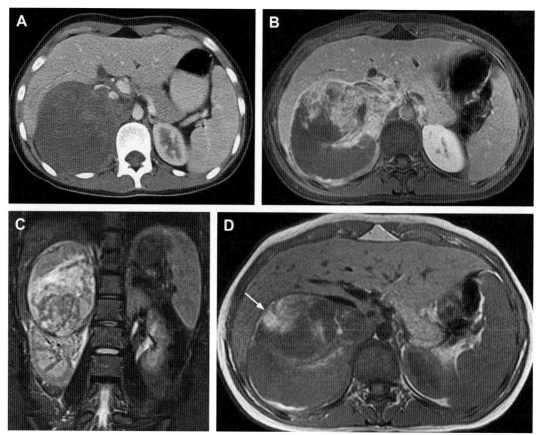

Fig. 15. MRT of the right adrenal gland in a16-year-old girl. (*A*) Contrast-enhanced CT; (*B*) contrast-enhanced, fat-suppressed, T1-weighted; (*C*) coronal, short inversion time, inversion-recovery (STIR); and (*D*) T1-weighted MR images show a large infiltrative right adrenal mass that also involves the diaphragm, the right psoas muscle, and adjacent retroperitoneum. The mass is heterogeneous, partially cystic, with areas of high signal intensity on T1-weighted image (*D*), suggestive of intralesional hemorrhage (*arrow*).

and abdominal distention, whereas vomiting and abdominal pain may be present at a later age. Imaging features include fatty components and/or calcifications in a well-defined mass in cases of mature teratomas (**Fig. 16**). Increased serum α-feto-protein is worrisome for malignant teratomas.[47]

NONNEOPLASTIC ADRENAL MASSES

Adrenal masses of nonneoplastic origin are rare beyond infancy and include hemorrhage, cyst, and infection. Adrenal hemorrhage typically occurs in the neonatal period (see **Fig. 9**) and the features that may help in its differentiation from neuroblastoma have been discussed in the section of neuroblastoma. When hemorrhage occurs in older children, a history of blunt trauma is often given. Other possible predisposing factors include bleeding diathesis, vasculitis, complications from meningococcal infection (Waterhouse-Friderichsen syndrome), and adrenal angiography.

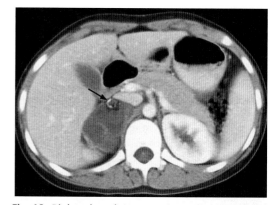

Fig. 16. Right adrenal teratoma in an 11-year-old girl. Axial contrast-enhanced CT image shows a heterogeneous right suprarenal mass with areas of solid and fluid attenuation. In the anterior aspect of the mass, small areas of calcification and fatty attenuation are noted (*arrow*).

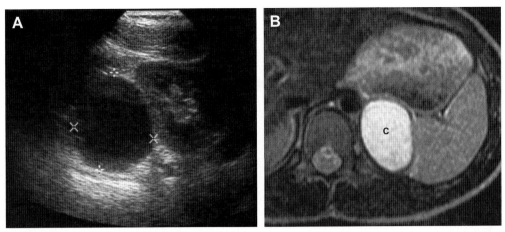

Fig. 17. A 15-year-old girl with left adrenal lymphatic malformation. (A) Transverse US image shows a 5.5-cm left adrenal cyst (between electronic cursors), medial to the upper pole of the left kidney. The cyst contains low-level echoes. (B) Transverse T2-weighted MR image shows a left adrenal cyst (C), which is hyperintense and slightly heterogeneous.

Adrenal cysts are in general rare, with an incidence of less than 2% of autopsies.[48] They are usually asymptomatic, and found incidentally. Most adrenal cysts are lymphatic malformations or hemorrhagic pseudocysts (39%).[48] Simple adrenal cyst, not associated with solid, masslike components, is rare in the pediatric age group, and is more commonly seen in older children.[49] Clinically, there is no evidence of endocrine dysfunction, hypertension, infection, or metastatic disease. Simple cysts are rounded, thin-walled lesions, with imaging features characteristic for fluid-containing structures. They are hypoechoic/anechoic on US, of fluid attenuation on CT, and with signal intensity characteristic of fluid on MR imaging (Fig. 17). They do not show internal enhancement with the administration of intravenous contrast material. Internal septa may be seen in the lymphatic malformations. US in the longitudinal plane and MR imaging in the coronal plane have been found to be most useful to document the extrarenal/extrahepatic location of these cysts.[49] Management depends on age and is usually conservative.

INCIDENTALLY DETECTED ADRENAL MASSES

Lesions of the adrenal gland depicted by any imaging modality performed for other indications are termed incidental adrenal masses. These

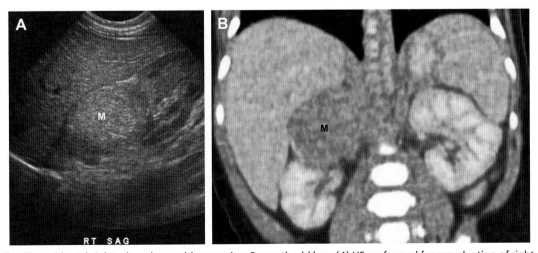

Fig. 18. Incidental right adrenal neuroblastoma in a 3-month-old boy. (A) US performed for reevaluation of right-sided grade IV vesicoureteral reflux shows a homogeneous hyperechoic right adrenal mass (M). (B) Contrast-enhanced CT image shows the homogeneous hypodense right adrenal mass (M).

lesions are rare, but their incidence is increasing.[50] This is because of the growing number of cross-sectional abdominal imaging examinations, and also because of the increasing sensitivity of imaging modalities, which can now easily detect lesions less than 1 cm in size.[51]

The most common incidental adrenal masses in adults are benign adenomas, the most common incidental adrenal masses in children are malignant neuroblastomas, and benign cortical adenomas account for less than 0.5% of all incidental adrenal masses in this age group (**Fig. 18**).[52] However, there are no specific, universally accepted guidelines to direct the management of incidental adrenal masses in children, and therefore the topic is controversial.

Tumor size and imaging appearance reportedly do not provide sufficient information for distinguishing with certainty between benign and malignant lesions.[53] It is also known that early surgical intervention has a high incidence of cure for neonatal and infantile neuroblastomas, and, as such, provides a significantly more favorable prognosis.[54]

Therefore, it has been recommended that all incidental adrenal masses detected before and after birth should be resected, because of the high proportion of malignant tumors.[53] An exception may be small lesions in children less than 3 months of age, for whom close, cautious observation including serial imaging studies may be permitted.[53]

Our experience has shown that many suprarenal masses in young infants may disappear spontaneously. Therefore, we highly recommend repeated imaging (primarily using US) at 3-week intervals, especially if the lesions are small, in young infants, if they remain stable or decrease in size on follow-up, and if the markers for neuroblastoma are absent.

REFERENCES

1. Boland GW, Blake MA, Holalkere NS, et al. PET/CT for the characterization of adrenal masses in patients with cancer: qualitative versus quantitative accuracy in 150 consecutive patients. AJR Am J Roentgenol 2009;192:956–62.
2. Murphy JJ, Tawfeeq M, Chang B, et al. Early experience with PET/CT scan in the evaluation of pediatric abdominal neoplasms. J Pediatr Surg 2008;43(12): 2186–92.
3. Roca I, Simó M, Sábado C, et al. PET/CT in paediatrics: it is time to increase its use! Eur J Nucl Med Mol Imaging 2007;34:628–9.
4. Shore RM. Positron emission tomography/computed tomography (PET/CT) in children. Pediatr Ann 2008; 37:404–12.
5. Kleis M, Daldrup-Link H, Matthay K, et al. Diagnostic value of PET/CT for the staging and restaging of pediatric tumors. Eur J Nucl Med Mol Imaging 2009;36:23–36.
6. Paterson A. Adrenal pathology in childhood: a spectrum of disease. Eur Radiol 2002;12:2491–508.
7. Hiorns MP, Owens CM. Radiology of neuroblastoma in children. Eur Radiol 2001;11:2071–81.
8. Rha SE, Byun JY, Jung SE, et al. Neurogenic tumors in the abdomen: tumor types and imaging characteristics. Radiographics 2003;23:29–43.
9. Ilias I, Pacak K. Diagnosis and management of tumors of the adrenal medulla. Horm Metab Res 2005;37: 717–21.
10. Tuchman M, Ramnaraine ML, Woods WG, et al. Three years of experience with random urinary homovanillic and vanillylmandelic acid levels in the diagnosis of neuroblastoma. Pediatrics 1987;79:203–5.
11. Brodeur GM, Pritchard J, Berthold F, et al. Revisions of the international criteria for neuroblastoma diagnosis, staging, and response to treatment. J Clin Oncol 1993;11:1466–77.
12. Monclair T, Brodeur GM, Ambros PF, et al. The International Neuroblastoma Risk Group (INRG) staging system: an INRG Task Force report. J Clin Oncol 2009;27:298–303.
13. Simon T, Hero B, Benz-Bohm G, et al. Review of image defined risk factors in localized neuroblastoma patients: results of the GPOH NB97 trial. Pediatr Blood Cancer 2008;50:965–9.
14. Evans AE, D'Angio GJ, Propert K, et al. Prognostic factor in neuroblastoma. Cancer 1987;59:1853–9.
15. Rubie H, Hartmann O, Michon J, et al. N-Myc gene amplification is a major prognostic factor in localized neuroblastoma: results of the French NBL 90 study. Neuroblastoma Study Group of the Société Française d'Oncologie Pédiatrique. J Clin Oncol 1997; 15:1171–82.
16. Mueller S, Matthay KK. Neuroblastoma: biology and staging. Curr Oncol Rep 2009;11:431–8.
17. McHugh K. Renal and adrenal tumours in children. Cancer Imaging 2007;7:41–51.
18. Daneman A, Navarro O, Haller JO. The adrenal and retroperitoneum. In: Slovis TL, editor. Caffey's pediatric diagnostic imaging. 11th edition. Philadelphia: Mosby Elsevier; 2008. p. 2214–33.
19. Wegner EA, Barrington SF, Kingston JE, et al. The impact of PET scanning on management of paediatric oncology patients. Eur J Nucl Med Mol Imaging 2005;32:23–30.
20. Jager PL, Slart RH, Corstens F, et al. PET-CT: a matter of opinion? Eur J Nucl Med Mol Imaging 2003;30:470–1.
21. Colavolpe C, Guedj E, Cammilleri S, et al. Utility of FDG-PET/CT in the follow-up of neuroblastoma which became MIBG-negative. Pediatr Blood Cancer 2008; 51:828–31.

22. Mc Dowell H, Losty P, Barnes N, et al. Utility of FDG-PET/CT in the follow-up of neuroblastoma which became MIBG-negative. Pediatr Blood Cancer 2009; 52:552.

23. Nuchtern JG. Perinatal neuroblastoma. Semin Pediatr Surg 2006;15:10–6.

24. Stevens MC. Neonatal tumours. Arch Dis Child 1988;63:1122–5.

25. Goodman SN. Neuroblastoma screening data. An epidemiologic analysis. Am J Dis Child 1991;145: 1415–22.

26. Kellnar S, Deindl C, Trammer A. Differential "adrenal gland tumor-adrenal gland hemorrhage" diagnosis. A sonographic follow-up. Monatsschr Kinderheilkd 1989;137:347–9 [in German].

27. Atkinson GO Jr, Zaatari GS, Lorenzo RL, et al. Cystic neuroblastoma in infants: radiographic and pathologic features. AJR Am J Roentgenol 1986;146:113–7.

28. Forman HP, Leonidas JC, Berdon WE, et al. Congenital neuroblastoma: evaluation with multimodality imaging. Radiology 1990;175:365–8.

29. Eklöf O, Mortensson W, Sandstedt B. Suprarenal haematoma versus neuroblastoma complicated by haemorrhage. A diagnostic dilemma in the newborn. Acta Radiol Diagn (Stockh) 1986;27:3–10.

30. Deeg KH, Bettendorf U, Hofmann V. Differential diagnosis of neonatal adrenal haemorrhage and congenital neuroblastoma by colour coded Doppler sonography and power Doppler sonography. Eur J Pediatr 1998;157:294–7.

31. Rosado-de-Christenson ML, Frazier AA, Stocker JT, et al. From the archives of the AFIP. Extralobar sequestration: radiologic-pathologic correlation. Radiographics 1993;13:425–41.

32. Curtis MR, Mooney DP, Vaccaro TJ, et al. Prenatal ultrasound characterization of the suprarenal mass: distinction between neuroblastoma and subdiaphragmatic extralobar pulmonary sequestration. J Ultrasound Med 1997;16:75–83.

33. Daneman A, Baunin C, Lobo E, et al. Disappearing suprarenal masses in fetuses and infants. Pediatr Radiol 1997;27:675–81.

34. Guo YK, Yang ZG, Li Y, et al. Uncommon adrenal masses: CT and MRI features with histopathologic correlation. Eur J Radiol 2007;62:359–70.

35. Ichikawa T, Ohtomo K, Araki T, et al. Ganglioneuroma: computed tomography and magnetic resonance features. Br J Radiol 1996;69:114–21.

36. Pacak K, Eisenhofer G, Ahlman H, et al. Pheochromocytoma: recommendations for clinical practice from the First International Symposium. October 2005. Nat Clin Pract Endocrinol Metab 2007;3:92–102.

37. Lenders JW, Eisenhofer G, Mannelli M, et al. Phaeochromocytoma. Lancet 2005;366:665–75.

38. Ross JH. Pheochromocytoma. Special considerations in children. Urol Clin North Am 2000;27: 393–402.

39. Bonfig W, Bittmann I, Bechtold S, et al. Virilising adrenocortical tumours in children. Eur J Pediatr 2003;162:623–8.

40. Daneman A, Chan HS, Martin J. Adrenal carcinoma and adenoma in children: a review of 17 patients. Pediatr Radiol 1983;13:11–8.

41. Agrons GA, Lonergan GJ, Dickey GE, et al. Adrenocortical neoplasms in children: radiologic-pathologic correlation. Radiographics 1999;19:989–1008.

42. Yaris N, Cobanoglu U, Dilber E, et al. Malignant rhabdoid tumor of adrenal gland. Med Pediatr Oncol 2002;39:128–31.

43. Haas JE, Palmer NF, Weinberg AG, et al. Ultrastructure of malignant rhabdoid tumor of the kidney. A distinctive renal tumor of children. Hum Pathol 1981;12:646–57.

44. Sotelo-Avila C, Gonzalez-Crussi F, deMello D, et al. Renal and extrarenal rhabdoid tumors in children: a clinicopathologic study of 14 patients. Semin Diagn Pathol 1986;3:151–63.

45. Luo CC, Huang CS, Chu SM, et al. Retroperitoneal teratomas in infancy and childhood. Pediatr Surg Int 2005;21:536–40.

46. Oguzkurt P, Ince E, Temiz A, et al. Prenatal diagnosis of a mass in the adrenal region that proved to be a teratoma. J Pediatr Hematol Oncol 2009; 31:350–1.

47. Kurman RJ, Scardino PT, McIntire KR, et al. Cellular localization of alpha-fetoprotein and human chorionic gonadotropin in germ cell tumors of the testis using and indirect immunoperoxidase technique. Cancer 1977;40:2136–51.

48. Rozenblit A, Morehouse HT, Amis ES Jr. Cystic adrenal lesions: CT features. Radiology 1996;201: 541–8.

49. Broadley P, Daneman A, Wesson D, et al. Large adrenal cysts in teenage girls: diagnosis and management. Pediatr Radiol 1997;27:550–2.

50. Copeland PM. The incidentally discovered adrenal mass. Ann Surg 1984;199:116–22.

51. Mayo-Smith WW. CT characterization of adrenal masses. Radiology 2003;226:289–90.

52. Xue H, Horwitz JR, Smith MB, et al. Malignant solid tumors in neonates: a 40-year review. J Pediatr Surg 1995;30:543–5.

53. Masiakos PT, Gerstle JT, Cheang T, et al. Is surgery necessary for incidentally discovered adrenal masses in children? J Pediatr Surg 2004;39:754–8.

54. Tsuchida Y, Ikeda H, Iehara T, et al. Neonatal neuroblastoma: incidence and clinical outcome. Med Pediatr Oncol 2003;40:391–3.

Imaging of Pediatric Pelvic Neoplasms

Ricki U. Shah, MD[a], Charles Lawrence, MD[b],*,
Kristin A. Fickenscher, MD[b], Lei Shao, MD[c],
Lisa H. Lowe, MD[b]

KEYWORDS
- Testicle • Ovary • Germinoma • Sacrococcygeal
- Teratoma • Bladder • Neoplasm

PRIMARY TESTICULAR NEOPLASMS

Testicular neoplasms represent approximately 1.0% to 1.5% of all childhood malignancies, with a peak incidence at 2 years of age.[1] Primary testicular tumors are classified by their tissue of origin and are divided into germ cell tumors, sex cord-stromal tumors, and mixed tumors. Germ cell tumors may differentiate into gonadal cell lines, in which case they are called seminomatous germ cell tumors. When they transform into undifferentiated totipotential cells they are termed nonseminomatous germ cell tumors.

A definitive diagnosis is not typically possible with radiological studies; however, imaging may be able to limit the differential diagnosis, especially when considered in the context of clinical history. Ultrasonography (US) is the initial modality of choice to image scrotal masses. Computed tomography (CT) is helpful for staging, but has the disadvantage of requiring ionizing radiation. Magnetic resonance (MR) imaging may be used for staging and as a problem-solving technique in some cases. The sensitivity of both sonography and MR imaging in differentiating between intratesticular and extratesticular lesion location is nearly 100%.[2] Testicular masses tend to have a nonspecific appearance of a solid mass on all cross-sectional imaging modalities. Useful generalizations are described as follows.

Intratesticular masses are more likely to be malignant than extratesticular masses. Aggressive tumors may invade the tunica albuginea, causing a more irregular appearance. Sonography may help distinguish simple versus reactive hydrocele, the latter being associated with testicular neoplasms in 15% to 25% of cases.[3–5] Reactive hydroceles (which may occur secondary to epididymitis, orchitis, testicular torsion, torsion of the appendix testis, trauma, or tumor) and invasion of the tunica albuginea suggest extratesticular involvement and are indications for further workup. Color Doppler sonography can determine the vascularity of a mass and may help to distinguish it from testicular torsion. Hypervascularity is present in 85% of neoplasms, although smaller tumors (<1.5 cm) are often avascular or hypovascular.[1,4] Unfortunately, hypervascularity on color Doppler US is a nonspecific finding seen in both malignancy and inflammation. Avascularity, an unusual finding in neoplasms, suggests a diagnosis of testicular torsion.

The metastatic workup of primary testicular masses includes CT of the chest, abdomen, and pelvis to screen for lung and lymph node involvement. It is also advisable to perform chest CT prior to surgery as postsurgical atelectasis may imitate metastatic lesions. Ultrasound should be used to screen the contralateral testicle for synchronous or metastatic lesions before and after orchiectomy.

Financial Disclosure: None.
[a] Department of Internal Medicine, University of Missouri Kansas City, Truman Medical Center, 2301 Holmes Street, Kansas City, MO 64108, USA
[b] Department of Radiology, Children's Mercy Hospital & Clinics, University of Missouri Kansas City, 2401 Gillham Road, Kansas City, MO 64108, USA
[c] Department of Pathology, Children's Mercy Hospital and Clinics, University of Missouri Kansas City, 2401 Gillham Road, Kansas City, MO 64108, USA
* Corresponding author.
E-mail address: calawrence@cmh.edu

Radiol Clin N Am 49 (2011) 729–748
doi:10.1016/j.rcl.2011.05.007

One condition, testicular microlithiasis (TM), has a controversial association with testicular neoplasms. Although the cause of TM is unknown, some believe that degeneration of cells in the seminiferous tubules may cause formation of microliths. TM has been described in patients with undescended or delayed testicular descent. Some argue that because TM and certain testicular neoplasms are associated with undescended testicles, periodic screening with US may be warranted. Specific disorders that have been associated with TM include Klinefelter syndrome, male pseudohermaphroditism, Down syndrome, and pulmonary alveolar microlithiasis (**Fig. 1**).[6,7]

Germ Cell Tumors

Germ cell tumors represent 70% to 90% of childhood testicular neoplasms.[1] These tumors are classified on a pathologic basis into seminomatous, which are rare in the pediatric population, and nonseminomatous subtypes. Nonseminomatous germ cell tumors are further subdivided into yolk sac tumors, teratoma/teratocarcinoma, embryonal, and choriocarcinoma varieties.

Seminomatous germ cell tumors

Seminomas are most common in adult patients (age in their 40s), presenting as a painless testicular mass. These tumors are rare in the pediatric population. Seminomas are very sensitive to chemotherapy and radiation, and therefore cure rates are high.[8] Seminomas tend to be uniformly hypoechoic, rarely undergoing necrosis or hemorrhage, and on MR imaging are homogeneously hypointense on T1-weighted and hyperintense on T2-weighted imaging (**Fig. 2**).[9]

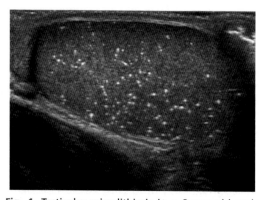

Fig. 1. Testicular microlithiasis in a 3-year-old male with scrotal pain. Longitudinal sonogram demonstrates innumerable foci of increased echogenicity with slight posterior shadowing scattered throughout the testicle. The contralateral testicle (not shown) had a similar appearance.

Nonseminomatous germ cell tumors

Yolk sac tumors Yolk sac tumors (endodermal sinus tumors) represent 80% to 90% of germ cell tumors in childhood, and up to 75% are diagnosed by the age of 2 years (**Table 1**).[10] Clinically, patients present with asymptomatic testicular enlargement and an elevated serum α-fetoprotein (AFP) level in 90% of cases.[9,11]

When used correctly, AFP levels can monitor the effectiveness of treatment, tumor recurrence, or presence of metastasis. However, infants younger than 6 months normally have elevated AFP. If the AFP does not normalize in a baby younger than 6 months after resection of the neoplasm, it is not necessarily an indication of persistent disease.

The majority of yolk sac tumors are confined to the scrotum at presentation, with the remainder having lymphatic metastases to regional/retroperitoneal lymph nodes or hematogenous spread to the lungs. Yolk sac tumors tend to be well circumscribed and heterogeneous in echogenicity on US, depending on the amount of internal hemorrhage, necrosis, and calcification. The appearance on color Doppler US has been described as chaotic and hypervascular (**Fig. 3**).[11] Patients older than 2 years often have a worse prognosis, and stage 1 yolk sac tumors have an 80% survival rate.[6]

Teratomas Testicular teratomas typically occur in boys younger than 4 years and are usually benign.[1] Up to a third of teratomas may metastasize to retroperitoneal lymph nodes within 5 years of diagnosis in postpubertal patients.[10] Postpubertal teratomas have a tendency to develop other components of germ cell tumors (such as choriocarcinoma, seminoma, and embryonal carcinoma), increasing the likelihood of malignancy. Therefore, orchiectomy is the treatment of choice in postpubertal teratomas. Testicular teratoma in a prepubertal patient is more likely to have a benign course, which may allow for tissue-sparing surgery. Metastatic disease from prepubertal teratomas (immature and mature) has not been reported.[12]

Testicular teratomas contain components of all 3 germ cell layers, including bony elements and adipose tissue. Their heterogeneity is reflected on US where they appear as complex masses with cystic and solid components. Bony elements (calcifications) are typically echogenic with posterior shadowing, and adipose tissue is echogenic without shadowing. In some cases superficial calcification will cause so much shadowing that the underlying lesion is hard to visualize. This US finding has been called "the tip of the iceberg" sign. Corresponding findings of mixed osseous, soft tissue, and fat attenuation are observed on CT and MR imaging.

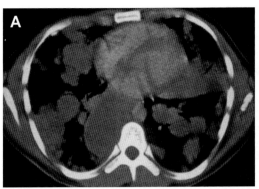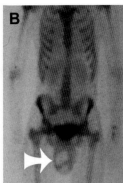

Fig. 2. Seminoma in an 18-year-old man with shortness of breath. (*A*) Axial chest CT reveals innumerable low-attenuation solid masses throughout both lungs. No scrotal examination was performed on physical examination, and bone scan was performed because of suspected metastatic disease. (*B*) Bone scan identifies enlarged scrotum with focal photopenic region (*arrow*). No further imaging was performed and right testicular mass confirmed at surgery.

Embryonal carcinoma and choriocarcinoma

Embryonal carcinomas and choriocarcinomas, although common in adults, are rarely seen in young children and therefore are not extensively discussed here. Embryonal carcinomas rarely occur in prepubertal males, usually presenting in the late teens and early adulthood (**Fig. 4**). These tumors are also more frequently seen in the mixed form, occurring in the pure form only in 2% to 3% of cases. Embryonal carcinomas have a nonspecific imaging appearance, often being heterogeneous and poorly marginated.[13] Patients with embryonal carcinoma may have elevated serum AFP and β-subunit of human chorionic gonadotropin (β-HCG) levels.[13]

Choriocarcinomas also tend to present later in life, usually between 20 and 40 years of age. Patients may present with gynecomastia (10%). Choriocarcinomas are heterogeneous in appearance with cystic and solid components, and may be hemorrhagic. Metastatic lesions may have indistinct borders due to hemorrhage (**Fig. 5**).[13]

Sex Cord-Stromal Tumors (Leydig, Sertoli, and Granulosa Thecal Cell)

Sex cord-stromal tumors, which include Leydig, Sertoli, and granulosa thecal cell subtypes, represent 10% to 30% of testicular tumors.[9,14] Leydig cell tumors arise from the stroma, and Sertoli cell tumors arise from the sex cords.[9] Leydig and Sertoli cell tumors are rare, accounting for 60% and 40% of sex cord tumors, respectively.[9] Ninety percent of Leydig and Sertoli cell tumors are benign.[9,14]

Sertoli cell tumors typically present with a painless testicular mass in the first year of life, and rarely gynecomastia due to estrogen production. Sertoli cell tumors are usually well circumscribed and hypoechoic. A rare subtype of Sertoli cell tumors, large-cell calcifying Sertoli cell tumor (LCCSCT), may be associated with the Carney complex (cardiac myxomas, skin pigmentation, and endocrine hyperactivity) and Peutz-Jeghers syndrome (gastrointestinal polyposis, mucocutaneous pigmentation). LCCSCT are well circumscribed and diffusely hyperechoic on US, with heavy acoustic shadowing due to calcification and moderate hypervascularity.[15]

Leydig cell tumors often secrete androgens, such as testosterone, which cause luteinizing hormone stimulation and precocious puberty. Occasionally they secrete estrogen, progesterone, and corticosteroids, which lead to gynecomastia or Cushing syndrome. Leydig cell tumors are most common in children aged 3 to 6 years and are more frequent in African American males.[3] On US, they are nonspecific and similar in appearance to Sertoli cell tumors, being well circumscribed and hypoechoic (**Fig. 6**).

Granulosa cell tumors of the testis are very rare in the pediatric population, but typically occur before 1 year of age (juvenile type). The adult type is rare and usually occurs in middle age. Biopsy shows follicular structures with surrounding granulosa cells. These tumors are typically hypoechoic, and the juvenile type has cystic and solid components visible on US (**Fig. 7**).[16]

Gonadoblastoma (Germ Cell Plus Stromal Cell Tumors)

Gonadoblastomas have both germ cell and stromal cell elements, and generally follow a benign course; however, approximately 10% can have components of any of the germ cell tumors such as yolk sac tumors.[10] Gonadoblastomas have a strong association with phenotypic females who have a male karyotype and dysgenetic gonads. These tumors are often bilateral and contain punctate

Table 1
Key clinical and imaging features of scrotal neoplasms

Neoplasm	Age	Key Clinical Features	Key Imaging Features
Intratesticular Neoplasms			
Germ Cell Tumors			
Seminomatous (seminoma)	30 y	Rare in pediatric population	Uniformly hypoechoic, hypointense on T1, hyperintense on T2
Nonseminomatous			
Yolk sac tumor (endodermal sinus tumor)	2 y	Most common pediatric testicular neoplasm, AFP elevation	Well circumscribed, heterogeneous echogenicity. Hypervascular
Teratoma	<4 y	Postpubertal more likely to be malignant	Heterogeneous due to cystic/solid components, calcifications, adipose tissue
Embryonal	Late teens, adulthood	Elevated AFP and β-HCG	Heterogeneous and poorly marginated
Choriocarcinoma	Late teens, adulthood	Elevated β-HCG, gynecomastia	Heterogeneous, cystic/solid components
Sex cord-stromal			
Sertoli cell tumor	<1 y	± Gynecomastia, Carney complex, Peutz-Jeghers syndrome	Nonspecific hypoechoic solid mass LCCSCT: heavy acoustic shadowing due to calcification
Leydig cell tumor	3–6 y	Secrete androgens or estrogens, precocious puberty, African American males	Well circumscribed, hypoechoic
Granulosa cell tumor	Juvenile: <1 y Adult: middle aged	Mixed cystic and solid mass	Hypoechoic, solid and cystic components
Mixed germ cell/sex cord			
Gonadoblastoma	5–10 y	Phenotypic females with male karyotype	Solid and hypoechoic
Secondary Testicular Neoplasms			
Leukemia/lymphoma	—	Bilateral testicular enlargement; treated leukemia/lymphoma	Decreased T2 signal intensity
Extratesticular Neoplasms			
Adenomatoid tumor	20–50 y	Nonspecific painless mass	Hyperechoic, homogeneous
Papillary cystadenoma	—	Von Hippel-Lindau, bilateral ~40%	Echogenic
Extratesticular lipoma	—	Fatty lesion	Hyperechoic, homogeneous, T1 hyperintense
Paratesticular rhabdomyosarcoma	2 peaks—ages 5 and 16 y	Solid extratesticular mass with variable heterogeneity	Hemorrhage and necrosis with increased flow on Doppler

Abbreviations: AFP, α-fetoprotein; HCG, human chorionic gonadotropin; LCCSCT, large-cell calcifying Sertoli cell tumor.

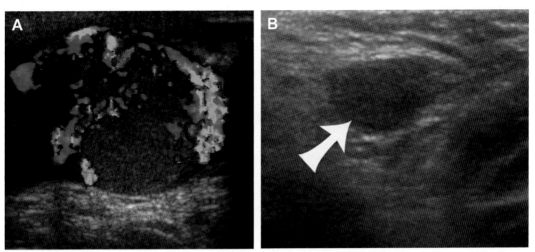

Fig. 3. Yolk sac tumor in a 5-month-old male with suspected orchitis that did not resolve. (*A*) Transverse Doppler sonogram shows a hypervascular, markedly enlarged hyperechoic right testis. (*B*) Compare with the normal left testis (*arrow*). Lung metastases were present on chest CT (not shown).

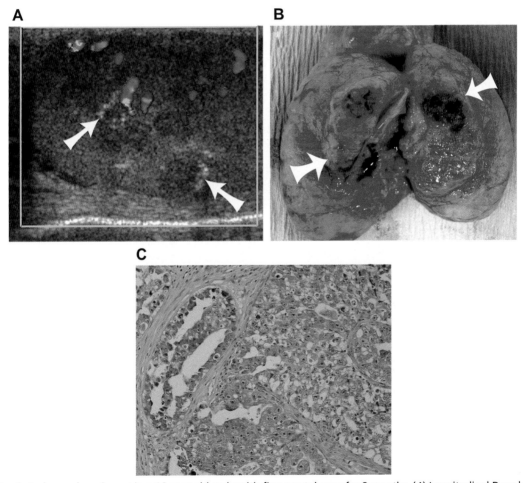

Fig. 4. Embryonal carcinoma in a 16-year-old male with firm scrotal mass for 2 months. (*A*) Longitudinal Doppler sonogram of the left testicle demonstrates a moderately vascular, poorly defined infiltrative mass with scattered calcifications (*arrows*). (*B*) Gross specimen confirms infiltrative mass (*arrows*) within the enlarged left testicle. (*C*) Histologic image shows pleomorphic epithelial cells arranged in solid sheets, trabeculae, or glands. The tumor cells contain slightly basophilic cytoplasm, and large hyperchromatic nuclei with prominent nucleoli (hematoxylin-eosin (H&E), original magnification ×200).

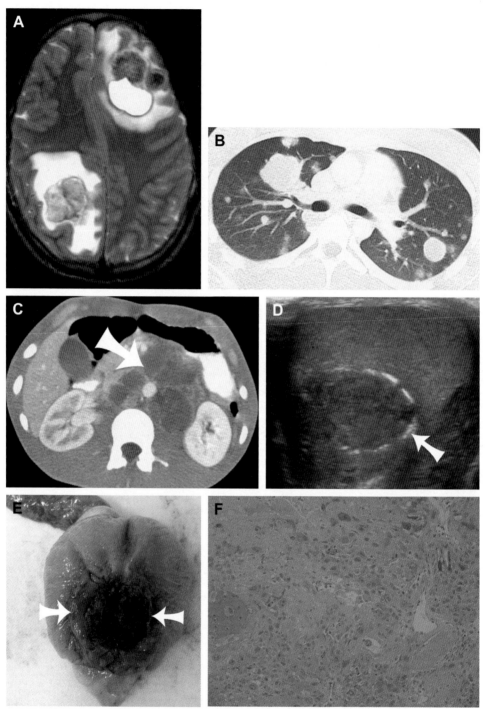

Fig. 5. Mixed germ cell tumor with choriocarcinoma elements in a 16-year-old male with seizures. (*A*) Axial T2 MR image of the brain demonstrates bilateral hypointense parenchymal masses surrounded by hyperintense edema. Metastatic disease was suspected and additional workup performed. (*B*) Axial CT image of the chest shows multiple, bilateral metastatic parenchymal nodules of varied size. Note that many of the lung nodules have hazy peripheral margins, a finding suggestive of hemorrhage, common in choriocarcinoma. (*C*) Axial contrast-enhanced CT of the abdomen identifies extensive low-attenuation retroperitoneal lymph nodes (*arrow*). (*D*) Transverse testicular sono-gram reveals a solid intratesticular mass with peripheral calcification (*arrow*). (*E*) Gross specimen demonstrates a left hemorrhagic intratesticular mass (*arrows*). (*F*) Histologic specimen shows a lesion composed of mixed trophoblasts with pronounced cytologic atypia, extensive necrosis, and hemorrhage. Trophoblasts were β-HCG positive (H&E, original magnification ×200).

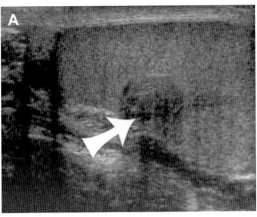
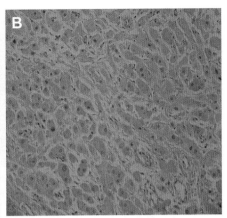

Fig. 6. Leydig cell tumor in a 15-year-old white male with testicular pain. (A) Longitudinal testicular sonogram demonstrates a well-defined hypoechoic mass (arrow). (B) Histologic specimen shows diffuse sheets of large polygonal neoplastic cells with abundant eosinophilic, slightly granular cytoplasm, and round nuclei (H&E, original magnification ×200).

dystrophic calcifications on imaging, and are often solid and hypoechoic.[4] The testis may appear hyperechoic in the center on US.[17]

Tumors of Supporting Tissues/Fascia

Leiomyoma, fibroma, hemangioma, and venolymphatic malformations (non-neoplastic tumor like condition) are rare, benign tumors originating from testicular supporting tissues. On imaging they are typically nonspecific solid masses, except for venolymphatic malformations, which are often multicystic with solid components, and may contain phleboliths (Fig. 8). Fibrosarcoma and leiomyosarcoma are rare malignant testicular lesions that arise from supporting structures, generally requiring biopsy for tissue-definitive diagnosis.[9]

Secondary Intratesticular Neoplasms

Secondary testicular neoplasms represent less than 10% of all testicular tumors.[9] Leukemia and lymphoma are the most common secondary intratesticular neoplasms, acute lymphoblastic leukemia being most common subtype. Because the blood-testes barrier may prevent toxic levels of chemotherapeutic drugs from being delivered to the testes during cancer treatment, neoplastic cells within the gonads remain unharmed, allowing the gonads to be a "sanctuary site" for malignant cells. These sanctuary sites serve as a source for future reactivation of lymphoma and leukemia. Patients with leukemia present with painless, usually bilateral, testicular enlargement. Sonography shows bilateral, or less often unilateral, homogeneous, hypoechoic testicular enlargement with disorganized hypervascular flow (Fig. 9). Leukemia, and especially lymphoma, have a distinctive decrease in T2 signal intensity on MR imaging that differs from most lesions, which are T2 hyperintense.[4,18]

Extratesticular Neoplasms

Extratesticular neoplasms arise from the epididymis, spermatic cord, and/or supporting tissue. These

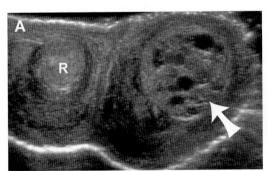
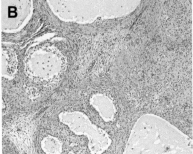

Fig. 7. Granulosa cell tumor in a 1-week-old male with an undescended testis. (A) Transverse sonogram exhibits a mixed echogenicity mass in the left testicle (arrow) compared with normal echogenicity of right (R) testicle. (B) Histologic image shows tumor composed of a nodular growth of granulosa cells, which focally form follicles of varying sizes and shapes (H&E, original magnification ×40).

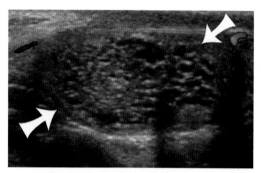

Fig. 8. Venolymphatic malformation in a 7-year-old male with right scrotal pain. Longitudinal Doppler sonogram shows the testicle has been replaced by a mixture of innumerable cystic foci separated by echogenic septations (*arrows*). Minimal peripheral flow is noted.

tumors are rare and generally benign. Only 3% of solid extratesticular neoplasms are malignant.[14] US is the modality of choice to localize scrotal masses as intratesticular or extratesticular. Benign epididymal neoplasms consist of adenomatoid tumors, lipoma, rhabdomyosarcoma, and papillary cystadenomas.

The adenomatoid tumor, which arises from the epididymis, is the most common extratesticular neoplasm. It is rare in children, usually presenting between 20 and 50 years of age with a painless scrotal mass.[19] Although the adenomatoid tumor has a wide variation of appearances on US, it is most often hyperechoic and homogeneous.

Papillary cystadenomas are associated with von Hippel-Lindau disease (60%), are bilateral in up to 40% of patients, and are echogenic on US.[14,19]

Extratesticular lipomas arise most frequently from the spermatic cord. Lipomas are hyperechoic and homogeneous on US. Findings on CT and MR imaging include a low attenuation and T1 bright signal fatty mass, respectively.[19]

Paratesticular rhabdomyosarcoma has two age peaks, 5 and 16 years.[14,19] Most patients present with a painless mass and 40% have metastasis most commonly to the lungs, cortical bone, or retroperitoneal lymph nodes.[4,19] Embryonal, alveolar, and pleomorphic are the most common histologic subtypes of rhabdomyosarcoma. Alveolar rhabdomyosarcoma occurs more frequently in the extremities and in older children, whereas the embryonal subtype occurs more frequently in the head, neck, and genitourinary tract. Hemorrhage and necrosis are common, giving it a wide spectrum of imaging appearances. Color Doppler US shows increased flow with a decreased resistance in the solid portions of the mass (**Fig. 10**). Tissue diagnosis requires biopsy, and CT is performed for staging.

Leiomyosarcoma and liposarcoma are very rare malignant neoplasms that may arise in the paratesticular tissue, and because of their infrequency are not further discussed here.

OVARIAN NEOPLASMS

About two-thirds of ovarian tumors in children are benign,[1,20] and one-third of ovarian neoplasms are malignant. The 3 main subtypes of primary ovarian neoplasms include germ cell tumors (60%–90%), sex cord-stromal tumors (10%–13%), and epithelial tumors (5%–11%) (**Table 2**).[1,21] Teratomas and cystadenomas are the most common benign ovarian neoplasms in children, with teratomas occurring more commonly than cystadenomas.

In general, ovarian neoplasms often have nonspecific imaging features, making them

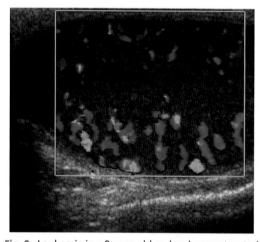

Fig. 9. Leukemia in a 9-year-old male who was treated for acute myelogenous leukemia 18 months prior. Doppler sonogram shows a homogeneously enlarged (8.6 mL volume), hypoechoic, hyperemic testicle. Normal-sized right testicle (volume 3.2 mL) is not shown.

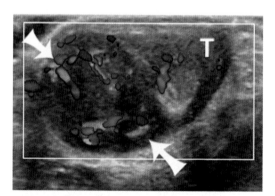

Fig. 10. Rhabdomyosarcoma of the epididymis in a 2-year-old male with scrotal swelling. Longitudinal sonogram reveals a well-defined, mixed-echogenicity, extratesticular mass (*arrows*) replacing the epididymis and displacing the testicle (T).

Table 2
Key clinical and imaging features of ovarian neoplasms

Tumor Type	Age	Key Clinical Features	Key Imaging Features
Germ Cell Tumors			
Mature teratoma	10–15 y	Asymptomatic pelvic mass or pain due to torsion/hemorrhage	Mixed calcium, fluid, fat, soft tissue attenuation
Immature teratoma	11–14 y	Asymptomatic pelvic mass or pain due to torsion/hemorrhage	Mixed calcium, fluid, fat, soft tissue attenuation
Dysgerminoma	16 y	Most common malignant ovarian neoplasm, radiosensitive	Nonspecific solid enhancing mass, enhancement of fibrovascular septae
Endodermal sinus tumor (yolk sac tumor)	18 y	Elevated AFP, rapidly growing and may have cystic degeneration	Large pelvic mass with cystic and solid components
Embryonal carcinoma	14 y	HCG elevated, Increased AFP, Various endocrine manifestations (precocious puberty)	Nonspecific
Sex Cord-Stromal			
Granulosa cell tumor	7.6 y	Isosexual precocity	Variable appearance: cystic to solid, heterogeneous due to hemorrhage
Sertoli-Leydig	25 y	Virilization/oligomenorrhea	Variable decrease in T1, T2 signal intensity
Mixed Germ Stromal Cell			
Gonadoblastoma	Perinatal	Dysgenetic gonads (see **Table 1**)	Circumscribed, mottled, or punctate calcifications
Epithelial			
Cystadenoma	Postpuberty (>20 y)	Nonspecific mass	Hypoechoic, thin walled, cystic
Mucinous cystadenocarcinoma	Rare in pediatrics	Large mass, presenting with a distended abdomen	Large, multicystic with septations

difficult to differentiate from one another. Familiarity with age of onset, clinical symptoms, laboratory data, and imaging features allow for a more narrow differential diagnosis. Useful general tendencies noted on imaging are discussed here.

US is the initial study of choice to screen for pelvic masses due to its widespread availability and ease of use. Although distinguishing benign versus malignant ovarian neoplasms is often difficult, US features suggesting malignancy include papillary projections, calcification, fluid in the cul-de-sac, tumors larger than 100 mm in largest diameter, lesions with irregular walls, and thickened irregular septae.[22]

The same features indicating malignancy on US are also present on CT. However, the mass may be better visualized in larger patients on CT. Predominance of soft tissue components (>50% by volume) increases the suspicion of malignancy.[1] Ascites, hepatic metastases, lymphadenopathy, and omental, mesenteric, or peritoneal implants suggest intra-abdominal spread. Extensive omental implants may occur, referred to as omental caking.

CT is the initial study of choice for staging, as it allows for visualization of spread into the chest, abdomen, and pelvis. MR imaging is superior to CT in some cases when evaluating the pelvic side wall and adjacent organs for invasion.[21]

Germ Cell Tumors

Germ cell tumors usually affect postpubertal females and present as painless pelvic or abdominal masses. Types of germ cell tumors include teratomas, dysgerminoma, endodermal sinus tumors (yolk sac tumor), embryonal carcinoma, and choriocarcinoma.

Teratomas

Teratomas, masses of germ cell origin, are more common in adolescence than in childhood. Though typically asymptomatic, patients may present with an abdominal or pelvic mass, or pain secondary to torsion or hemorrhage. Teratomas are bilateral in 10% to 25% of cases and undergo torsion in up to 30% of cases.[20]

The sonographic findings of teratomas are variable depending on the contents of the lesion present, such as sebum, serous fluid, calcium, hair, and fat. Teratomas are often complex, ranging from purely cystic to completely solid with echogenic calcifications and/or fat, mural nodules, floating debris, fluid levels, or any combination of the aforementioned components. Mural nodules are seen in up to 70% of postpubertal females, the so-called Rokitansky nodule, and 40% of prepubertal females (Fig. 11).[9,23] Acoustic shadowing on US occurs in up to 50% of teratomas secondary to calcified material or a matted mixture of sebum and hair.[23]

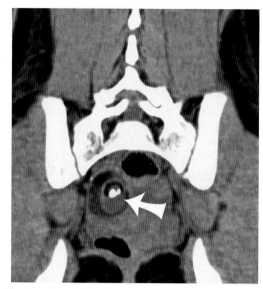

Fig. 11. Mature ovarian teratoma in a 15-year-old female with abdominal pain. Axial unenhanced CT image shows a right ovarian mass with intermixed fat, soft tissue, and calcification (*arrow*). Note internal nodule of material, the so-called Rokitansky nodule.

As with testicular teratomas, shadowing can be extensive enough to prevent visualization of much of the underlying lesion termed the "tip of the iceberg sign."[23] Only 2% to 10% of ovarian teratomas are malignant.[24] Imaging finding of malignant germ cell tumors are nonspecific overall, but some findings tend to suggest malignancy.[24] Specifically, central necrosis within a solid mass, thickened irregular septae, and papillary projections are suggestive of malignancy (Fig. 12).[9]

On CT, ovarian teratomas reveal a variable mixture of internal fat, fluid, and calcification, which can be characterized by Hounsfield units. Mural nodules, fat-fluid levels, and floating debris may also be seen. CT is usually adequate to characterize ovarian masses and define tumor extension. Teratomas rarely rupture into the peritoneal cavity, bladder, small bowel, rectum, sigmoid colon, vagina, or through the abdominal wall. Acute peritonitis and chronic granulomatous peritonitis due to a chronically leaking teratoma are exceedingly rare. Multiple small peritoneal implants and variable ascites may simulate carcinomatosis or tuberculous peritonitis.[25]

MR imaging may be helpful when CT is equivocal. MR is particularly able to identify pelvic side wall invasion and involvement of adjacent pelvic structures in malignant ovarian masses, including teratomas. Like US and CT, MR imaging reveals a heterogeneous lesion of variable signal intensity. Serous fluid is of low intensity on T1-weighted and bright on T2-weighted sequences, whereas

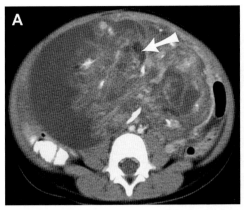
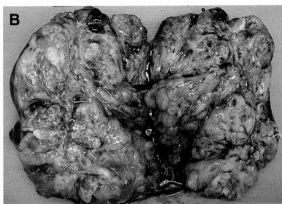

Fig. 12. Immature teratoma in a 3-year-old female with abdominal pain and distension. (*A*) Axial contrast-enhanced CT image through the pelvis shows a mixed-attenuation mass containing soft tissue, fat (*arrow*), and numerous scattered calcifications. (*B*) Gross image reveals a heterogeneous, nodular left ovarian mass.

intralesional fat is of high signal intensity on T1-weighted and T2-weighted sequences. Fat-suppressed sequences are useful to distinguish between intratumoral nonsuppressing hyperintense blood products and suppressing lipid material. Calcified structures, such as bone and teeth, as well as hair demonstrate low T1 and T2 signal intensity. Contrast administration shows variable enhancement of the solid portions of the lesion and the cyst walls. Other findings seen on CT and US, such as fat-fluid levels, floating debris, dependent layering, calcifications, and rounded mural nodules (dermoid plugs), may also be seen with MR imaging.[1,20,21]

The mainstay of treatment for ovarian teratomas is complete surgical resection, which is curative in the vast majority of cases. Malignant degeneration of mature into immature teratoma is rare, occurring in approximately 1% to 2% of cases.[26]

Ovarian dysgerminoma

Although rare, ovarian dysgerminoma is the most common malignant ovarian germ cell tumor in the pediatric population. The average age of presentation is 19 years, and tumor markers include lactate dehydrogenase and β-HCG.[27,28] Because it has a nonspecific imaging appearance, it is difficult to differentiate from other ovarian masses. Cross-sectional imaging of ovarian dysgerminomas shows a solid, encapsulated mass, which may have fine stippled calcifications (**Fig. 13**). Enhancement of fibrovascular septae after contrast administration is also present. It is bilateral in 10% to 15% of cases and is the only ovarian malignancy that spreads via the lymphatic system. Dysgerminoma has a good prognosis, with greater than 80% survival. It is treated with surgical resection of the involved ovary only and is highly radiosensitive.[21]

Endodermal sinus tumors (yolk sac tumors)

Ovarian endodermal sinus tumors are rare in the pediatric population, and are typically large at the time of diagnosis. The average age at presentation is between 18 and 19 years.[29] Patients often have an elevated AFP with endodermal sinus tumors (75%). AFP, as stated in the section on testicular endodermal sinus tumor, can be a useful marker for evaluation of tumor recurrence.[9,23] Cross-sectional imaging with US, CT, and MR show a large nonspecific pelvic mass with cystic and solid components (**Fig. 14**). Extension into peritoneum and adjacent structures, including the spinal canal, is not uncommon. Surgical resection of the involved ovary followed by chemotherapy has a reported range of survival of from 92% to 39%.[29,30]

Embryonal carcinoma

Ovarian embryonal carcinomas are also rare in the pediatric population, accounting for only 3% of primitive ovarian germ cell tumors.[31] The median age at presentation is 14 years.[23,31] Embryonal carcinomas can secrete AFP and 50% have an elevated β-HCG level.[23,31] Various endocrine manifestations such as precocious puberty, vaginal bleeding, amenorrhea, and hirsutism may be present. Cross-sectional imaging features are nonspecific. Intraperitoneal spread is not uncommon. Treatment of embryonal carcinoma includes surgery and chemotherapy. Survival rates are similar to those for yolk sac tumors.[30]

Sex Cord-Stromal Tumors

The most common sex cord-stromal tumors are granulosa cell (75%) and Sertoli-Leydig cell tumors (15%).[1] Sex cord-stromal tumors metastasize by lymphogenous spread to regional or distant lymph nodes, and/or hematogenous dissemination to the lungs and liver.

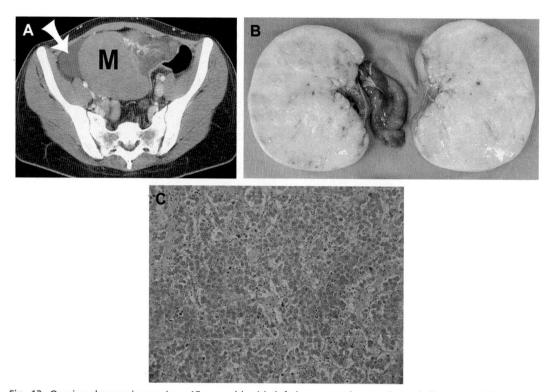

Fig. 13. Ovarian dysgerminoma in a 15-year-old with left lower quadrant pain and distention. (*A*) Contrast-enhanced axial CT of the pelvis shows a homogeneous enhancing soft tissue mass (M) with a small amount of adjacent ascites (*arrow*). (*B*) Gross specimen of the right ovary confirms a homogeneous infiltrative ovarian mass. (*C*) Histologic specimen reveals nests of uniform tumor cells outlined by fibrous bands. Tumor cells have clear cytoplasm, well-defined cell borders, large central nuclei, and clumped chromatin. Sparse nonneoplastic lymphocytic infiltrate is present within the fibrous tissue (H&E, original magnification ×200).

Granulosa cell tumors

Granulosa cell tumors are rare in children, presenting at a median age of 7.6 years.[32] Children with granulosa cell tumors typically present with isosexual precocity (appropriate secondary sexual characteristics prior to puberty) due to estrogen secretion. Patients may also have endometrial bleeding and uterine enlargement. These neoplasms are highly variable in appearance on cross-sectional imaging with US, CT, and MR imaging, ranging from cystic to solid, often being heterogeneous because of internal hemorrhage and infarct (**Fig. 15**).[33] Surgical resection is the mainstay of therapy, usually followed by radiation or chemotherapy.[34] Juvenile forms of granulosa cell tumor have the best prognosis. Unfortunately a tendency for late tumor recurrence is well documented, thus follow-up is required.[35]

Sertoli-Leydig cell tumors

Sertoli-Leydig cell tumors are very rare in children (mean age 25 years), accounting for only 0.5% of all ovarian masses.[36] Patients with Sertoli-Leydig

cell tumors (arrhenoblastoma) may present with virilization or oligomenorrhea due to androgen production. These tumors range from solid to cystic and may have a papillary component. On cross-sectional imaging, the mass is usually well defined and solid. On MR imaging, they may be hypointense on T1-weighted and T2 weighted sequences, often containing multiple cystic areas (**Fig. 16**).[33] Treatment includes surgical resection of the ovary, usually followed by chemotherapy. The prognosis of Sertoli-Leydig tumors depends on the stage of disease. In one study, the 5- and 10-year survival rates were both 92%.[37]

Gonadoblastoma

Gonadoblastomas are mixed germ cell and sex cord-stromal tumors. These tumors originate in the perinatal period, but may present from age 1 year into adulthood. Gonadoblastomas are often found in patients with dysgenetic gonads of phenotypic females with an XY genotype.[38] Although gonadoblastomas are mostly benign, they frequently contain components of other germ cells,

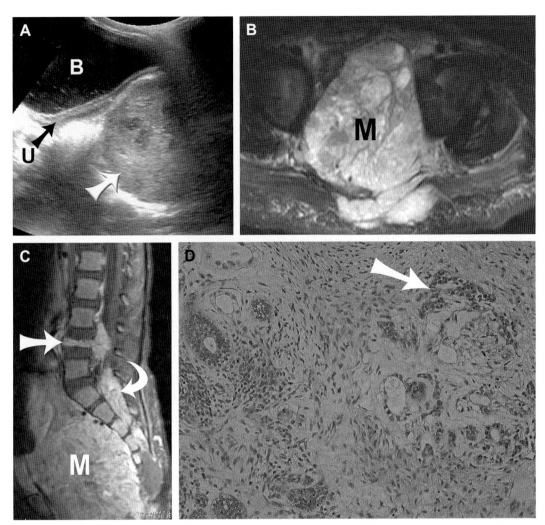

Fig. 14. Yolk sac tumor in a 2-year-old female with perineal skin changes. (*A*) Longitudinal sonogram of the pelvis demonstrates a heterogeneous echogenicity mass (*white arrow*). Also noted are the compressed bladder (B) and small prepubertal uterus (U, [*black arrow*]). (*B*) Axial and (*C*) Sagittal contrast-enhanced fat-suppressed T1-weighted MR images reveal a heterogeneous, mixed cystic and solid, enhancing pelvic mass (M). Spine involvement is causing vertebra plana (*arrow*) and epidural extension (*curved arrow*). (*D*) Histologic section shows mature and immature tissues derived from all 3 germ layers. In 15% of the sampled tissue, the neoplastic cells are in ribbons, or lining irregular cystic spaces as seen in the right side and upper left corner of the picture. The tumor cells contain clear cytoplasm and large nucleoli with fine chromatin and small nucleoli. Tumor cells were also positive for α-fetoprotein (H&E, original magnification ×200).

which put them at risk for malignant degeneration in approximately 50% to 60% of patients.[38] Gonadoblastomas are bilateral in 30% to 50% of cases[39]; they may develop circumscribed, mottled, or punctate calcifications visible on plain radiographs and CT.[40]

Epithelial Tumors (Cystadenomas and Cystadenocarcinomas)

Epithelial neoplasms of the ovary, including cystadenomas and cystadenocarcinomas, represent about 10% to 17% of all ovarian neoplasms in children.[41,42] Cystadenomas are divided into serous and mucinous subtypes. Cystadenomas present after puberty, with the lesions being rare before 20 years of age. Presenting symptoms include nonspecific abdominal pain or a painless abdominal mass.[42] On sonography, ovarian cystadenomas appear as thick-walled smoothly marginated cystic masses with hypoechoic or anechoic contents. These tumors have a variable appearance on MR imaging, but are typically large cystic pelvic or abdominal masses ranging from 4 to 20 cm in size.[9,18] Gadolinium contrast agents show enhancement of the papillary projections and cyst wall.[6,12]

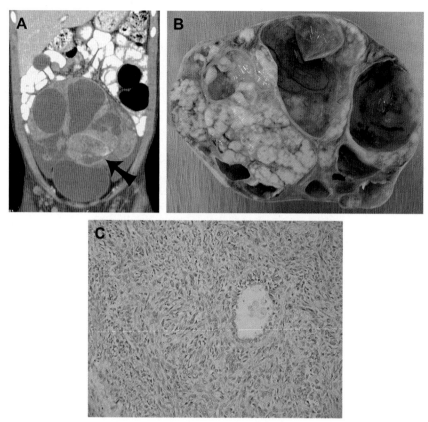

Fig. 15. Juvenile granulosa cell tumor in a 7-year-old female with abdominal pain. (*A*) Reformatted coronal contrast-enhanced CT image of the abdomen and pelvis demonstrates a mixed-attenuation cystic and solid mass with foci of internal calcification (*arrow*). (*B*) Gross specimen of the left ovary confirms a multicystic mass with internal septations. (*C*) Histologic specimen reveals a cellular neoplasm with follicle formation. The tumor cells, which are cytologically distinct from the adult granulosa cell tumor, show round or oval hyperchromatic nuclei that lack nuclear grooves. Abundant eosinophilic cytoplasm, varying nuclear atypia, and mitotic activity are seen (H&E, original magnification ×100).

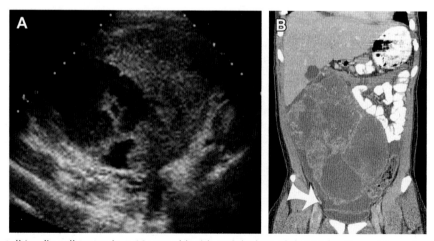

Fig. 16. Sertoli-Leydig cell tumor in a 14-year-old with weight loss, abdominal pain, and irregular menses. (*A*) Longitudinal sonogram shows a heterogeneous, mixed solid and cystic mass in the right adnexa. (*B*) Contrast-enhanced CT image confirms a heterogeneous solid mass with low-attenuation cystic areas. A small amount of free fluid is seen adjacent to the mass (*arrow*).

Mucinous cystadenomas rarely occur in the pediatric population, occurring more frequently in postpubertal females. Mucinous cystadenomas have the potential to be malignant mucinous cysta-denocarcinomas, and may metastasize through peritoneal/omental seeding. Patients typically present with a distended abdomen. On US, CT, and MR imaging, they appear as large multicystic ovarian masses with septations.[41] Treatment is usually surgical, and because of the large size, ovary-sparing surgery may be difficult (**Fig. 17**).

Secondary Ovarian Neoplasms

Secondary ovarian neoplasms include leukemia and lymphoma (**Fig. 18**). The gonads, as discussed in the section on testicles, may act as sanctuary sites for surviving tumor cells after chemotherapy administration.[43] On cross-sectional imaging, one sees unilaterally or bilaterally enlarged, often hyperemic, variably enhancing ovaries. History of treated neoplasm is important for suggesting this diagnosis.[23,43]

UTERINE/VAGINAL TUMORS

Uterine and vaginal tumors are rare in the pediatric population, and are more likely to be malignant in children than in adults. The most common uterine/vaginal tumors are rhadomyosarcomas, which arise from the anterior vagina near the cervix or the cervix itself. Endodermal sinus tumor of the vagina, and clear cell adenocarcinoma, arise from the vagina (**Table 3**).

Children with rhabdomyosarcoma frequently present with vaginal bleeding and/or protrusion of a polypoid mass from the vaginal introitus. Three histologic subsets of rhabdomyosarcoma are described, including embryonal (which includes embryonal, botryoid, and spindle cell), alveolar,

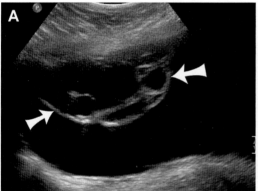
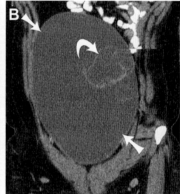
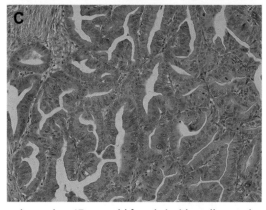

Fig. 17. Mucinous cystadenocarcinoma in a 17-year-old female incidentally noted on plain radiograph performed before surgery. (*A*) Longitudinal sonogram of the pelvis shows a large cystic mass with a septated mural nodule (*arrows*). (*B*) Coronal reformatted contrast-enhanced CT image reveals a cystic midline pelvic mass (*arrows*) with several internal septations (*curved arrow*). At surgery the lesion originated from the left ovary. (*C*) Histologic specimen shows a multilocular lesion with focal areas of florid papillary and glandular epithelial proliferation, nuclear stratification, and increased mitotic activity, consistent with well-differentiated mucinous cystadenocarcinoma. The majority of the tumor reveals cysts lined by intestinal-type mucinous epithelium without cytologic atypia (not shown) (H&E, original magnification ×200).

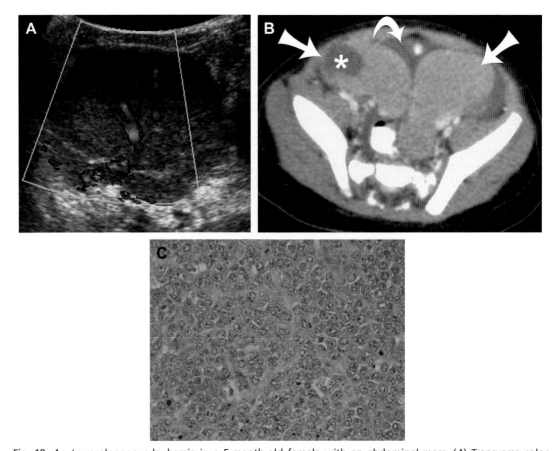

Fig. 18. Acute myelogenous leukemia in a 5-month-old female with an abdominal mass. (A) Transverse color Doppler sonogram demonstrates an enlarged, homogeneous, hypervascular right ovary. The contralateral ovary (not shown) had the same appearance. (B) Axial contrast-enhanced CT image of the pelvis confirms bilateral ovarian enlargement (*arrows*) with some cystic change on the right (*asterisk*), and pelvic ascites (*curved arrow*). (C) Histologic specimen reveals sheets of monomorphic cells with large nuclei, high cellular turnover with atypical mitoses, and foci of cellular necrosis (H&E, original magnification ×400).

and pleomorphic/anaplastic. Embryonal and bo-tryoid variants are typically found in the vagina or genitourinary region in females. The embryonal type has the best prognosis, with a 5-year survival rate of 69%.[44] Rhabdomyosarcomas may be locally aggressive, invading the uterus and adjacent pelvic structures.

US is the initial screening tool used to detect pelvic masses, and CT or MR imaging is used to evaluate tumor extent. Rhabdomyosarcomas usually have central areas of decreased echogenicity seen within the uterus/vagina, due to necrosis or ulceration (Fig. 19). On T1-weighted MR imaging, rhabdomyosarcomas have intensity slightly greater than muscle and less than fat. On T2, the signal intensity increases. On CT and MR imaging, areas of central necrosis are commonly seen. CT and MR are used to assess for local invasion and distant metastases including evaluation for retroperitoneal lymphadenopathy, liver, lung,

and bone metastases. Treatment of rhabdomyosarcoma includes a combination of chemotherapy for 4 to 5 months followed by surgical excision and/or radiation therapy.

Endodermal sinus tumor and clear cell adenocarcinoma of the vagina often become very large and fill the vagina at the time of diagnosis. Clear cell adenocarcinoma is associated with maternal use of diethylstilbestrol during pregnancy. These tumors are indistinguishable from rhabdomyosarcoma.

BLADDER MASSES

A variety of bladder masses occurs in children. Benign lesions, most of which are rare, include fibromas, hemangiomas, schwannomas, hematomas, ureteroceles, leiomyomas, endometriomas, and pseudotumoral cystitis of chronic granulomatous disease. Malignant lesions include rhabdomyosarcomas, leiomyosarcomas, and transitional

Table 3
Key clinical and imaging features of uterine/vaginal neoplasms

Tumor Type	Key Clinical Features	Key Imaging Features
Rhabdomyosarcoma	Cluster of grapes, central necrosis, locally aggressive	Central areas of decreased echogenicity due to necrosis
Clear cell	Maternal diethylstilbestrol use	Nonspecific imaging findings

cell carcinomas. Secondary involvement may also occur rarely, with lesions such as lymphoma (**Fig. 20**). Although most of these neoplasms are nonspecific in appearance and cannot be distinguished from one another with imaging, one helpful general sign of malignancy is invasion of the adjacent soft tissues. Presenting symptoms may be related to vesicoureteral reflux, pelvic pain, or hematuria.

Bladder lesions are initially characterized by US and voiding cystourethrogram (VCUG), with VCUG showing a filling defect. Color Doppler US evaluation may be helpful for further evaluation, as entities such as hematoma will show a lack of Doppler flow. MR imaging is a helpful tool to detect disruption of the bladder wall and extension into the adjacent pelvic side wall and soft tissues. CT is particularly useful to assess for lung metastasis; however, one must always be cognizant of the associated radiation exposure in children who will potentially require repetitive preoperative and postoperative/follow-up imaging.

Rhabdomyosarcoma is by far the most common malignant bladder lesion. It occurs in several histologic subtypes with the most common, as stated earlier, being the embryonal type. The appearance on MR imaging, CT, and US is highly variable, as one can see hemorrhagic, cystic, and solid components (**Fig. 21**).

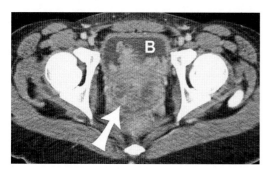

Fig. 19. Rhabdomyosarcoma in a 2-year-old female with a vulvar mass. Axial contrast-enhanced CT image of the pelvis demonstrates bladder (B) invasion from the vulvar origin mass (*arrow*). The mass is predominately solid with subtle internal areas of low attenuation.

When assessing the extent of the lesion (staging) it is important to address local and distant spread to nodes (including size), soft tissue extension, and adjacent organ invasion with CT or MR imaging. Distant metastases are often seen in cortical bone, lung, and lymph nodes. These points are well addressed with MR imaging, as soft tissue extension and disruption of a solid organ's wall are readily evaluated by checking for interruption of the normal low signal within the walls of organs such as the rectum and bladder. MR imaging suffers from the same limitations as do other cross-sectional imaging modalities in lymph node evaluation. Interpretation is limited to the size of the node when assessing for potential underlying involvement, as metastatic normal-sized nodal disease will go undetected.

SACROCOCCYGEAL TERATOMA

Sacrococcygeal teratoma is a complex lesion with a varied differential diagnosis in the neonate. Included in the list of differentials are lesions such as neuroblastoma, chordoma, rhabdomyosarcoma, anterior meningocele, and neurenteric cysts. These lesions are often quite heterogeneous in nature with foci of soft tissue, cysts, and calcifications.

Sacrococcygeal teratomas usually present in neonates and are often seen in utero on US as a large mass protruding from the sacrum/buttock. Other findings include vertebral body erosion, or a soft tissue mass with areas of calcification seen on radiographs. The classification of sacrococcygeal teratomas includes 4 types, depending on the degree to which they are intrapelvic or extrapelvic in location. Type 1 is external in nature, protruding from the sacral region. Type 2 has both internal and external abdominal components, but is mostly external. Type 3 is mostly intrapelvic (internal) but has an external component. Type 4 is entirely internal or intrapelvic (presacral) in location. Sacrococcygeal teratomas are complex and may be associated with sacral and anorectal abnormalities, which is referred to as the Currarino triad (sacral defect, anorectal malformation, and presacral anomaly such as anterior meningocele, teratoma, or cyst). Type 4 presacral lesions are

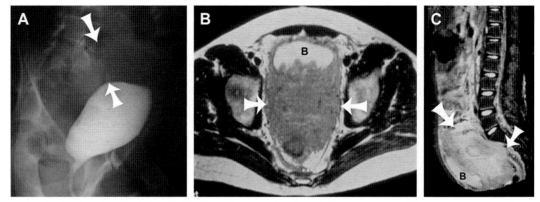

Fig. 20. Burkitt lymphoma of the bladder in a 15-year-old male with frequency. (*A*) Oblique image from a fluoroscopic voiding cystourethrogram reveals a thickened bladder wall (*arrows*). (*B*) Axial contrast-enhanced T1-weighted MR image of the pelvis demonstrates a large mass (*arrows*) along the posterior bladder (B) wall. (*C*) Sagittal T2-weighted MR image confirms a mass (*arrows*) along the posterior bladder wall. Note that the bladder (B) is displaced anteriorly.

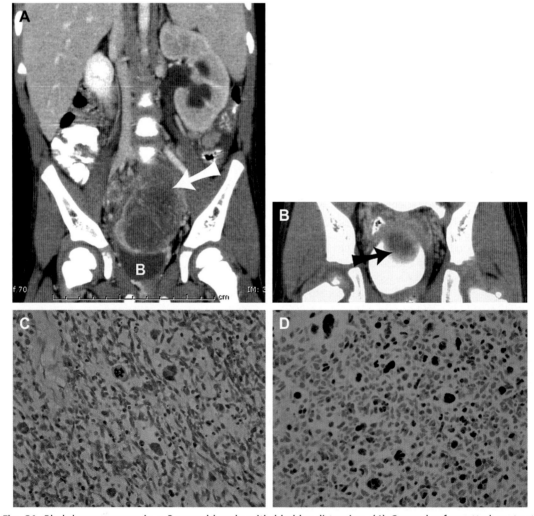

Fig. 21. Rhabdomyosarcoma in a 3-year-old male with bladder distension. (*A*) Coronal reformatted contrast-enhanced CT image of the pelvis show a heterogeneous mass (*arrow*) extending from the bladder (B). (*B*) Delayed contrast-enhanced CT image of the pelvis shows contrast surrounding the bladder mass (*arrow*). (*C*) Histologic specimen of anaplastic embryonal rhabdomyosarcoma reveals pleomorphic tumor cells with bright eosinophilic cytoplasm in a myxoid stroma. Some tumor cells contain enlarged, or multiple, hyperchromatic nuclei with atypical mitotic figures (H&E, original magnification ×200). (*D*) Myogenin immunohistochemistry shows patchy nuclear positivity, typical for embryonal rhabdomyosarcoma (H&E, original magnification ×200).

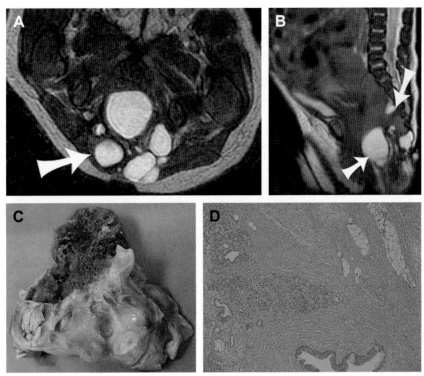

Fig. 22. Sacrococcygeal teratoma in a 1-day-old girl with a buttock mass. (*A*) Axial and (*B*) Sagittal T2 MR images through the pelvis show a heterogeneous mixed signal intensity cystic and solid mass (*arrows*) that is mostly extrapelvic with some intrapelvic (presacral) extension. (*C*) Gross specimen demonstrates the varied appearance of soft tissue, fat, and calcification. (*D*) Histologic specimen identifies cells from all 3 germ layers. There are islands of glandular tissue (endoderm), adipose tissue (mesoderm), and glial tissue (ectoderm). No immature or malignant tissue is present in the tumor (H&E, original magnification ×40).

associated with sacral anomalies and rectal stenosis, so contrast enema may be helpful for evaluation. With regard to lesion type and detection, those with type 3 and 4 designation are often detected later because of their internal nature. Lesions detected later are at higher risk of malignant potential. It is important to note if a lesion is cystic, because cystic lesions tend to have a better prognosis than solid ones. In addition, females have a better prognosis than males.

Lesions diagnosed after 2 months of age are more likely to contain malignant tissue. These lesions are best evaluated with CT and/or MR imaging (**Fig. 22**). Sacrococcygeal teratomas may metastasize to the liver, lungs, and lymph nodes. Following treatment, they may revert to a mature teratoma or be seen as fibrotic masses. It is interesting that recurrence has been seen at up to 40 years after resection, which can be heralded by rising AFP levels.

REFERENCES

1. Siegel MJ. Pelvic tumors in childhood. Radiol Clin North Am 1997;35:1455–75.

2. Tessler FN, Tublin ME, Rifkin MD. Ultrasound assessment of testicular and paratesticular masses. J Clin Ultrasound 1996;24:423–36.

3. Kaplan GW, Cromie WC, Kelalis PP, et al. Prepubertal yolk sac testicular tumors–report of the testicular tumor registry. J Urol 1988;140:1109–12.

4. Coley BS, Siegel MJ. Pediatric sonography. Philadelphia: Lippincott Williams and Wilkins; 2002.

5. Taskinen S, Fagerholm R, Aronniemi J, et al. Testicular tumors in children and adolescents. J Pediatr Urol 2008;4:134–7.

6. McEniff N, Doherty F, Katz J, et al. Yolk sac tumor of the testis discovered on a routine annual sonogram in a boy with testicular microlithiasis. AJR Am J Roentgenol 1995;164:971–2.

7. Janzen DL, Mathieson JR, Marsh JI, et al. Testicular microlithiasis: sonographic and clinical features. AJR Am J Roentgenol 1992;158:1057–60.

8. Neill M, Warde P, Fleshner N. Management of low-stage testicular seminoma. Urol Clin North Am 2007;34:127–36 [abstract vii–viii].

9. Siegel MJ, Hoffer FA. Magnetic resonance imaging of nongynecologic pelvic masses in children. Magn Reson Imaging Clin N Am 2002;10:325–44, vi.

10. Slovis T, editor. Caffey's pediatric diagnostic imaging. Philadelphia (PA): Mosby Elsevier; 2008.

11. Xu HX, Yi XP. Sonographic appearance of a testicular yolk sac tumor in a 2-year-old boy. J Clin Ultrasound 2007;35:55–7.

12. Pohl HG, Shukla AR, Metcalf PD, et al. Prepubertal testis tumors: actual prevalence rate of histological types. J Urol 2004;172:2370–2.

13. Kundra V. Testicular cancer. Semin Roentgenol 2004; 39:437–50.

14. Woodward PJ, Schwab CM, Sesterhenn IA. From the archives of the AFIP: extratesticular scrotal masses: radiologic-pathologic correlation. Radiographics 2003;23:215–40.

15. Gierke CL, King BF, Bostwick DG, et al. Large-cell calcifying Sertoli cell tumor of the testis: appearance at sonography. AJR Am J Roentgenol 1994;163:373–5.

16. Hisano M, Souza FM, Malheiros DM, et al. Granulosa cell tumor of the adult testis: report of a case and review of the literature. Clinics (Sao Paulo) 2006;61:77–8.

17. Papaioannou G, Sebire NJ, McHugh K. Imaging of the unusual pediatric 'blastomas'. Cancer Imaging 2009;9:1–11.

18. Boechat MI. MR imaging of the pediatric pelvis. Magn Reson Imaging Clin N Am 1996;4:679–96.

19. Akbar SA, Sayyed TA, Jafri SZ, et al. Multimodality imaging of paratesticular neoplasms and their rare mimics. Radiographics 2003;23:1461–76.

20. Garel L, Dubois J, Grignon A, et al. US of the pediatric female pelvis: a clinical perspective. Radiographics 2001;21:1393–407.

21. Siegel MJ. Magnetic resonance imaging of the adolescent female pelvis. Magn Reson Imaging Clin N Am 2002;10:303–24, vi.

22. Timmerman D, Testa AC, Bourne T, et al. Simple ultrasound-based rules for the diagnosis of ovarian cancer. Ultrasound Obstet Gynecol 2008;31: 681–90.

23. Siegel M. Pediatric sonography. Philadelphia: Lippincott Williams and Wilkins; 2002.

24. Stranzinger E, Strouse PJ. Ultrasound of the pediatric female pelvis. Semin Ultrasound CT MR 2008; 29:98–113.

25. Fibus TF. Intraperitoneal rupture of a benign cystic ovarian teratoma: findings at CT and MR imaging. AJR Am J Roentgenol 2000;174:261–2.

26. Outwater EK, Siegelman ES, Hunt JL. Ovarian teratomas: tumor types and imaging characteristics. Radiographics 2001;21:475–90.

27. Brewer M, Gershenson DM, Herzog CE, et al. Outcome and reproductive function after chemotherapy for ovarian dysgerminoma. J Clin Oncol 1999;17:2670–5.

28. Chisholm JC, Darmady JM, Kohler JA. Dysgerminoma in mother and daughter: use of lactate dehydrogenase as a tumor marker in the child. Pediatr Hematol Oncol 1995;12:305–8.

29. Levitin A, Haller KD, Cohen HL, et al. Endodermal sinus tumor of the ovary: imaging evaluation. AJR Am J Roentgenol 1996;167:791–3.

30. Morris HH, La Vecchia C, Draper GJ. Endodermal sinus tumor and embryonal carcinoma of the ovary in children. Gynecol Oncol 1985;21:7–17.

31. Singh N. The pathology of ovarian embryonal carcinoma. CME J Gynecol Oncol 2002;7:215–8.

32. Calaminus G, Wessalowski R, Harms D, et al. Juvenile granulosa cell tumors of the ovary in children and adolescents: results from 33 patients registered in a prospective cooperative study. Gynecol Oncol 1997;65:447–52.

33. Jung SE, Rha SE, Lee JM, et al. CT and MRI findings of sex cord-stromal tumor of the ovary. AJR Am J Roentgenol 2005;185:207–15.

34. Lee IW, Levin W, Chapman W, et al. Radiotherapy for the treatment of metastatic granulosa cell tumor in the mediastinum: a case report. Gynecol Oncol 1999;73:455–60.

35. Schumer ST, Cannistra SA. Granulosa cell tumor of the ovary. J Clin Oncol 2003;21:1180–9.

36. Tandon R, Goel P, Saha PK, et al. A rare ovarian tumor - Sertoli-Leydig cell tumor with heterologous element. MedGenMed 2007;9:44.

37. Zaloudek C, Norris HJ. Sertoli-Leydig tumors of the ovary. A clinicopathologic study of 64 intermediate and poorly differentiated neoplasms. Am J Surg Pathol 1984;8:405–18.

38. Pauls K, Franke FE, Buttner R, et al. Gonadoblastoma: evidence for a stepwise progression to dysgerminoma in a dysgenetic ovary. Virchows Arch 2005; 447:603–9.

39. De Backer A, Madern GC, Oosterhuis JW, et al. Ovarian germ cell tumors in children: a clinical study of 66 patients. Pediatr Blood Cancer 2006;46: 459–64.

40. Seymour EQ, Hood JB, Underwood PB Jr, et al. Gonadoblastoma: an ovarian tumor with characteristic pelvic calcifications. AJR Am J Roentgenol 1976; 127:1001–2.

41. Karaman A, Azili MN, Boduroglu EC, et al. A huge ovarian mucinous cystadenoma in a 14-year-old premenarchal girl: review on ovarian mucinous tumor in premenarchal girls. J Pediatr Adolesc Gynecol 2008;21:41–4.

42. Morowitz M, Huff D, von Allmen D. Epithelial ovarian tumors in children: a retrospective analysis. J Pediatr Surg 2003;38:331–5 [discussion: 331–5].

43. Kim JW, Cho MK, Kim CH, et al. Ovarian and multiple lymph nodes recurrence of acute lymphoblastic leukemia: a case report and review of literature. Pediatr Surg Int 2008;24:1269–73.

44. Sultan I, Qaddoumi I, Yaser S, et al. Comparing adult and pediatric rhabdomyosarcoma in the surveillance, epidemiology and end results program, 1973 to 2005: an analysis of 2,600 patients. J Clin Oncol 2009;27:3391–7.

Imaging Pediatric Bone Sarcomas

Sue C. Kaste, DO[a,b,c,*]

KEYWORDS

- Osteosarcoma • Ewing sarcoma • Chondrosarcoma
- Pediatric bone tumors

Primary malignant bone tumors are rare (8.7 cases per million annual incidence), and account for about 6% of all new pediatric cancer cases per year in the United States.[1] Osteosarcoma and Ewing Sarcoma Family of Tumors (ESFT) comprise the majority of cases (400 and 250 cases per year, respectively).[2] Patients typically present with pain and/or swelling. Identification of the lesion not uncommonly occurs as a result of imaging performed for trauma. Diagnosis is frequently delayed for several weeks to months, due in part to the rarity of such tumors and that the presence of a malignancy in an otherwise healthy adolescent is unexpected. Continuous evolution of chemotherapy regimens, surgical techniques, and imaging technology has contributed to improved overall survival. Thus tumor management and patient care should be provided by a multidisciplinary team of health care professionals that includes radiology, oncology, orthopedic surgery, radiation oncology, and physical therapy.[3]

Bone tumors are classified according to the proliferating cell type. Each of the elements of which bone is composed—cartilage, osteoid, fibrous tissue, and marrow—can give rise to benign or malignant tumors. Clinical and standard imaging (radiographs, technetium-99m methylene diphosphonate [[99mTc]MDP] bone scan, computed tomography [CT]) characteristics of the various tumor types have been previously published and have not appreciably changed over the decades.[4,5] However, imaging recommendations evolve in concert with treatment advancements and clinical trial regimens.[6] This article reviews the 3 most common pediatric bone sarcomas—osteosarcoma, Ewing sarcoma, and chondrosarcoma—and their imaging as applicable to contemporary disease staging and monitoring, and explores the roles of evolving imaging techniques such as magnetic resonance (MR) and positron emission tomography (PET)-CT.

PEDIATRIC BONE SARCOMAS
Osteosarcoma

Osteosarcoma is the most common primary malignant bone tumor. Osteosarcoma occurs primarily during puberty and has been associated with rapid patient growth.[7] In females, the peak age is earlier than in males (12 years vs 16 years, respectively).[7,8] A second peak is seen in adults older than 60 years. The reported incidence of osteosarcoma from the 2009 report of the Surveillance, Epidemiology, and End Results (SEER) Program is 4.4 cases per million in patients up to 24 years of age, more prevalent in blacks than whites (4.2 vs 5.0, respectively), and more prevalent in females than males.

This work was supported in part by grants P30 CA-21765 and P01 CA-20180 from the National Institutes of Health, a Center of Excellence grant from the State of Tennessee, and the American Lebanese Syrian Associated Charities (ALSAC).

[a] Department of Radiological Sciences, St. Jude Children's Research Hospital, MSN #220, 262 Danny Thomas Place, Memphis, TN 38105, USA
[b] Department of Oncology, St. Jude Children's Research Hospital, MSN #220, 262 Danny Thomas Place, Memphis, TN 38105, USA
[c] Department of Radiology, University of Tennessee School of Health Science Center, 910 Madison Avenue, Memphis, TN 38163, USA
* Department of Radiological Sciences, St. Jude Children's Research Hospital, MSN #220, 262 Danny Thomas Place, Memphis, TN 38105.
E-mail address: sue.kaste@stjude.org

Radiol Clin N Am 49 (2011) 749–765
doi:10.1016/j.rcl.2011.05.006

The current 5-year relative survival rate of pediatric cases is 61.6%.[8] Advances in therapy improved survival from 15% to 20% when surgery alone was used for therapy to 55% to 80% by the 1980s with the addition of chemotherapy.[7,9] However, no significant improvement in survival rates has occurred between 1994 and 2003.[8] Survival has been associated with age at diagnosis, race, anatomic site of the primary tumor (highest survival in bones of the hands or feet and poorest survival seen in pelvic primary tumors), pathologic subtypes (best in chondroblastic osteosarcoma and worst in small cell osteosarcoma), and stage of disease (localized disease best survival; those with distant metastatic disease the poorest), and response to chemotherapy[7,8,10] determined at the time of definitive tumor resection. Two-dimensional tumor size relative to the patient's body surface area[11] and/or absolute tumor size[12] may have prognostic roles.

Osteosarcoma is histologically composed of mesenchymal stem cells that produce osteoid. In addition to the "classic" central medullary osteosarcoma, histologically distinct variants are also recognized: surface (parosteal, periosteal, and high-grade) and low-grade intraosseous osteosarcomas.[9,13] With the exception of the high-grade surface osteosarcoma, these variants are associated with an overall more favorable prognosis.

Treatment is determined by tumor histology. Classic osteosarcoma is treated with neoadjuvant multiagent chemotherapy followed by surgery and additional chemotherapy.[13] Both parosteal and periosteal osteosarcoma require surgical resection. Chemotherapy is not typically indicated for parosteal osteosarcoma, and its role in treating periosteal osteosarcoma is controversial.[14] As osteosarcoma is radiation resistant, radiation therapy is typically reserved for axial unresectable lesions and for palliative care.[9] The roles of vascular endothelial growth factor (VEGF)[15] and other signaling pathways are under investigation as potential factors to be integrated into risk-adapted therapy.[15,16] In response to the incorporation of new treatment agents into clinical regimens, the imaging assessment of the effectiveness of therapy must now reflect the biological response of tumor with robust sensitivity and accuracy.

Ewing Sarcoma

Ewing sarcoma (a member of the ESFT) is the second most common malignant bone tumor in pediatrics.[8,13,17] These tumors are small, round, blue cell tumors, thought to originate in neural crest cells.[17] The ESFT is estimated to have an annual incidence in the United States of 2.1 cases per million children, accounting for about 2% of all pediatric and young adult cancers.[17] These tumors may arise in either bone or soft tissue, occur more frequently in males than in females, and are associated with increased incidence in white and Hispanic children than in black or Asian children.[17] The vast majority of ESFT cases are associated with a t[11;22] [q24;q12] translocation.[1,17]

Several prognostic factors are considered in newly diagnosed patients with Ewing sarcoma. The recent SEER report based on more than 1600 cases of Ewing sarcoma registered between 1973 and 2005 indicates that independently significant variables include distant disease, stage, primary location of the axial skeleton, and primary tumor size exceeding 8 cm as independent predictors of worse overall survival.[18] These investigators found no significant prognostic significance of race or age at diagnosis. However, among Caucasian patients female sex was identified as an independent predictor of improved survival ($P = .031$).[18] Notable is the incidence of Ewing sarcoma in Caucasians being 9 times higher than in African Americans, and over the course of this study (1973–2005) the incidence of Ewing sarcoma increased only among Caucasians.[18] Pre-teens have improved outcome compared with adolescents, and both groups show improved survival when compared with adults.[19] Event-free survival of patients with pelvic tumors has been reported to range from 43%[20] to 50% compared with 61% in patients with proximal, 68% distal extremity primary ($P = .003$),[21] and 60.6% extremity tumors in general.[20] More recently, Lin and colleagues[22] demonstrated that centrally located primary disease ($P = .002$) and tumor response to therapy ($P = .007$) are independent predictors of local disease recurrence. Histologic response of less than 90% necrosis was associated with increased risk of local disease recurrence. Patients diagnosed with metastatic disease have a considerably worse outcome than those with nonmetastatic disease, and those with metastasis limited to the lungs fare better than those with either bone metastasis alone or both bone and lung metastasis, as reported by the European Intergroup Cooperative Ewing Sarcoma Study Group.[23] As with the aforementioned factors, patients with larger tumors have a worse survival when compared with those with smaller tumors.[19,21,24] A more recent study of 21 pediatric patients who underwent both static and dynamic enhanced MR found that tumor volume, width, and depth, but not length or dynamic enhancement variables, at diagnosis correlate with the risk of metastatic disease.[25]

Chondrosarcoma

Chondrosarcoma is a rare heterogeneous group of tumors that may arise from bone or soft tissue. Those arising from bone account for approximately 3.6% of all primary bone malignancies in the United States.[26] The incidence of chondrosarcoma is estimated to be 1 in 200,000 per year, with survival ranging from 0% to 93% depending on histologic subtype.[27] From the National Cancer database, Damron and colleagues[28] reported the 5-year relative survival of all forms of chondrosarcoma to be about 75% (range, 52%–87% depending on histologic subtype). Survival over the past 30 years has remained static.[27] Prognostic predictors of outcome include grade and size of tumor and uncontaminated, wide surgical margins. The development of local disease recurrence also seems to portend development of distant metastases and ultimately poor survival.[29] These tumors have a predilection for the proximal femur and pelvis.[30] The incidence of chondrosarcoma increases with increasing age. Though most often seen in middle-aged patients, chondrosarcoma arises in adolescents and young adults as primary or secondary lesions.

In an estimated 0.5% to 5% of cases,[31] chondrosarcomas may arise in a preexisting lesion, most notably osteochondroma or enchondroma. Both the radiologic and histologic distinctions between a benign osteochondroma or enchondroma and malignant chondrosarcoma (grade 1) are difficult to delineate and are associated with high interobserver variability.[13,26,32,33] Clinically, low-grade chondrosarcoma should be considered if a patient with enchondroma complains of pain, especially night pain.[33] Factors associated with increased risk of malignant dedifferentiation include the presence of multiple osteochondromas or enchondromas,[13,34] axial location, and size exceeding 5 cm.[32] Ahmed and colleagues[35] reported an institutional incidence of sarcomatous dedifferentiation of 7.6% in single osteochondromas and 36.3% in cases of multiple osteochondromas. These investigators also found dedifferentiation of lesions to be associated with flat bone locations and male gender, and to develop in patients 10 to 20 years earlier than primary chondrosarcoma.

Reported radiologic signs of sarcomatous dedifferentiation include heterogeneous mineralization, presence of a soft tissue mass, poorly defined lesion margination, and destruction of the cartilaginous cap.[35,36] Several investigators have associated the presence of peritumoral edema with chondrosarcoma but not with enchondromas.[35,37–39] However, this association occurred in only 20% of cases of clear cell variant of chondrosarcoma reported by Janzen and colleagues.[39]

Clinical and radiologic techniques for differentiating between benign and malignant cartilaginous tumors are under development. Using the onset and rate of contrast enhancement, reports indicate a potential role for dynamic enhanced MR in differentiating between osteochondromas or enchondromas and chondrosarcomas, but this technique was less helpful in patients whose growth plates were not yet fused.[40] Feldman and colleagues[41] have shown [^{18}F]fluorodeoxyglucose ([^{18}F]FDG) PET imaging to distinguish between benign enchondromas and chondrosarcomas, with 90.9% sensitivity, 100% specificity, and 96.6% accuracy when using maximum standard uptake value (SUV) of 2.0 to distinguish between benign and malignant cartilaginous tumors. However, the role of PET or PET-CT in differentiating between benign enchondromas and chondrosarcoma has not yet been established. Recent identification of integrin-linked kinase expression patterns may be able to serve as biomarkers capable of distinguishing between enchondromas and chondrosarcomas.[42]

Chondrosarcomas are classified as grade 1 to 3, based on clinical behavior and likelihood of metastasizing; central (arising from the intramedullary space) versus peripheral (arising from the surface of bone); and primary or secondary.[26,33,34] Between 85% and 90% of chondrosarcomas are classified as conventional chondrosarcoma,[26,32,34] most of which are further classified as grade 1 or 2 (low or intermediate grade), and behave in an indolent manner with low potential to metastasize. The remaining 5% to 10% of conventional lesions are classified as grade 3 lesions and possess high metastatic potential.[26] Rare variants of chondrosarcoma include dedifferentiated chondrosarcoma, a low-grade tumor that degenerates into a high-grade sarcoma. Mesenchymal chondrosarcoma accounts for about 3% to 10% of primary chondrosarcomas, is highly malignant, occurs in a population younger than for conventional chondrosarcoma, and is associated with late local and distant disease recurrence.[30,43,44] The clear cell variant of chondrosarcoma accounts for about 2% to 5% of all chondrosarcomas, is seen in younger patients, has a predilection for involving the epiphysis of femur or humerus,[30,37] and may clinically be confused with chondroblastoma.[30] Myxoid chondrosarcoma is a slow-growing tumor associated with frequent local recurrence and metastases; it is seen in younger patients.[26,44] Periosteal chondrosarcoma is a very rare form that accounts for less than 2% of chondrosarcomas. Unlike the lesions discussed above, this variant arises from the cortical surface, most commonly of the metaphysis,[45] and is covered by a fibrous sheath that is contiguous with the periosteum.[4,32,45] As it typically is found in patients in the second to fourth decades of life, this lesion may be seen in adolescents; there is a predilection for males.[45]

Overall, the prognosis for patients with chondrosarcoma is favorable. From nearly 3000 cases captured in the SEER database, only tumor grade and stage were found to be independent predictors of survival. Patients surviving 10 years from diagnosis were unlikely to die of disease-related causes.[27] Surgical resection is the primary means of local tumor control.[34,44] Prognosis and the likelihood of local recurrence are correlated with the adequacy of surgical resection.[33,46] Radiation therapy may be useful for treatment of positive surgical margins, but its role has been controversial in treating chondrosarcoma because of the relative resistance of the tumor to radiation therapy.[46] Chemotherapy for advanced or metastatic disease and its utility in variant forms of chondrosarcoma has been of inconsistent value.[30,32,33] As these tumors are relatively resistant to radiation therapy, development of novel therapies is needed to improve disease control, particularly in cases of metastatic disease.[34] Recent genetic and molecular biological studies have identified a variety of gene expressions, signaling pathways, receptors, oncogene mutations, and hormones that may provide targets for the development of novel and specific therapeutic targets.[15,26,31,47,48]

THE ROLE OF IMAGING

Diagnostic imaging provides information critical to local disease staging, identification of distant metastases, monitoring response to therapy, and detecting recurrent disease. Imaging techniques adhering to the ALARA principle (As Low As Reasonably Achievable) must be used that optimize the accuracy of diagnosis and staging while minimizing patient exposure to ionizing radiation.[49–53] Initial evaluation is based on radiographs. MR imaging is typically performed following demonstration of a bone tumor; definitive diagnosis requires histologic analysis.

Staging workup of the primary tumor should ideally be performed prior to biopsy for several reasons.[5,6,54] Postoperative changes can complicate imaging interpretation, therefore the usefulness of postoperative imaging as staging information may be limited. Biopsy is directed by imaging, and the biopsy approach should be coordinated with the surgical approach planned for the

definitive surgical procedure. Such a practice limits the risk of contaminating soft tissues with tumor cells in a region that would not ordinarily be resected. Biopsy from an approach not included in the planned surgical field risks expanding the volume of tissues, ultimately requiring surgical resection.[3] An incisional biopsy is usually performed when malignancy is suspected, to obtain adequate tissue for histologic diagnosis and biological studies. The results of such studies are now incorporated into treatment protocols. Even in experienced hands, the histopathologic diagnosis of these tumors is difficult to achieve from fine-needle aspiration.[55]

Staging evaluation requires identification of all disease sites. Treatment protocols often stratify therapy based on tumor histology, size and location of the primary tumor, involvement of other structures, presence or absence of metastatic sites, and skip lesions. Bone sarcomas metastasize hematogenously primarily to lungs and later to bone. As bone lacks lymphatics, only rarely has involvement of regional lymph nodes been reported, and such a finding is associated with a poor prognosis.[56] Delineation of the primary bone tumor and any involvement of adjacent soft tissues, bony structures, and vascular structures is important not only for disease staging but for monitoring treatment response and planning surgery and, when appropriate, radiation therapy. The entire length of the involved bone must be imaged to accurately define its extent and to detect any skip lesions. Skip lesions represent embolic micrometastasis within marrow sinusoids of the same bone that are discontinuous from the primary tumor (**Fig. 1**).[57] Transarticular skip metastases occur within the joint adjacent to the primary tumor. Skip lesions are usually seen with high-grade sarcomas and are prognostic of poor survival.[56,57] A preliminary report by Bruland and colleagues[58] suggests that at the time of primary diagnosis the presence of micrometastatic bone marrow disease determined by immunomagnetic isolation correlates with clinical stage and disease progression. However, such a technique is not currently in widespread clinical use.

Preliminary diagnosis is based on radiographic findings coupled with the clinical history.[59] Contemporary imaging includes MR of the primary site of disease. The multiplanar capabilities of MR coupled with inherent tissue signal characteristics optimize tumor characterization, define involvement of adjacent soft tissues, delineate intramedullary extent of disease (**Fig. 2**), and determine local or regional metastases. In some cases, MR may redirect clinical management by distinguishing between malignant (**Fig. 3**) and nonmalignant

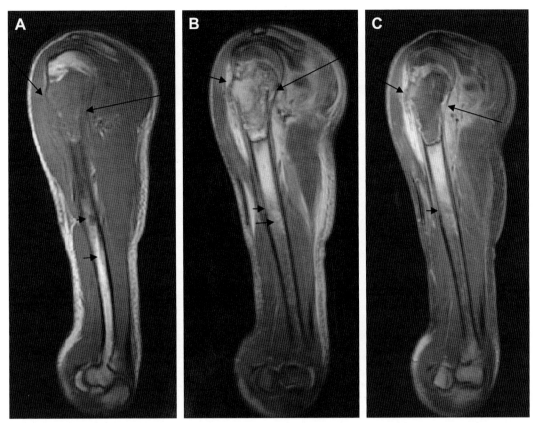

Fig. 1. Skip lesions in a 15-year-old boy with osteosarcoma (*arrows*) of right humerus at diagnosis. Sagittal mid-humeral MR images with (*A*) noncontrast T1-weighted, (*B*) STIR (short-tau inversion recovery), and (*C*) post-contrast fat-saturated T1-weighted sequences. Note mid-humeral diaphyseal focus of tumor (*short arrows*), histologically proven to be a skip metastasis. This lesion is most conspicuous on noncontrast T1-weighted sequence and becomes indistinguishable from adjacent edema in STIR sequence. With contrast enhancement, the skip lesion becomes intense with enhancing edema.

(**Fig. 4**) disease. Dynamic enhanced MR techniques obtained at the time of diagnosis provide baseline information for following tumor response to therapy (**Fig. 5**).[60–62] Thus far, a prognostic role for such techniques based on findings at the time of diagnosis has not been established.[25]

CT of the chest is used for determination of pulmonary metastases. Unfortunately, even with the current quality of technology, the number of CT-determined pulmonary nodules correlates poorly with the number detected surgically, underestimating the number of lesions detected at surgery by 35%.[63] Only rarely can CT characteristics of these nodules be definitive for metastatic disease (**Fig. 6**). Histologic diagnosis is frequently required, as the presence of pulmonary metastases elevates disease staging in bone sarcomas and, thus, alters therapy. CT is helpful in these cases in directing surgical biopsy. Monitoring of response of pulmonary metastases and identification of new lesions is routinely performed with chest CT.

Historically, [99mTc]MDP bone scans were used for delineating sites of distant bone metastases and for monitoring tumor response to therapy (see **Fig. 2**). However, [18F]FDG (a surrogate of glucose metabolism) PET/PET-CT is now being investigated to determine its role in staging and monitoring tumor response and in detecting recurrent and metastatic disease (**Fig. 7**).[64–70] Preliminary results show that [18F]FDG PET/PET-CT may be a sensitive and promising modality for patients with bone sarcomas.[41,66,67,71–73] Investigation by Franzius and colleagues[67] also found that [18F]FDG PET had superior specificity, sensitivity, and accuracy in detecting skeletal metastases compared with bone scintigraphy, but when they analyzed these parameters by histologic diagnosis (ie, osteosarcoma vs Ewing sarcoma), the superiority of [18F]FDG PET varied. Identification of bone metastases by [18F]FDG PET was superior to [99mTc]MDP bone scintigraphy in patients with Ewing sarcoma (sensitivity, specificity, accuracy of [18F]PET, and bone scintigraphy

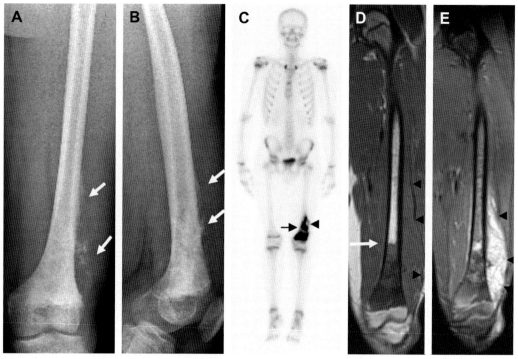

Fig. 2. A 16 year-old boy with osteosarcoma of distal left femur; intramedullary tumor extent is best shown on T1-weighted sequence. Anteroposterior (*A*) and (*B*) lateral views of the left femur show aggressive periosteal reaction (*arrows*) in distal left femur. (*C*) Coronal whole-body [^{99m}Tc]MDP bone scan shows intensive metabolic activity within the intramedullary portion of the tumor (*arrow*) but relative paucity around the periphery of the extracortical extent laterally (*arrowhead*). (*D*) Coronal noncontrast T1-weighted MR sequence exquisitely demonstrates the intramedullary extent of disease. The arrow indicates the sharp transition from normal bright fatty marrow to dark tumor marrow. Arrowheads delineate the soft tissue portion of disease. (*E*) With contrast administration, the soft tissue mass becomes well delineated but the intramedullary transition enhances heterogeneously with marrow enhancement.

of 1.00, 0.96, 0.97 vs 0.68, 0.87, 0.82, respectively). However, in cases of osteosarcoma the investigators found bone scintigraphy to be superior to [^{18}F]FDG PET, having identified 5 metastatic bone lesions not demonstrated by [^{18}F]FDG PET. The ability of [^{18}F]FDG PET/PET-CT to predict tumor grade (particularly with chondrosarcomas) is under investigation.[64,73] The information provided by [^{18}F]FDG PET/PET-CT is particularly useful as a means of assessing metabolic treatment response coupled with anatomic and histologic tumor response.

IMAGING STRATEGY

Regardless of the type of bone sarcoma, imaging is critical to the establishment of diagnosis, staging, and surgical planning, assessment of therapeutic response, and off-therapy monitoring.

Imaging at Diagnosis

Imaging performed at the time of diagnosis must define and characterize the primary bone lesion and its impact on adjacent soft tissues, and determine the presence of metastatic disease. Radiographs provide the primary imaging investigation[3] followed by MR of the primary site of disease. MR imaging must encompass the primary tumor site and the entire bone in which the tumor resides in order to identify any potential skip lesions.[3,5] Though rare (occurring in about 2% to 6.5% of cases of high-grade osteosarcoma and even fewer in Ewing sarcoma), skip lesions impart a significantly worse patient outcome[74–76] and necessitate modification of the surgical procedure (see **Fig. 1**).[75,77] Skip lesions are distinctly separate from the primary tumor, and may occur in proximity to or distal from the primary tumor in the same bone or across the joint.[75,77] [^{99m}Tc] MDP bone scintigraphy has not been shown to be reliable in demonstrating skip metastases[75–77] or other multifocal bone lesions when compared with MR.[78] MR sequences typically comprise noncontrast T1-weighted, fat-saturated T2-weighted, short-tau inversion recovery (STIR), and postcontrast fat-saturated T1-weighted sequences. These

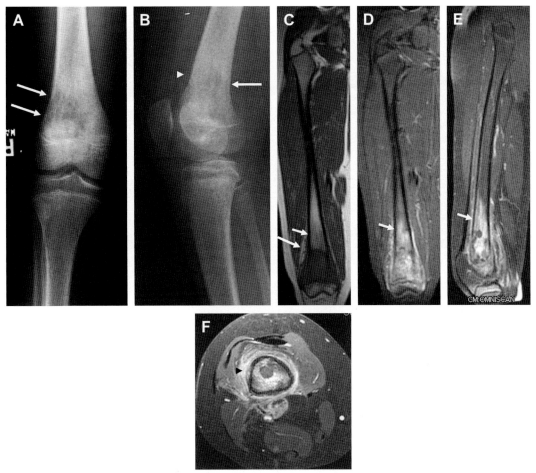

Fig. 3. A 13-year-old girl with a 3-month history of right knee pain, histologically proven to be Ewing sarcoma. Anteroposterior (*A*) and lateral (*B*) radiographs of the right knee show a poorly defined, irregular region of metaphyseal demineralization (*arrows*) with minimal anterior cortical scalloping (*B, arrowhead*). (*C*) Coronal noncontrast T1-weighted MR shows the intramedullary line of demarcation of the tumor (*long arrow*) with mild adjacent poorly defined intramedullary edema (*short arrow*). Coronal STIR (*D*) and sagittal postcontrast T1-weighted image with fat suppression (*E*) demonstrate the extent of the intramedullary enhancing edema (*short arrows*). On these 2 sequences, the increased signal of the edema silhouettes the intramedullary tumor, making delineation of tumor from surrounding edema difficult. The axial postcontrast T1-weighted image with fat saturation (*F*) confirms these findings but also shows tumor extension through the medial cortex (*black arrowhead*). Note the similarities in the appearance of the radiographs, soft tissue, and intramedullary edema in this case with those in **Fig. 4.**

sequences should be performed in at least 2 and preferably 3 planes, with one longitudinal imaging sequence visualizing the entire bone.[5,6,25] Measurement of intramedullary tumor may be difficult in the presence of peritumoral edema. Noncontrast T1-weighted sequence,[79] dynamic enhanced imaging,[38,80] or combining T1-weighted with STIR sequence can be helpful (see **Figs. 1, 3,** and **5**)[81] and may aid in distinguishing tumor from surrounding edema. Most reports of skip lesions address their significance in osteosarcoma. However, the same considerations for imaging and surgical planning apply to the rarely reported cases

of Ewing sarcoma in which skip lesions occur; the reported prognosis of such patients is dismal.[82]

Accurate determination of tumor size is predictive of outcome in osteosarcoma. Absolute (but not relative) tumor volume is associated with a predictive value of overall survival ($P = .018$) and event-free survival ($P = .036$) in pediatric nonmetastatic osteosarcoma of the extremity.[12] Measurement of intramedullary tumor extent is best demonstrated using a longitudinal T1-weighted noncontrast sequence of the involved bone (see **Figs. 2** and **3**).[79] Of particular importance in planning surgical procedures is determination of

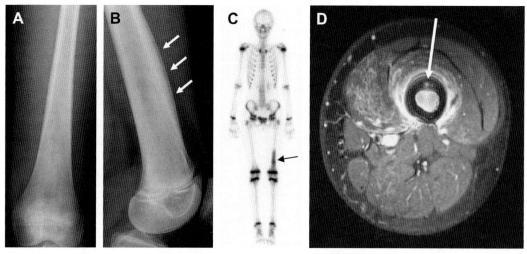

Fig. 4. A 9-year-old girl underwent evaluation for left thigh pain of several weeks' duration with presumed diagnosis of Ewing sarcoma family of tumors. Anteroposterior (*A*) and (*B*) lateral radiographs of the left femur demonstrate subtle heterogeneous mineralization and layered periosteal reaction along the anterior diaphysis (*arrows*). These findings correlate with increased metabolic activity shown on the corresponding [99mTc]MDP bone scan (*C*). Within the increased activity, the left distal femur is a focus of more intense activity (*arrow*). (*D*) This focus correlates with the tiny cortical abscess demonstrated on axial contrast-enhanced MR (*arrow*) with fat saturation, indicating osteomyelitis and confirmed by biopsy.

tumor extension across the physis and into the epiphysis. Similarly, tumor size at the time of diagnosis of Ewing sarcoma is prognostically significant for patient outcome; volumetrically smaller tumors are associated with improved disease-free survival.[25]

Dynamic enhanced MR of the primary site of disease serves as an indicator of tumor perfusion, microcirculation, and tumor interstitium. It serves as a surrogate variable for assessing drug delivery[60–62,72] but is not currently available for routine clinical use. This technique is an additional prognostic factor predictive of disease-free survival in patients receiving chemotherapy for osteosarcoma (P = .035).[60,62] A higher initial regional access of contrast was associated with greater disease-free survival.[61] With growing investigation of antiangiogenesis factors as therapeutic agents, the use and value of dynamic enhancement may become a key imaging technique in routine monitoring of chemotherapy perfusion of tumor and treatment response.

A prognostically significant role of [18F]FDG PET/PET-CT based on the intensity of metabolic activity in the primary tumor at the time of diagnosis has been suggested. Franzius and colleagues[66] found that the maximum intensity of tumor to nontumor uptake in osteosarcoma was statistically significantly correlated with overall ($P<$.05) and event-free survival ($P<$.005); high metabolic activity correlated with poor outcome. Large prospective studies are needed to further

define the role of [18F]FDG PET/PET-CT in the management of patients with osteosarcoma.

In addition to defining the primary tumor, metastatic disease must also be determined for complete staging. Chest CT is used for detection of pulmonary metastatic disease. Chest CT is considerably more sensitive than chest radiography for detecting small pulmonary metastases.[6] PET/PET-CT shows strong promise for detecting distant metastases in cases of bone sarcoma (see **Fig. 7**), but is not without limitations. It has been shown to have up to 100% sensitivity in detecting distant metastatic sites, but detection of pulmonary lesions smaller than 5 mm in diameter typically fall below the resolution threshold of PET/PET-CT.[83,84] Pulmonary nodules between 5 and 9 mm in size are often undetectable with PET-CT.[83] In addition, metabolic activity in benign lesions, in sites of infection, and in normal structures, particularly in pediatric patients, may complicate interpretation of FDG activity.[83,85–87] Thus, spiral CT remains the most sensitive modality currently available for detection of pulmonary metastases.[83,86]

Detection of distant skeletal metastases has historically been performed with bone scintigraphy, preferably using the single-photon emission CT technique.[6] However, the use of [18F]FDG PET or PET-CT has grown over the past several years for staging bone sarcomas.[3,6,88] In comparison with CT and MR, PET/PET-CT has been shown to be superior in detecting skeletal and soft tissue

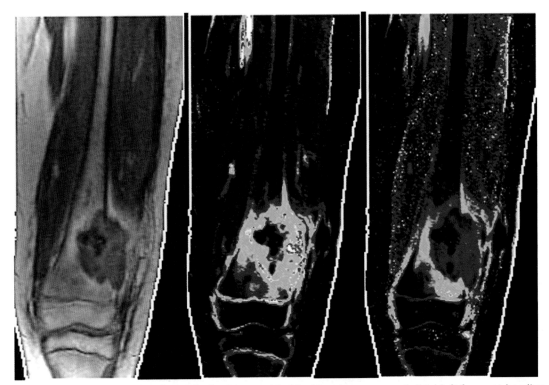

Fig. 5. Dynamic enhanced MRI (DEMRI) of a 14-year-old girl with osteosarcoma of distal left femur at baseline evaluation. The left-hand image is the final T1-weighted contrast-enhanced dynamic set. Quantitative T1 relaxation measures before contrast (*middle image*) and dynamic contrast-enhanced MR (*right-hand image*) were both acquired as 16-slice 3-dimensional acquisitions with 5-mm thick sections covering the full extent of the tumor. A representative section from the center of the imaging volume is shown. The middle image is the K_{trans} (transfer rate constant for contrast transfer from plasma to extracellular space [min^{-1}]) image. The right-hand image is *ve* (fractional extracellular/extravascular space). (*Courtesy of* Wilburn E. Reddick, PhD.)

metastases.[6,68,84,89,90] PET/PET-CT may also be valuable in detecting skeletal metastases that demonstrate no abnormal activity by [^{99m}Tc]MDP bone scans.[88]

Whole-body MR techniques are currently under investigation for the detection of skeletal metastases. Daldrup-Link and colleagues[65] studied 39 pediatric patients ranging in age from 2 to 19 years (osteosarcoma n = 3, Ewing sarcoma n = 20, other n = 16). Using whole-body spin-echo MR, they found MR to have a higher sensitivity than [^{99m}Tc]MDP bone scans but lower sensitivity than [^{18}F]FDG PET/PET-CT in detecting bone metastases.

Imaging During Therapy

Because most pediatric patients are treated according to established therapeutic protocols, imaging timing is standardized by tumor type and treatment protocol. Additional imaging may be performed for clinical indications that arise outside of the protocol study design. Key factors to be addressed include change in size of the primary tumor, change in tumor imaging characteristics such as extent of necrosis, ossification, and vascularity, response of metastases identified at the time of diagnosis, determination of new metastatic sites, and identification of treatment sequelae. Establishment of new disease and/or progression of existing disease may prompt a change in planned therapy.

Static MR imaging provides the backbone for monitoring disease response to therapy for pediatric bone sarcomas. The clinical significance of a change in size depends on the primary tumor type. Osteosarcoma decreases little in size during therapy,[91] due to the dense osteoid. Historically, radiographic demonstration of increased ossification and improved demarcation of the soft tissue component indicated a favorable therapeutic response. However, neither radiographs nor CT are able to delineate viable residual from nonviable disease.[91]

In contrast to osteosarcoma, therapeutic response of Ewing sarcomas is indicated by a decrease in

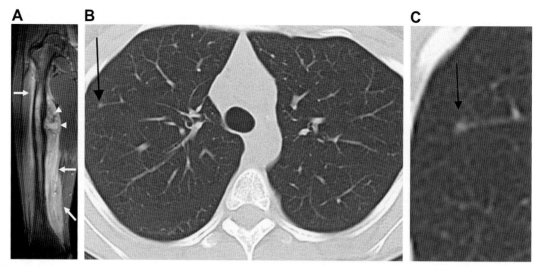

Fig. 6. A 14-year-old girl underwent evaluation of a 2-month history of right thigh pain and swelling. She was diagnosed with high-grade right femoral periosteal osteosarcoma (*arrowheads*). (*A*) Coronal STIR image of the right thigh demonstrates massive edema (*arrows*) extensively involving the adductor muscles and to a lesser extent, abductor muscles. (*B, C*) Staging chest CT revealed a nonspecific 4-mm nodule in the right upper lobe (*arrow*), which was histologically proved to be acute necrotizing granuloma with bronchiolitis but with no evidence of malignancy.

tumor volume.[91,92] A reduction of less than 25% in tumor size and/or residual soft tissue mass correlated with a poor response.[92] Investigators found no correlation with signal intensity or its change during chemotherapy and histopathologic response.[92]

A change in the extent and pattern of peritumoral edema has been explored as another imaging variable in assessing tumor response to therapy. MR demonstration of a decrease in peritumoral edema has been suggested as a favorable sign of chemotherapeutic response in cases of osteosarcoma[38,93–95] and Ewing sarcoma[92] alike.

Dynamic enhanced MR sequences demonstrating and quantifying the degree of tumor necrosis as an indicator of biological response is also now possible (see **Fig. 5**).[60–62,96] The slope of linear regression of the regional access of contrast is predictive of disease-free survival. After preoperative chemotherapy, Reddick and colleagues[61] showed that a lower regional access of contrast to tumor was predictive of better outcome in primary osteosarcoma. Similar findings have been reported in series of both osteosarcoma and Ewing sarcoma.[96] MR-determined percentage of tumoral necrosis in both osteosarcoma and Ewing sarcoma correlates well with histopathologic determination of tumor necrosis.[92,96]

Also undergoing assessment of its role in determining biological response to therapy in bone sarcomas is PET/PET-CT.[72,97] The greatest experience with this technique in bone sarcomas is

using [^{18}F]FDG. A favorable response to therapy is indicated by a decrease in metabolic activity in tumor sites that correlates with reduced tumor cell viability.[41,71,72,97] Brenner and colleagues[71] found that patients at increased risk for local disease recurrence or development of metastatic disease could be identified by combining the pretreatment SUV and histopathologic tumor grade. Other investigators found that a reduction in tumor to nontumor ratios of [^{18}F]FDG PET exceeding 30% was associated with good response to chemotherapy and that [^{18}F]FDG PET was superior to [^{99m}Tc]MDP bone scans in determining histologic response to therapy in pediatric cases.[97] Similarly, Hawkins and colleagues[98] found that the initial response to therapy may be predictive of outcome as measured by a decrease in SUV after induction chemotherapy in Ewing sarcoma. These investigators failed to find the same prognostic significance in cases of osteosarcoma.[99] More recently the sensitivity, specificity, and accuracy of PET-CT was found to be superior to PET alone in staging and following patients with Ewing sarcoma.[68] The long-term prognostic value of such information has yet to be fully established.

The roles for disease staging, tumor grading, and assessment of therapeutic response of additional radiopharmaceutical agents such as [^{11}C]methionine[72,100] and 3'-deoxy-3'-[^{18}F]fluoro-thymidine ([^{18}F]FLT) are currently under investigation.[41,72,101–104] Preliminary work by Buck

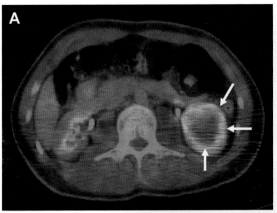
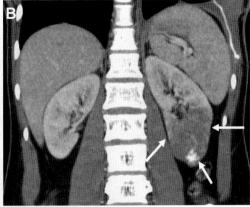
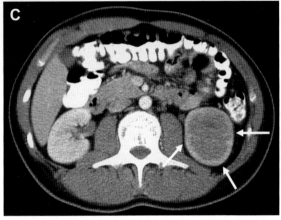

Fig. 7. An 18-year-old man treated 6 years earlier for osteosarcoma of the right tibia underwent surveillance PET-CT for monitoring of disease recurrence. (A) Fused PET-CT image showing metabolically active metastatic osteosarcoma of the lower pole left kidney (arrows). (B) Coronal and (C) axial reformatted images from a contrast-enhanced diagnostic abdominal CT scan show the large left lower pole renal mass with tumor calcifications (arrows).

and colleagues[102] found that [^{18}F]FLT identified all malignant bone and soft tissue tumors and effectively discriminated between low-grade and high-grade tumors when a maximum SUV of 2.0 was used as the cutoff value. As already discussed, noninvasive assessment and monitoring of disease is optimized by merging biological tumor activity with anatomic characteristics. Under development is merging of biological information of PET with the refined anatomic and dynamic imaging of MR, resulting in PET-MR (Fig. 8).[105–107]

Imaging During Follow-Up

Despite advances in staging and treatment of bone sarcomas, approximately 30% of patients with osteosarcoma will develop disease relapse, most often involving the lungs.[17,108] Local relapse in patients with nonmetastatic extremity osteosarcoma is independently associated with tumor

response to therapy, inadequacy of surgical margins,[109] tumor volume, age at diagnosis, and histologic subtype.[10] Most instances of disease relapse develop within 2 to 3 years of diagnosis but relapse beyond 4 years does occur.[10,70,110]

Of patients treated for Ewing sarcoma, 30% to 40% can be expected to develop local and/or distant recurrent disease typically occurring between 2 and 10 years after diagnosis. However, rare cases of delayed recurrence at 16 and 19 years after diagnosis have been reported.[111] More than half of these patients will have pulmonary or skeletal disease.[23] The recent report from the Childhood Cancer Survivor Study found that survivors of pediatric Ewing sarcoma had the highest 20-year cumulative incidence of recurrent disease amongst 8 pediatric tumor categories, estimated at 13% (95% confidence interval 9.4–16.5).[110] Local recurrent disease from chondrosarcoma is not uncommon, but distant metastases are rare and may develop years after initial

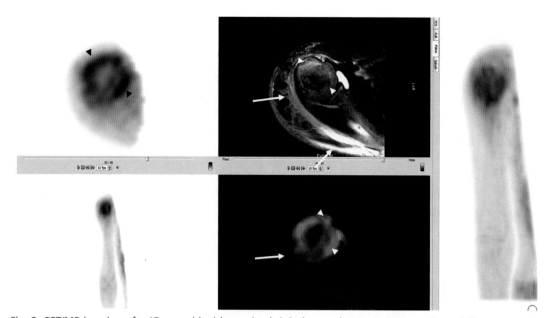

Fig. 8. PET/MR imaging of a 15-year-old with proximal right humeral osteosarcoma at time of diagnosis. Multi-planar PET-CT images through the right humerus and axial fat-saturated T2-weighted image through the proximal humeral osteosarcoma merged with a comparable image from reconstructed PET-CT study shows intense abnormal metabolic activity, most prominent around the periphery of the tumor (*arrowheads*). Note the relative absence of metabolic activity in the associated soft tissue edema (*arrows*). (*Courtesy of* Barry S. Shulkin, MD, MBA.)

treatment.[9] Thus patients with bone sarcomas are monitored for at least 5 years after diagnosis.[9] Recent guidelines from the Children's Oncology Group Bone Tumor Committee suggest 10 years of follow-up for the monitoring of primary and metastatic disease.[6]

Local disease recurrence is often suspected clinically because the patient returns with pain or development of a mass. Radiographs remain the front-line imaging study of the primary skeletal disease site and of those suspected of metastatic involvement, providing important information regarding prosthesis integrity in patients who have undergone limb-sparing procedures.[112] Further, radiographs are useful for demonstrating processes that may symptomatically mimic disease recurrence, such as fractures. Imaging with MR, CT, PET/PET-CT, and even [99mTc]MDP bone scans provide information important for disease characterization and detection of distant metastases. Asymmetric weight bearing related to prior surgery, radiation therapy, or the use of a prosthesis make

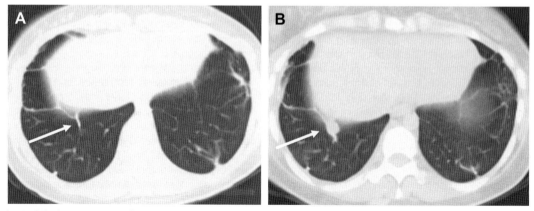

Fig. 9. (*A*) Chest CT was performed 2 months after thoracotomy for pulmonary metastectomy and revealed tumor recurrence in right lower lobe scar (*arrow*). (*B*) Note nodular expansion within the scar. (*Courtesy of* M. Beth McCarville, MD.)

interpretation of PET/PET-CT and [^{99m}Tc]MDP bone scans more difficult.[9] Sensitivity, specificity, and accuracy of PET detection of bone sarcoma recurrence are reported to be 0.96, 0.81, and 0.90, respectively, and exceed those of conventional imaging techniques (1.00, 0.56, and 0,82, respectively).[113]

Interpretation of the imaging findings may be complicated by prior treatment. The usefulness of CT and MR in detecting new or assessing known recurrence may be compromised in the presence of a metallic prosthesis that creates significant artifact. Metallic artifact can be decreased in MR by using T1-weighted turbo spin echo and turbo STIR with high bandwidth and short echo times.[114] Chest CT is performed serially for several years after diagnosis. The frequency varies somewhat by treatment protocol and tumor type, and are typically performed every 4 to 6 months for several years followed subsequently by less frequent monitoring.[9] CT is unable to distinguish between benign and metastatic pulmonary nodules in children with known malignant solid tumors.[115] A similar dilemma occurs in patients who have previously undergone a thoracotomy (Fig. 9). In one series of pediatric osteosarcoma patients, pulmonary nodules recurred in 32 of 35 patients with a history of prior thoracotomy. The only finding consistently found to indicate recurrent metastatic disease was progression of pleural thickening. The investigators also found that the development of a pulmonary nodule in the lung contralateral to the prior thoracotomy was most often malignant.[116]

SUMMARY

Diagnostic imaging is a critical component in the multidisciplinary management of pediatric bone sarcomas. From diagnosis through post-therapy monitoring, imaging identifies disease, monitors tumor response to therapy, and guides follow-up intervention. The evolution of imaging techniques that combine biological and anatomic information is ongoing and should further augment pediatric oncologic care.

ACKNOWLEDGMENTS

The author thanks Dr Stephen F. Miller for critical review of the manuscript and Sandra Gaither for manuscript preparation.

REFERENCES

1. Caudill JS, Arndt CA. Diagnosis and management of bone malignancy in adolescence. Adolesc Med State Art Rev 2007;18(1):62–78, ix.

2. Ludwig JA. Ewing sarcoma: historical perspectives, current state-of-the-art, and opportunities for targeted therapy in the future. Curr Opin Oncol 2008;20(4):412–8.

3. Federman N, Bernthal N, Eilber FC, et al. The multidisciplinary management of osteosarcoma. Curr Treat Options Oncol 2009;10(1–2):82–93.

4. Murphey MD, Walker EA, Wilson AJ, et al. From the archives of the AFIP: imaging of primary chondrosarcoma: radiologic-pathologic correlation. Radiographics 2003;23(5):1245–78.

5. Wootton-Gorges SL. MR imaging of primary bone tumors and tumor-like conditions in children. Magn Reson Imaging Clin N Am 2009;17(3):469–87, vi.

6. Meyer JS, Nadel HR, Marina N, et al. Imaging guidelines for children with Ewing sarcoma and osteosarcoma: a report from the Children's Oncology Group Bone Tumor Committee. Pediatr Blood Cancer 2008;51(2):163–70.

7. Longhi A, Errani C, De Paolis M, et al. Primary bone osteosarcoma in the pediatric age: state of the art. Cancer Treat Rev 2006;32(6):423–36.

8. Mirabello L, Troisi RJ, Savage SA. Osteosarcoma incidence and survival rates from 1973 to 2004: data from the Surveillance, Epidemiology, and End Results Program. Cancer 2009;115(7):1531–43.

9. Link MP, Gebhardt MC, Mark PC. Osteosarcoma. In: Pizzo PA, Poplack DG, editors. Principles & practice of pediatric oncology. 5th edition. Philadelphia: Lippincott Williams & Wilkins; 2010.

10. Ferrari S, Bertoni F, Mercuri M, et al. Predictive factors of disease-free survival for non-metastatic osteosarcoma of the extremity: an analysis of 300 patients treated at the Rizzoli Institute. Ann Oncol 2001;12(8):1145–50.

11. Lee JA, Kim MS, Kim DH, et al. Relative tumor burden predicts metastasis-free survival in pediatric osteosarcoma. Pediatr Blood Cancer 2008;50(2):195–200.

12. Kaste SC, Liu T, Billups CA, et al. Tumor size as a predictor of outcome in pediatric non-metastatic osteosarcoma of the extremity. Pediatr Blood Cancer 2004;43(7):723–8.

13. Pahade J, Sekhar A, Shetty SK. Imaging of malignant skeletal tumors. Cancer Treat Res 2008;143:367–422.

14. Kaste SC, Fuller CE, Saharia A, et al. Pediatric surface osteosarcoma: clinical, pathologic, and radiologic features. Pediatr Blood Cancer 2006;47(2):152–62.

15. Papachristou DJ, Papavassiliou AG. Osteosarcoma and chondrosarcoma: new signaling pathways as targets for novel therapeutic interventions. Int J Biochem Cell Biol 2007;39(5):857–62.

16. Lewis VO. What's new in musculoskeletal oncology. J Bone Joint Surg Am 2009;91(6):1546–56.

17. Heare T, Hensley MA, Dell'Orfano S. Bone tumors: osteosarcoma and Ewing's sarcoma. Curr Opin Pediatr 2009;21(3):365–72.

18. Jawad MU, Cheung MC, Min ES, et al. Ewing sarcoma demonstrates racial disparities in incidence-related and sex-related differences in outcome: an analysis of 1631 cases from the SEER database, 1973–2005. Cancer 2009;115(15):3526–36.

19. Leavey PJ, Collier AB. Ewing sarcoma: prognostic criteria, outcomes and future treatment. Expert Rev Anticancer Ther 2008;8(4):617–24.

20. Bacci G, Ferrari S, Bertoni F, et al. Prognostic factors in nonmetastatic Ewing's sarcoma of bone treated with adjuvant chemotherapy: analysis of 359 patients at the Istituto Ortopedico Rizzoli. J Clin Oncol 2000;18(1):4–11.

21. Grier HE, Krailo MD, Tarbell NJ, et al. Addition of ifosfamide and etoposide to standard chemotherapy for Ewing's sarcoma and primitive neuroectodermal tumor of bone. N Engl J Med 2003; 348(8):694–701.

22. Lin PP, Jaffe N, Herzog CE, et al. Chemotherapy response is an important predictor of local recurrence in Ewing sarcoma. Cancer 2007;109(3):603–11.

23. Cotterill SJ, Ahrens S, Paulussen M, et al. Prognostic factors in Ewing's tumor of bone: analysis of 975 patients from the European Intergroup Cooperative Ewing's Sarcoma Study Group. J Clin Oncol 2000;18(17):3108–14.

24. Bacci G, Longhi A, Ferrari S, et al. Prognostic factors in non-metastatic Ewing's sarcoma tumor of bone: an analysis of 579 patients treated at a single institution with adjuvant or neoadjuvant chemotherapy between 1972 and 1998. Acta Oncol 2006;45(4):469–75.

25. Miller SL, Hoffer FA, Reddick WE, et al. Tumor volume or dynamic contrast-enhanced MRI for prediction of clinical outcome of Ewing sarcoma family of tumors. Pediatr Radiol 2001;31(7):518–23.

26. Chow WA. Update on chondrosarcomas. Curr Opin Oncol 2007;19(4):371–6.

27. Giuffrida AY, Burgueno JE, Koniaris LG, et al. Chondrosarcoma in the United States (1973 to 2003): an analysis of 2890 cases from the SEER database. J Bone Joint Surg Am 2009;91(5):1063–72.

28. Damron TA, Ward WG, Stewart A. Osteosarcoma, chondrosarcoma, and Ewing's sarcoma: National Cancer Data Base Report. Clin Orthop Relat Res 2007;459:40–7.

29. Puri A, Shah M, Agarwal MG, et al. Chondrosarcoma of bone: does the size of the tumor, the presence of a pathologic fracture, or prior intervention have an impact on local control and survival? J Cancer Res Ther 2009;5(1):14–9.

30. Riedel RF, Larrier N, Dodd L, et al. The clinical management of chondrosarcoma. Curr Treat Options Oncol 2009;10(1–2):94–106.

31. Bovee JV. Multiple osteochondromas. Orphanet J Rare Dis 2008;3:3.

32. Gelderblom H, Hogendoorn PC, Dijkstra SD, et al. The clinical approach towards chondrosarcoma. Oncologist 2008;13(3):320–9.

33. Ryzewicz M, Manaster BJ, Naar E, et al. Low-grade cartilage tumors: diagnosis and treatment. Orthopedics 2007;30(1):35–46.

34. Hallor KH, Staaf J, Bovee JV, et al. Genomic profiling of chondrosarcoma: chromosomal patterns in central and peripheral tumors. Clin Cancer Res 2009;15(8):2685–94.

35. Ahmed AR, Tan TS, Unni KK, et al. Secondary chondrosarcoma in osteochondroma: report of 107 patients. Clin Orthop Relat Res 2003;411: 193–206.

36. Littrell LA, Wenger DE, Wold LE, et al. Radiographic, CT, and MR imaging features of dedifferentiated chondrosarcomas: a retrospective review of 174 de novo cases. Radiographics 2004;24(5): 1397–409.

37. Collins MS, Koyama T, Swee RG, et al. Clear cell chondrosarcoma: radiographic, computed tomographic, and magnetic resonance findings in 34 patients with pathologic correlation. Skeletal Radiol 2003;32(12):687–94.

38. James SL, Panicek DM, Davies AM. Bone marrow oedema associated with benign and malignant bone tumours. Eur J Radiol 2008;67(1):11–21.

39. Janzen L, Logan PM, O'Connell JX, et al. Intramedullary chondroid tumors of bone: correlation of abnormal peritumoral marrow and soft-tissue MRI signal with tumor type. Skeletal Radiol 1997;26(2): 100–6.

40. Geirnaerdt MJ, Hogendoorn PC, Bloem JL, et al. Cartilaginous tumors: fast contrast-enhanced MR imaging. Radiology 2000;214(2):539–46.

41. Feldman F, Van HR, Saxena C, et al. 18FDG-PET applications for cartilage neoplasms. Skeletal Radiol 2005;34(7):367–74.

42. Papachristou DJ, Gkretsi V, Rao UN, et al. Expression of integrin-linked kinase and its binding partners in chondrosarcoma: association with prognostic significance. Eur J Cancer 2008;44(16):2518–25.

43. Cesari M, Bertoni F, Bacchini P, et al. Mesenchymal chondrosarcoma. An analysis of patients treated at a single institution. Tumori 2007;93(5):423–7.

44. Dantonello TM, Int-Veen C, Leuschner I, et al. Mesenchymal chondrosarcoma of soft tissues and bone in children, adolescents, and young adults: experiences of the CWS and COSS study groups. Cancer 2008;112(11):2424–31.

45. Chaabane S, Bouaziz MC, Drissi C, et al. Periosteal chondrosarcoma. AJR Am J Roentgenol 2009; 192(1):W1–6.

46. Weber KL. What's new in musculoskeletal oncology. J Bone Joint Surg Am 2005;87(6):1400–10.

47. Schrage YM, Machado I, Meijer D, et al. COX-2 expression in chondrosarcoma: a role for celecoxib treatment? Eur J Cancer 2010;46(3):616–24.

48. Wunder JS, Nielsen TO, Maki RG, et al. Opportunities for improving the therapeutic ratio for patients with sarcoma. Lancet Oncol 2007;8(6):513–24.

49. Hall EJ. Radiation biology for pediatric radiologists. Pediatr Radiol 2009;39(Suppl 1):S57–64.

50. King MA, Kanal KM, Relyea-Chew A, et al. Radiation exposure from pediatric head CT: a bi-institutional study. Pediatr Radiol 2009;39(10):1059–65.

51. Paterson A, Frush DP. Dose reduction in paediatric MDCT: general principles. Clin Radiol 2007;62(6): 507–17.

52. Semelka RC, Armao DM, Elias J Jr, et al. Imaging strategies to reduce the risk of radiation in CT studies, including selective substitution with MRI. J Magn Reson Imaging 2007;25(5):900–9.

53. Voss SD, Reaman GH, Kaste SC, et al. The ALARA concept in pediatric oncology. Pediatr Radiol 2009; 39(11):1142–6.

54. Brisse HJ. Staging of common paediatric tumours. Pediatr Radiol 2009;39(Suppl 3):482–90.

55. Pohar-Marinsek Z. Difficulties in diagnosing small round cell tumours of childhood from fine needle aspiration cytology samples. Cytopathology 2008; 19(2):67–79.

56. Brennan MF, Singer S, Maki RG, et al. Soft tissue sarcoma. In: DeVita VT Jr, Lawrence TS, Rosenberg SA, editors. Devita, Hellman & Rosenberg's cancer: principles & practice of oncology. 8th edition. Philadelphia: Lippincott Williams & Wilkins; 2010.

57. Kager L, Zoubek A, Kastner U, et al. Skip metastases in osteosarcoma: experience of the Cooperative Osteosarcoma Study Group. J Clin Oncol 2006;24(10):1535–41.

58. Bruland OS, Hoifodt H, Hall KS, et al. Bone marrow micrometastases studied by an immunomagnetic isolation procedure in extremity localized non-metastatic osteosarcoma patients. Cancer Treat Res 2010;152:509–15.

59. Bielack SS, Carrle D. State-of-the-art approach in selective curable tumors: bone sarcoma. Ann Oncol 2008;19(Suppl 7):vii155–60.

60. Reddick WE, Bhargava R, Taylor JS, et al. Dynamic contrast-enhanced MR imaging evaluation of osteosarcoma response to neoadjuvant chemotherapy. J Magn Reson Imaging 1995;5(6):689–94.

61. Reddick WE, Taylor JS, Fletcher BD. Dynamic MR imaging (DEMRI) of microcirculation in bone sarcoma. J Magn Reson Imaging 1999;10(3):277–85.

62. Reddick WE, Wang S, Xiong X, et al. Dynamic magnetic resonance imaging of regional contrast access as an additional prognostic factor in pediatric osteosarcoma. Cancer 2001;91(12): 2230–7.

63. Kayton ML, Huvos AG, Casher J, et al. Computed tomographic scan of the chest underestimates the number of metastatic lesions in osteosarcoma. J Pediatr Surg 2006;41(1):200–6.

64. Charest M, Hickeson M, Lisbona R, et al. FDG PET/CT imaging in primary osseous and soft tissue sarcomas: a retrospective review of 212 cases. Eur J Nucl Med Mol Imaging 2009;36(12):1944–51.

65. Daldrup-Link HE, Franziuss C, Link TM, et al. Whole-body MR imaging for detection of bone metastases in children and young adults: comparison with skeletal scintigraphy and FDG PET. AJR Am J Roentgenol 2001;177(1):229–36.

66. Franzius C, Bielack S, Flege S, et al. Prognostic significance of (18)F-FDG and (99m)Tc-methylene diphosphonate uptake in primary osteosarcoma. J Nucl Med 2002;43(8):1012–7.

67. Franzius C, Sciuk J, Daldrup-Link HE, et al. FDG-PET for detection of osseous metastases from malignant primary bone tumours: comparison with bone scintigraphy. Eur J Nucl Med 2000;27(9):1305–11.

68. Gerth HU, Juergens KU, Dirksen U, et al. Significant benefit of multimodal imaging: PET/CT compared with PET alone in staging and follow-up of patients with Ewing tumors. J Nucl Med 2007;48(12):1932–9.

69. Mar WA, Taljanovic MS, Bagatell R, et al. Update on imaging and treatment of Ewing sarcoma family tumors: what the radiologist needs to know. J Comput Assist Tomogr 2008;32(1):108–18.

70. Stauss J, Franzius C, Pfluger T, et al. Guidelines for 18F-FDG PET and PET-CT imaging in paediatric oncology. Eur J Nucl Med Mol Imaging 2008; 35(8):1581–8.

71. Brenner W, Conrad EU, Eary JF. FDG PET imaging for grading and prediction of outcome in chondrosarcoma patients. Eur J Nucl Med Mol Imaging 2004;31(2):189–95.

72. Landa J, Schwartz LH. Contemporary imaging in sarcoma. Oncologist 2009;14(10):1021–38.

73. Lee FY, Yu J, Chang SS, et al. Diagnostic value and limitations of fluorine-18 fluorodeoxyglucose positron emission tomography for cartilaginous tumors of bone. J Bone Joint Surg Am 2004;86(12): 2677–85.

74. Jeon DG, Kim MS, Cho WH, et al. Clinical outcome of osteosarcoma with primary total femoral resection. Clin Orthop Relat Res 2007;457:176–82.

75. Leavey PJ, Day MD, Booth T, et al. Skip metastasis in osteosarcoma. J Pediatr Hematol Oncol 2003; 25(10):806–8.

76. Sajadi KR, Heck RK, Neel MD, et al. The incidence and prognosis of osteosarcoma skip metastases. Clin Orthop Relat Res 2004;426:92–6.

77. Bhagia SM, Grimer RJ, Davies AM, et al. Scintigraphically negative skip metastasis in osteosarcoma. Eur Radiol 1997;7(9):1446–8.

78. Mentzel HJ, Kentouche K, Sauner D, et al. Comparison of whole-body STIR-MRI and ^{99m}Tc-methylene-diphosphonate scintigraphy in children with suspected multifocal bone lesions. Eur Radiol 2004;14(12):2297–302.

79. Onikul E, Fletcher BD, Parham DM, et al. Accuracy of MR imaging for estimating intraosseous extent of osteosarcoma. AJR Am J Roentgenol 1996;167(5):1211–5.

80. Iwasawa T, Tanaka Y, Aida N, et al. Microscopic intraosseous extension of osteosarcoma: assessment on dynamic contrast-enhanced MRI. Skeletal Radiol 1997;26(4):214–21.

81. Hoffer FA, Nikanorov AY, Reddick WE, et al. Accuracy of MR imaging for detecting epiphyseal extension of osteosarcoma. Pediatr Radiol 2000;30(5):289–98.

82. Jiya TU, Wuisman PI. Long-term follow-up of 15 patients with non-metastatic Ewing's sarcoma and a skip lesion. Acta Orthop 2005;76(6):899–903.

83. Franzius C, Daldrup-Link HE, Sciuk J, et al. FDG-PET for detection of pulmonary metastases from malignant primary bone tumors: comparison with spiral CT. Ann Oncol 2001;12(4):479–86.

84. Kumar R, Chauhan A, Vellimana AK, et al. Role of PET/PET-CT in the management of sarcomas. Expert Rev Anticancer Ther 2006;6(8):1241–50.

85. Bestic JM, Peterson JJ, Bancroft LW. Pediatric FDG PET/CT: Physiologic uptake, normal variants, and benign conditions [corrected]. Radiographics 2009;29(5):1487–500.

86. Franzius C, Juergens KU. PET/CT in paediatric oncology: indications and pitfalls. Pediatr Radiol 2009;39(Suppl 3):446–9.

87. Shammas A, Lim R, Charron M. Pediatric FDG PET/CT: physiologic uptake, normal variants, and benign conditions. Radiographics 2009;29(5):1467–86.

88. Benz MR, Tchekmedyian N, Eilber FC, et al. Utilization of positron emission tomography in the management of patients with sarcoma. Curr Opin Oncol 2009;21(4):345–51.

89. Kleis M, Daldrup-Link H, Matthay K, et al. Diagnostic value of PET/CT for the staging and restaging of pediatric tumors. Eur J Nucl Med Mol Imaging 2009;36(1):23–36.

90. Volker T, Denecke T, Steffen I, et al. Positron emission tomography for staging of pediatric sarcoma patients: results of a prospective multicenter trial. J Clin Oncol 2007;25(34):5435–41.

91. Shapeero LG, Vanel D. Imaging evaluation of the response of high-grade osteosarcoma and Ewing sarcoma to chemotherapy with emphasis on dynamic contrast-enhanced magnetic resonance imaging. Semin Musculoskelet Radiol 2000;4(1):137–46.

92. van der Woude HJ, Bloem JL, Holscher HC, et al. Monitoring the effect of chemotherapy in Ewing's sarcoma of bone with MR imaging. Skeletal Radiol 1994;23(7):493–500.

93. Fletcher BD. Response of osteosarcoma and Ewing sarcoma to chemotherapy: imaging evaluation. AJR Am J Roentgenol 1991;157(4):825–33.

94. Holscher HC, Bloem JL, Vanel D, et al. Osteosarcoma: chemotherapy-induced changes at MR imaging. Radiology 1992;182(3):839–44.

95. Pan G, Raymond AK, Carrasco CH, et al. Osteosarcoma: MR imaging after preoperative chemotherapy. Radiology 1990;174(2):517–26.

96. Dyke JP, Panicek DM, Healey JH, et al. Osteogenic and Ewing sarcomas: estimation of necrotic fraction during induction chemotherapy with dynamic contrast-enhanced MR imaging. Radiology 2003;228(1):271–8.

97. Franzius C, Sciuk J, Brinkschmidt C, et al. Evaluation of chemotherapy response in primary bone tumors with F-18 FDG positron emission tomography compared with histologically assessed tumor necrosis. Clin Nucl Med 2000;25(11):874–81.

98. Hawkins DS, Schuetze SM, Butrynski JE, et al. [^{18}F] Fluorodeoxyglucose positron emission tomography predicts outcome for Ewing sarcoma family of tumors. J Clin Oncol 2005;23(34):8828–34.

99. Hawkins DS, Conrad EU III, Butrynski JE, et al. [F-18]-fluorodeoxy-D-glucose-positron emission tomography response is associated with outcome for extremity osteosarcoma in children and young adults. Cancer 2009;115(15):3519–25.

100. Ghigi G, Micera R, Maffione AM, et al. ^{11}C-methionine vs. ^{18}F-FDG PET in soft tissue sarcoma patients treated with neoadjuvant therapy: preliminary results. In Vivo 2009;23(1):105–10.

101. Arvanitis C, Bendapudi PK, Tseng JR, et al. (18)F and (18)FDG PET imaging of osteosarcoma to non-invasively monitor in situ changes in cellular proliferation and bone differentiation upon MYC inactivation. Cancer Biol Ther 2008;7(12):1947–51.

102. Buck AK, Herrmann K, Buschenfelde CM, et al. Imaging bone and soft tissue tumors with the proliferation marker [^{18}F]fluorodeoxythymidine. Clin Cancer Res 2008;14(10):2970–7.

103. Cobben DC, Elsinga PH, Suurmeijer AJ, et al. Detection and grading of soft tissue sarcomas of the extremities with (18)F-3'-fluoro-3'-deoxy-L-thymidine. Clin Cancer Res 2004;10(5):1685–90.

104. Leyton J, Latigo JR, Perumal M, et al. Early detection of tumor response to chemotherapy by 3'-deoxy-3'-[^{18}F]fluorothymidine positron emission tomography: the effect of cisplatin on a fibrosarcoma tumor model in vivo. Cancer Res 2005;65(10):4202–10.

105. Wehrl HF, Judenhofer MS, Wiehr S, et al. Pre-clinical PET/MR: technological advances and new perspectives in biomedical research. Eur J Nucl Med Mol Imaging 2009;36(Suppl 1):S56–68.

106. Wehrl HF, Sauter AW, Judenhofer MS, et al. Combined PET/MR imaging—technology and applications. Technol Cancer Res Treat 2010;9(1): 5–20.

107. Zaidi H, Montandon ML, Alavi A. The clinical role of fusion imaging using PET, CT, and MR imaging. Magn Reson Imaging Clin N Am 2010;18(1): 133–49.

108. Ferrari S, Briccoli A, Mercuri M, et al. Postrelapse survival in osteosarcoma of the extremities: prognostic factors for long-term survival. J Clin Oncol 2003;21(4):710–5.

109. Bacci G, Forni C, Longhi A, et al. Local recurrence and local control of non-metastatic osteosarcoma of the extremities: a 27-year experience in a single institution. J Surg Oncol 2007;96(2):118–23.

110. Wasilewski-Masker K, Liu Q, Yasui Y, et al. Late recurrence in pediatric cancer: a report from the Childhood Cancer Survivor Study. J Natl Cancer Inst 2009;101(24):1709–20.

111. Hanna SA, David LA, Gikas PD, et al. Very late local recurrence of Ewing's sarcoma—can you ever say 'cured'? A report of two cases and literature review. Ann R Coll Surg Engl 2008; 90(7):W12–5.

112. Costelloe CM, Kumar R, Yasko AW, et al. Imaging characteristics of locally recurrent tumors of bone. AJR Am J Roentgenol 2007;188(3):855–63.

113. Franzius C, Daldrup-Link HE, Wagner-Bohn A, et al. FDG-PET for detection of recurrences from malignant primary bone tumors: comparison with conventional imaging. Ann Oncol 2002;13(1): 157–60.

114. Viano AM, Gronemeyer SA, Haliloglu M, et al. Improved MR imaging for patients with metallic implants. Magn Reson Imaging 2000;18(3): 287–95.

115. McCarville MB, Lederman HM, Santana VM, et al. Distinguishing benign from malignant pulmonary nodules with helical chest CT in children with malignant solid tumors. Radiology 2006;239(2): 514–20.

116. McCarville MB, Kaste SC, Cain AM, et al. Prognostic factors and imaging patterns of recurrent pulmonary nodules after thoracotomy in children with osteosarcoma. Cancer 2001;91(6):1170–6.

Leukemia and Lymphoma

R. Paul Guillerman, MD[a],*, Stephan D. Voss, MD, PhD[b],
Bruce R. Parker, MD[a]

KEYWORDS

- Lymphoma • Leukemia • Hodgkin lymphoma
- Non-Hodgkin lymphoma • Acute lymphoblastic leukemia
- Acute myeloid leukemia

Leukemia and lymphoma are the most common and third most common pediatric malignancies, respectively, and together account for nearly half of all cases of childhood cancer. Although childhood leukemia and lymphoma share similar cell lineage origins and both are treated with risk-stratified protocols entailing cytotoxic chemotherapy, the clinical manifestations and imaging indications for these malignancies vary substantially, with some overlap. Advances in imaging have played a particularly important role in improving the assessment of lymphoma at the time of diagnosis, during treatment, and following therapy. Imaging has also helped guide the design of clinical trials evaluating novel treatment strategies.

Along with providing relevant details on current classification, epidemiology, and treatment, this article reviews the current roles of imaging in the management of pediatric patients with leukemia and lymphoma, with attention to diagnosis, staging, risk stratification, therapy response assessment, and surveillance for disease relapse and adverse effects of therapy. Advances in functional imaging and integration of clinical imaging research into cancer cooperative group study protocols are also discussed to provide insights into future applications of imaging in the management of pediatric leukemia and lymphoma patients.

LEUKEMIA
Classification and Epidemiology

Leukemia is the most common childhood malignancy, accounting for one-quarter to one-third of childhood malignancy cases. Nearly all childhood leukemia cases are the acute form. Acute leukemia is classified by the morphology, immunophenotype, and cytogenetics of the leukemic cells into acute lymphoblastic leukemia (ALL) and acute myeloid leukemia (AML). ALL and AML account for three-quarters and one-fifth of childhood leukemia cases, respectively. Chronic myelogenous leukemia (CML) accounts for less than 5% of cases of childhood leukemia, whereas juvenile myelomonocytic leukemia (JMML), a myelodysplastic-myeloproliferative syndrome, accounts for less than 1% of cases of childhood leukemia.[1] There is a sharp peak in ALL incidences among children 2 to 3 years of age, with evidence that ALL initiates in utero[2] AML rates are highest in the first 2 years of life, decline to a nadir at 6 years of age, and slowly increase during the adolescent years.[3]

ALL is subtyped by the World Health Organization (WHO) by immunophenotype as B-lymphoblastic or T-lymphoblastic.[4] Precursor B-cell ALL accounts for 80% to 85% of childhood ALL. About 12% of ALL is T-cell lineage, which is associated with older age, male gender, leukocytosis, and a mediastinal

[a] Department of Pediatric Radiology, Texas Children's Hospital, 6701 Fannin Street, Suite 470, Houston, TX 77030, USA
[b] Department of Radiology, Children's Hospital Boston, Harvard Medical School, 300 Longwood Avenue, Boston, MA 02115, USA
* Corresponding author.
E-mail address: rpguille@texaschildrens.org

Radiol Clin N Am 49 (2011) 767–797
doi:10.1016/j.rcl.2011.05.004
0033-8389/11/$ – see front matter © 2011 Elsevier Inc. All rights reserved.

mass. T-cell lineage ALL may be regarded as a disseminated form of T-cell lymphoblastic lymphoma in terms of malignant phenotype, approach to therapy, and patterns of relapse. About 2% of ALL is mature B-cell and the disseminated form of Burkitt or Burkitt-like lymphoma.[1] AML has traditionally been subtyped into M0 to M7 forms according to the French-American-British (FAB) Cooperative Group morphologic-immunohisto-chemical classification system. Acute promyelo-cytic leukemia (APL), the M3 subtype of AML, is notable for bleeding complications related to severe coagulopathy. A newer classification of AML by the WHO incorporates cytogenetic abnormalities and specific gene mutations and provides more reliable prognostic information.[4]

An increased risk of leukemia is associated with certain genetic disorders, including trisomy 21, monosomy 7, and neurofibromatosis type 1 (partic-ularly JMML), and DNA repair disorders such as ataxia-telangiectasia. Of special interest to the radiologist is the reported increased risk of leukemia from prenatal or postnatal radiation expo-sure, although the magnitude of the risk is subject to considerable uncertainty and debate.[5]

Treatment

Risk-based treatment assignment is used in chil-dren with leukemia so that those children who have a good outcome with modest therapy can be spared more intensive and toxic treatment, whereas a more aggressive, and potentially more toxic, therapeutic approach can be provided for patients who have a lower probability of long-term survival. The 10-year event-free survival (EFS) rate is 67% to 78% for standard and higher risk childhood ALL with risk-adapted combination chemotherapy and central nervous system (CNS) prophylactic therapy (intrathecal chemotherapy with or without cranial radiation).[6] More intensive chemotherapy regimens or hematopoietic stem cell transplantation (HSCT) may be pursued for certain high-risk ALL groups and marrow relapse.

Children with AML have a wide range in outcome depending on specific biologic factors, with a 5-year EFS rate of 40% to 58%.[7] Infection, severe hemorrhage, hyperleukocytosis-related leukosta-sis, and resistant leukemia lead to the high mortality. The mainstay of AML treatment is systemic combi-nation chemotherapy, with some form of CNS-directed therapy incorporated into most protocols. Induction of profound bone marrow aplasia is generally necessary to achieve remission, and leukocyte growth factors such as G-CSF or GM-CSF are often administered to reduce the duration of neutropenia, but have no significant effect on

mortality. The duration of remission is prolonged by chemotherapy intensification and/or HSCT, although HSCT may not be necessary in those with complete remission and favorable prognostic factors.[8,9]

Imaging Features

Fever, petechiae, lethargy, and pallor caused by bone marrow suppression by leukemic cells are common at presentation. These symptoms and signs often prompt a chest radiograph. Chest radi-ography may reveal a mediastinal mass (especially from thymic infiltration in T-cell ALL), cardiomegaly and pulmonary vascular plethora (related to anemia), pulmonary air space opacification (related to infection, hemorrhage, or leukostasis), pleural thickening (especially in JMML), splenomegaly (present in 75%), or skeletal abnormalities.[10]

More than a third of children with leukemia present with limping, bone pain, arthralgia, or other complaints referable to the extremities or spine. Approximately 40% of children presenting with acute leukemia have at least 1 radiographic skeletal abnormality.[11,12] The number of bones involved on radiographs correlates with bone pain severity, but symptoms correlate poorly with the location of skeletal lesions on radiographs and asymptomatic involvement is common, especially in non–weight-bearing areas.[12,13] Findings of leukemia on skeletal radiographs include transverse lucent metaphyseal bands, diffuse demineralization, subperiosteal cortical bone erosion, periosteal reaction, lytic bone lesions, osteosclerosis, and pathologic frac-tures. Transverse metaphyseal lucent bands, also known as leukemic lines, are attributable to distur-bance of endosteal mineralization resulting in abnormally small trabeculae adjacent to the zone of provisional calcification. In preschool-aged chil-dren, transverse lucent metaphyseal bands are more specific for leukemia than for other diseases and are most conspicuous at sites of rapid skeletal growth such as the distal femur, proximal tibia, proximal humerus, and distal radius (Fig. 1).[12] Diffuse demineralization is common, particularly after therapy, whereas osteosclerosis is uncommon and usually a late manifestation after therapy. Path-ologic fractures are most commonly observed as vertebral compression deformities in the setting of diffuse demineralization. Lytic bone lesions are usually metadiaphyseal and geographic or perme-ative. Subperiosteal resorption of the medial cortex of the proximal humerus is commonly visible on chest radiographs at the time of presentation, but is nonspecific and can also be observed in the setting of Gaucher disease, sickle cell disease, neuroblastoma, or lymphoma (Fig. 2).[14]

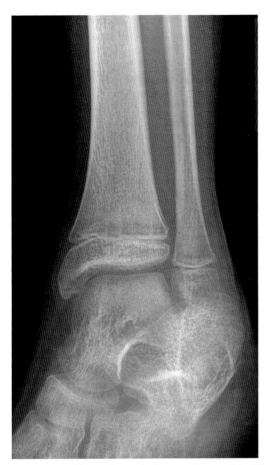

Technetium (Tc)-99m phosphonate–based bone scintigraphy is abnormal in 75% of patients with ALL at diagnosis. The most common abnormality is symmetric increased uptake in the metadiaphyses of the lower limbs (Fig. 3). Other patterns include diffuse increased uptake in a superscan pattern with accentuation of the long bone metaphyses, focal increased uptake at sites of cortical bone destruction or pathologic fracture, and focal decreased uptake at sites of osteonecrosis.[15] The addition of early phase whole-body scintigraphy may increase the sensitivity for detection of abnormal uptake from leukemia in the long bone metadiaphyses, spine, and pelvis compared with that of delayed-phase whole-body scintigraphy alone.[16] The number of regions with abnormal uptake is positively correlated with age. There is only modest correlation between the sites of abnormal uptake, radiographic abnormalities, and clinical signs and symptoms.[17]

On magnetic resonance (MR) imaging, malignant infiltration of the bone marrow by leukemia typically manifests as increased signal intensity on fat-suppressed T2-weighted and short-tau inversion recovery (STIR) sequences and decreased signal intensity on T1-weighted images.[18] Prolongation of the T1 relaxation time correlates with the proportion of blast cells in the marrow.[19] The infiltration is usually diffuse, including involvement of the epiphyses (Fig. 4). The findings are less conspicuous in hematopoietic marrow than in fatty marrow and consequently are more difficult to appreciate in younger children before the physiologic conversion of hematopoietic to fatty marrow.[20] ALL and AML cannot be reliably

Fig. 1. An ankle radiograph from a 7-year-old girl with precursor B-cell ALL shows transverse lucent bands (leukemic lines) along the distal tibial and fibular metaphyses just proximal to the zones of provisional calcification.

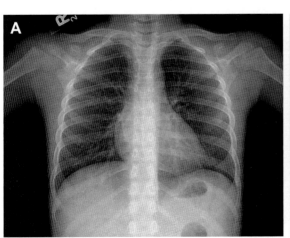
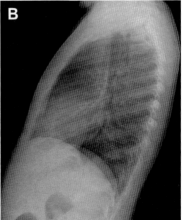

Fig. 2. Anteroposterior (A) and lateral (B) chest radiographs of a 7-year-old boy with precursor B-cell ALL reveal subperiosteal resorption of the medial cortex and subtle transverse lucent metaphyseal bands of the proximal humeri, as well as diffuse demineralization of the vertebral bodies.

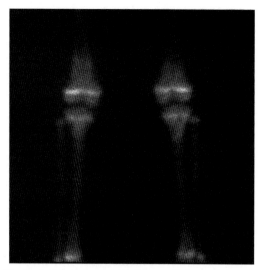

Fig. 3. A delayed-phase Tc-99m methylene diphosph-onate bone scintigraphy image of the lower extremi-ties of a child with precursor B-cell ALL depicts symmetric increased radiopharmaceutical uptake in the long bone metadiaphyses.

distinguished from MR imaging or MR spectros-copy. The MR imaging appearance associated with marrow infiltration by acute leukemia is not specific and can also be seen in settings of hema-topoietic marrow hyperplasia and infiltrative metastases from solid tumors such as neuroblas-toma, rhabdomyosarcoma, and Ewing sarcoma.[21]

Leukemic involvement of the solid viscera, especially the spleen and thymus, is common, and manifests as organomegaly from diffuse infil-tration or as focal masses. Diffuse infiltration of the thymus is characteristic of T-cell ALL (Fig. 5). Splenomegaly and a mediastinal mass from thymic infiltration at presentation of childhood ALL are independent predictors of tumor lysis syndrome.[22] The constellation of splenomegaly, hepatomegaly, lymphadenopathy, and skin rash is characteristic of JMML.[23] Nephromegaly at presentation is usually caused by leukemic cell infiltration, but can also be caused by renal vein thrombosis from intravascular leukostasis.[24] Focal renal leukemic masses at presentation are usually multifocal, bilateral, low attenuation on computed tomography (CT), and hypoechoic on ultrasound, and must be differentiated from lymphoma, nephroblastomatosis, and infection. Renal infiltra-tion is most frequent with T-cell ALL and the M4 and M5 subtypes of AML, and is often accom-panied by extramedullary involvement at other sites.[25] Leukemic infiltration of the kidneys is rarely associated with acute renal failure or renal tubular dysfunction at presentation.[26,27] Pancre-atic enlargement from leukemic infiltration is unusual.[28]

Brain atrophy, at least borderline in degree and of unclear cause, can be seen by CT in 40% of children with ALL at diagnosis.[29] Even in the pres-ence of neurologic symptoms, CNS imaging find-ings other than atrophy are uncommon. Head CT or MR imaging can reveal hemorrhage or infarction

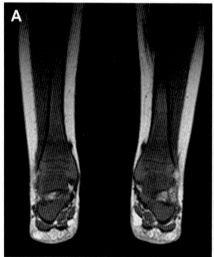
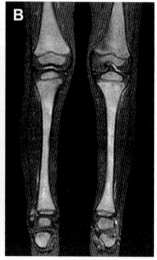

Fig. 4. An MR imaging examination of the lower extremities performed on a 3-year-old boy with refusal to walk shows diffuse abnormal low signal intensity of the bone marrow on a T1-weighted image (A) and diffuse abnormal high intensity of the bone marrow on a STIR (B) image caused by marrow infiltration by precursor B-cell ALL.

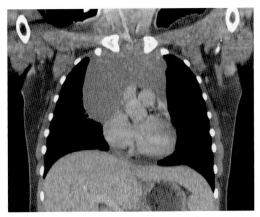

Fig. 5. A coronal chest CT image of 13-year-old patient with T-cell ALL shows a characteristic mediastinal mass from diffuse leukemic infiltration of the thymus.

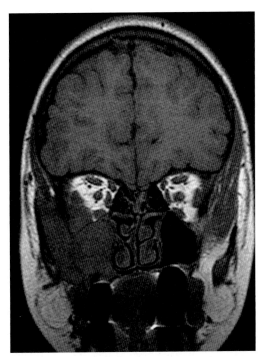

Fig. 6. A coronal T1-weighted image from an MR imaging examination in an 11-year-old girl with AML shows a soft tissue mass of the right maxillary sinus, zygoma, and inferior orbit that is isointense to the marrow of the diploe of the skull, consistent with a chloroma.

caused by intravascular leukostasis or thrombocytopenia.[30] Cerebral hemorrhage is more common than subdural or subarachnoid hemorrhage. Abnormal enhancement of the meninges or nerve roots in a child with leukemia suggests leptomeningeal involvement, even if CSF cytologic studies are negative. As many as half of all cases of acute leukemia involve ocular manifestations, and the most frequent finding is retinal hemorrhage. Retinal hemorrhages related to leukemia are usually bilateral and located in the posterior pole.[31]

A potential diagnostic pitfall is aleukemic or subleukemic leukemia. From one-quarter to one-third of cases of leukemia present with anemia and thrombocytopenia but no leukocytosis or leukemic blasts on peripheral blood smear.[11,32,33] Many of these patients have bone or joint pain that can masquerade clinically as osteomyelitis or arthritis for several months and prompt referral for musculoskeletal MR imaging examinations. Appropriate recognition of bone marrow infiltration on MR imaging can suggest the correct diagnosis of leukemia before leukocytosis or blasts in the peripheral blood are noted.[34]

Extramedullary leukemia (EML), also known as granulocytic sarcoma or chloroma, describes a mass of leukemic cells outside the bone marrow. EML is more common in infants than in older children and can precede the blast phase by up to 4 years.[35] The skin, orbits, CNS, and spine are the most common sites, and symptoms relate to mass effect. On CT, EML masses show variable enhancement and can be confused with other neoplasms, hematoma, or abscess. On MR imaging, EML masses show isointensity to hypercellular bone marrow (**Fig. 6**). EML is most commonly associated with AML and is rare, occurring as an isolated finding in less than 1% of cases of AML and in 11% of cases along with marrow disease at the time of diagnosis.[36]

A definitive diagnosis of leukemia is usually established by bone marrow aspiration or biopsy revealing malignant cells of myeloid or lymphoid lineage. Definitive diagnosis can also be established by biopsy of an extramedullary mass of leukemic cells.

Staging and Risk Stratification

Leukemia is conceptualized as a disseminated malignancy of the hematopoietic system and there is no role for traditional staging based on imaging findings as for lymphoma and solid tumors, even for children with isolated EML who must be treated as if there is systemic disease. ALL is classified as low risk, standard risk, high risk, and very high risk from clinical and biologic features and early treatment response. Higher risk ALL groups include infants, adolescents, those with high leukocyte counts, those with CNS disease, those with initial induction failure or high levels of end-induction minimal residual disease (MRD), and those with

T-cell lineage, hypodiploidy or certain chromosome translocations.[37] In AML, risk category definitions are in evolution. Adolescent and obese patients are in a poorer outcome group and leukocyte count at diagnosis is inversely related to survival, whereas trisomy 21, APL subtype, and early response to therapy are favorable factors.[38]

The prognostic significance of radiographic and scintigraphic bone abnormalities is uncertain, relating to conflicting reports in the literature. It has been reported that multiple bone involvement on radiographs portends a shorter duration of remission and survival[39]; that there is no correlation of radiological or scintigraphic extent of bone disease and duration of remission or survival[13,17]; that children without radiographic abnormalities have an aggressive form of leukemia, whereas those with a few bone lesions have an indolent form[40]; and that those with radiographic bone lesions represent a subset with a better prognosis.[33]

Nephromegaly at the time of presentation is reportedly an adverse prognostic factor for ALL.[41] Nephromegaly in childhood ALL is also correlated with subsequent renal damage detectable by renal MAG-3 or dimercaptosuccinic acid (DMSA) scintigraphy.[42] Overt testicular involvement at diagnosis has been considered an adverse prognostic factor for ALL, but this may no longer be the case with aggressive initial therapy. Neither the presence of a mediastinal mass at the time of diagnosis nor an incomplete response with a residual mediastinal mass on chest radiograph at day 35 or 70 of therapy predicts a worse prognosis in T-cell ALL.[43]

Therapy Response Evaluation

Imaging is not currently relied on to evaluate response to therapy for childhood leukemia. However, some trends may be observed on skeletal radiographs. The transverse metaphyseal lucent bands usually resolve quickly with treatment, whereas periostitis, cortical erosion, and lytic bone lesions resolve more slowly, and osteopenia may worsen, related to steroids. Bone sclerosis and osteonecrosis may also develop after therapy.

The high sensitivity of MR imaging for bone marrow abnormalities has led to investigation of MR imaging as a method for therapy response evaluation. During chemotherapy for leukemia, the bone marrow becomes hypocellular and edematous. Following chemotherapy, there is progressive regeneration of normal hematopoietic cells and fat. Marked increase in the marrow fat fraction is observed by chemical shift MR imaging in the marrow of patients responding to chemotherapy,

whereas a low marrow fat fraction persists in the setting of unresponsive disease. In children with ALL who enter remission, marrow T1 relaxation time normalizes, whereas the marrow T1 relaxation time remains prolonged in those who do not enter remission. However, the specificity of MR imaging is limited by the difficulty in differentiating viable neoplasm from effects of therapy, including hematopoietic marrow regeneration (particularly with G-CSF or GM-CSF therapy), hematopoietic marrow reconstitution following stem cell transplantation, marrow iron overload from transfusional hemosiderosis, and marrow infarction and fibrosis.[44–46] Because of these limitations, MR imaging has not replaced marrow aspirate or biopsy for assessment of therapeutic response in leukemia.[47]

Surveillance for Relapse

The most common site of ALL relapse is the marrow, followed by the CNS and testes. Isolated marrow involvement occurs in 48% of cases of relapsed ALL in children at a median time of 26 months, whereas the incidence of isolated CNS relapse is less than 5% and the incidence of isolated testicular relapse is less than 2%. Outcome of ALL is poorer with early relapse and with isolated bone marrow relapse than with later relapse and combined marrow and testicular or CNS relapse.[48] Most AML relapses occur in the marrow, with CNS relapse being uncommon. Survival is substantially lower in those with shorter remissions, and relapsed leukemia is still the primary cause of death in patients with AML.[49]

In some instances, relapse of leukemia in the vertebral marrow can be detected by MR imaging several weeks before relapse is detected by iliac bone marrow aspirate or biopsy, reflecting the patchy nature of relapsed leukemia and effects of sampling bias.[50] Unlike the diffuse marrow abnormality typical of leukemia on MR imaging at presentation, early relapsed ALL can manifest as well-defined nodules of low signal intensity on T1-weighted sequences and high signal intensity on T2-weighted and STIR sequences. In this setting, directed marrow lesional biopsy may be required to avoid false-negative iliac marrow sampling.[51] Although time to relapse is an important predictor of outcome, evidence that early detection of relapse by frequent surveillance improves outcome is lacking.[52]

Extramedullary involvement is more common at relapse than at presentation. Sanctuary sites for leukemic cells during therapy, where relapse can occur even in the presence of bone marrow remission, include the CNS, testes, and kidneys. CNS prophylaxis has greatly reduced the incidence of CNS relapse, and surveillance imaging of the CNS is not warranted. A possible exception is EML, for which relapse is extramedullary in nearly 40% of cases and most often in the CNS.[36] Patients with suspected testicular relapse generally go to biopsy without imaging, but occasionally ultrasound is requested and may show hypoechoic, enlarged testicles with or without focal lesions (**Fig. 7**). Isolated testicular relapse is rare and testicular biopsy at the end of therapy has failed to show a survival benefit for patients with early detection of occult disease,[53] arguing against a role for surveillance imaging of the testes.

Surveillance chest radiographs are sometimes obtained to evaluate for mediastinal relapse in patients with T-cell ALL with a prior mediastinal mass. However, a beneficial impact of this practice on outcome has not been established.

LYMPHOMA
Classification and Epidemiology

Pediatric lymphoma, including Hodgkin lymphoma (HL) and non-Hodgkin lymphoma (NHL), is the third most common malignant neoplasm in childhood and adolescence. HL is unusual in patients younger than 4 years of age, and typically occurs in older children and adolescents.[3] In patients younger than 10 years of age, there is a male predominance of HL; beyond this age the relative incidence begins to equilibrate between the genders and patients older than 15 years of age have an approximately equal incidence between boys and girls.[54] There are some studies suggesting an association between chronic Epstein-Barr virus (EBV) and HL and this has led some investigators to propose a distinction between the childhood and adolescent/young adult forms of HL.[54,55]

HL is characterized by a variable number of characteristic clonal multinucleated giant cells (Reid-Sternberg [RS] cells) in an inflammatory milieu. The WHO classification separates the uncommon nodular lymphocyte-predominant form of HL (NLPHL) from the common form, designated classic HL. WHO subtypes of classic HL are nodular sclerosis (NS), lymphocyte rich (LR), mixed cellularity (MC), and lymphocyte depleted (LD).[56] The NS subtype of HL accounts for greater than 85% of pediatric HL and is characterized by lymph nodes that have thickened capsules and dense collagenous bands that separate the nodes into macronodules. The presence of collagen and fibrous stroma contributes to the presence of residual mediastinal soft tissue that is commonly seen early after completion of therapy, even after no viable disease remains. The MC subtype accounts for 30% of the cases in young children and can be confused for NHL.

The characteristic RS cell in classic HL is believed to arise from preapoptotic germinal center B-cells that cannot synthesize immunoglobulin and show constitutive activation of the nuclear factor κ-B pathway, conferring resistance to apoptotic stimuli. EBV is associated with 15% to 25% of HL in developed countries and up to 90% in developing countries, most commonly in younger patients with MC histology. Despite this, EBV serologic status does not seem to be a prognostic factor in pediatric patients with HL,[57] in contrast with patients with NHL.

NHL of childhood is a heterogeneous collection of lymphoid neoplasms that are not classified as HL. Although a large number of forms of NHL are recognized, the 4 most commonly occurring in children include Burkitt lymphoma (BL), diffuse large B-cell lymphoma (DLBCL), anaplastic large

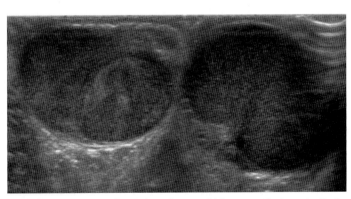

Fig. 7. Testicular relapse of precursor B-cell ALL in a 3-year-old boy manifests as testicular enlargement by ill-defined masses on ultrasonography.

cell lymphoma (ALCL), and precursor T-cell and B-cell lymphoblastic lymphoma (LL). In contrast with HL, NHL is more common in children younger than 10 years of age. There is also a male predominance, particularly in older patients.[58] Age-specific incidence also varies according to disease classification, with LL occurring with a fairly constant rate across all age groups, whereas ALCL and DLBCL predominate in older adolescents. Although the cause of NHL is uncertain, there is an increased incidence of lymphomas in immunosuppressed patients. Other studies have shown a role for EBV in the pathogenesis of lymphoproliferative disease and NHL. Taken together, these findings suggest that disordered immunoregulation, with resultant clonal proliferation of immature cells that have failed to differentiate, contributes to malignant transformation in NHL.[59]

Each NHL subtype has characteristic pathologic features, and recent molecular and translational investigations have led to new understanding of the pathobiology of NHL.[54,59] BL and DLBCL are believed to derive from lymph node germinal center regions where proliferating B-cell lymphoblasts normally differentiate. The activation of proto-oncogenes and/or disruption of tumor suppressor genes or hypermutation of proto-oncogenes are believed to result in the malignant transformation of these germinal center lymphoblasts. Consistent with this interpretation, B-lineage cell surface antigen CD20 shows increased expression on both BL and DLBCL. ALCL shows expression of CD30 and is characterized by overexpression of the anaplastic lymphoma kinase (ALK) tyrosine kinase, which is believed to play a role in ALCL tumor genesis. LL, in contrast with the other pediatric NHL subtypes, predominantly arises from immature T-cells, corresponding to defined stages of thymocyte differentiation. Less than 10% of LL is of B-cell origin.[58] When greater than 25% of the bone marrow is infiltrated with lymphoblasts, the disease is termed ALL rather than LL. Posttransplant lymphoproliferative disease (PTLD) is seen in the setting of both solid organ and bone marrow transplantation, and results directly from host immunosuppression.[60,61] PTLD, which is usually EBV-related, is not initially classified as a malignant lymphoma and frequently responds to reduction in immunosuppression. However, the lymphoproliferative disease may progress to an aggressive B-cell lymphoma, resulting in widespread malignant disease.[62]

Treatment

With current treatment approaches, the 5-year survival rate for children and adolescents diagnosed with HL is around 95%.[7] This high cure rate has led to renewed interest in the role that treatment-related toxicities and long-term consequences of therapy play in overall morbidity and mortality.[63,64] The risk of death caused by disease at 20 years from diagnosis almost equals the risk of death from other causes, including treatment-related effects.[63]

In the 1960s and 1970s, extended field radiation therapy improved disease-free and overall survival rates amongst patients with HL.[55] However, this so-called mantle radiation resulted in significant late effects in the irradiated tissues. Subsequent development of a combination of chemotherapy regimens showed that disease-free survival could be improved with lower dose radiation therapy regimens, and, in certain patients with HL, elimination of radiation therapy altogether. In patients with low-stage HL, overall survival was no different for patients whose initial therapy was chemotherapy alone, because of effective salvage regimens.[65,66] In patients with advanced-stage HL, EFS was higher for those who received initial chemotherapy and radiation therapy compared with those with chemotherapy alone.[54,67] As with current standard regimens, these early treatment regimens were risk adapted: those with favorable-risk disease, defined by low stage and low bulk disease, typically receive 2 to 4 cycles of multiagent chemotherapy with either low-dose involved field radiation or no radiation, whereas those patients with higher risk disease are stratified to receive more intensive chemotherapy before involved field radiotherapy.[55]

These risk-adapted approaches do not take into account initial disease response, in contrast with response-adapted approaches, in which the overall treatment intensity is modulated during the course of therapy based on initial response. This latter approach is emerging as a potential means of further reducing therapy and potentially reducing late effects for those patients with HL in whom cure is likely, while maintaining high cure rates and aggressive treatment of those patients at higher risk of relapse.[64,67]

Patients with NHL have lower overall survival rates compared with HL. With current treatment approaches, more than 85% of children and 75% of adolescents with NHL survive at least 5 years.[7] Treatment of childhood NHL depends on localized versus disseminated disease. Localized disease is typically defined as stage I or II disease, whereas stage III or IV disease is generally considered to be disseminated. In most children, NHL is widely disseminated from the outset, and systemic treatment with aggressive combination chemotherapy is usually recommended for most patients.[54,58]

Children with refractory or relapsed NHL have a worse outcome than newly diagnosed patients, and thus aggressive up-front therapy and early remission remain the goal of new treatment regimens.[68]

The outcome for LL is excellent, with longer leukemialike therapy consisting of induction, consolidation, and maintenance therapy. In contrast, nonlymphoblastic NHL has superior outcome with short, intensive pulse therapy. For recurrent or refractory B-lineage NHL or LL, survival is low (10%–20%), emphasizing the importance of achieving cure during the initial therapy. For recurrent or refractory ALCL, as many as 60% of patients can ultimately be salvaged and achieve long-term survival.[69] PTLD can involve multiple organs and systems, and responds variably to conventional lymphoma therapies.[60–62]

Radiation therapy plays little role in the routine management of pediatric NHL, in contrast with HL.[58] Mediastinal radiation is not commonly used for patients with mediastinal masses, except in the emergent treatment of symptomatic superior vena cava obstruction or airway obstruction. Even in this instance, low-dose radiation is usually used.

Imaging Features

In HL, chest radiographs obtained for upper respiratory symptoms and/or vague constitutional symptoms, such as fever or night sweats, often prompt the initial diagnosis. At the time of diagnosis, a mediastinal mass is present in more than two-thirds of patients with HL (**Figs. 8** and **9**).[70]

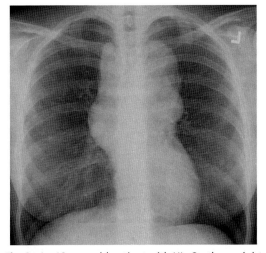

Fig. 8. An 18-year-old patient with HL. On the upright posteroanterior (PA) chest radiograph, the transverse width of the mediastinal mass exceeds one-third of the thoracic diameter, meeting the criterion for bulk disease.

The diagnostic evaluation should always include imaging of the chest and neck up to the level of the Waldeyer ring. Large neck and mediastinal masses may compress the airway and central vascular structures. Care must therefore be taken in sedating these patients before imaging.[71] After a careful physiologic and radiographic evaluation of the patient has been performed, the least invasive procedure should be used to establish the diagnosis. If possible, peripheral lymph node biopsy is preferable. Aspiration cytology is not sufficient because of the absence of stromal tissue, and core needle biopsies are necessary. Surgical staging has been largely replaced by imaging; however, mediastinoscopy or thoracoscopy may be needed when other modalities fail to establish the diagnosis or if questionable areas of involvement result in upstaging the patient and histologic confirmation is required.

Lung involvement is seen in less than 5% of children younger than 10 years of age and 15% of adolescents with HL.[70,72] Nodules greater than 1 cm are the most common pulmonary finding during staging of patients with HL, although diffuse interstitial thickening and lobar or segmental consolidation are other pulmonary manifestations of disease. The presence of pulmonary disease usually occurs in association with ipsilateral hilar or mediastinal lymphadenopathy (**Fig. 10**). The most common mechanisms of disease spreading into the lungs are hematogenous and lymphangitic spread, and less frequent, direct invasion. Pleural and pericardial effusions are infrequent findings in HL and usually result from lymphatic obstruction.[70] Pleural effusions are typically transudative and usually negative for malignant cells. Pericardial effusion, when present, may suggest tumor involvement of the pericardium from direct extension of the adjacent mediastinal mass. Where pericardial involvement is suspected, MR imaging may be superior to CT, particularly with the advent of respiratory and cardiac gated MR imaging.

Liver involvement by HL is almost always associated with splenic involvement, and splenic involvement without associated para-aortic lymphadenopathy is unusual (**Fig. 11**). Splenic involvement occurs in 30% to 40% of Hodgkin disease (HD). Splenic size is unreliable for predicting splenic HD involvement.[73]

At diagnosis, bone marrow involvement is unusual in HL. MR imaging and [^{18}F]fluorodeoxyglucose (FDG)–positron emission tomography (PET) are more sensitive than conventional CT for detecting bone marrow involvement.[72] Cortical bone involvement is similarly rare in HL. When present, lesions are typically lytic and may have accompanying periosteal reaction.[70]

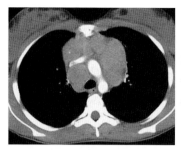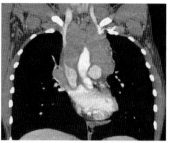

Fig. 9. Chest CT images of an 18-year-old girl (see chest radiograph in **Fig. 8**) with HL depict characteristic conglomerate lobular mediastinal lymphadenopathy.

Historically, gallium (^{67}Ga) scintigraphy was the mainstay of functional imaging in lymphoma but has now usually been replaced by FDG-PET. FDG-PET has been shown to be more sensitive than gallium scintigraphy for determining lung, bone, and nodal involvement and has a much lower radiation dose than gallium scintigraphy.[74–76] Gallium has prolonged retention in the bowel, further limiting its usefulness in evaluating intra-abdominal disease. Although gallium scintigraphy approaches the sensitivity of FDG-PET for diagnosis and staging of neck and mediastinal/chest nodal disease in pediatric HL, nearly all institutions have access to FDG-PET scanning and there is currently little justification for gallium scanning.

FDG-PET has been studied extensively in adult lymphoma[77] and, to a lesser extent, in pediatric populations.[72,78] The overall consensus from multiple studies is that FDG-PET is more sensitive than CT for involvement of normal-sized lymph nodes and extranodal disease, including the spleen, liver, and bone marrow (see **Fig. 11**; **Fig. 12**).[79–84] Combined FDG-PET/CT imaging retains the high sensitivity of FDG-PET for detecting disease, but improves the specificity, with coregistered fused images resulting in the highest sensitivity and specificity at detecting disease and correlating sites of abnormal FDG uptake with specific anatomic regions.[80,82,85,86]

False-positive FDG uptake is well recognized and can result from rebound thymic hyperplasia, hypermetabolic brown fat, muscle, hyperplastic/recovering marrow and/or spleen, gonadal and breast cyclic hormonal stimulation, and sites of recent surgery or infection (**Fig. 13**).[87,88] The characteristic patterns of nonspecific uptake are well recognized by experienced radiologists and nuclear medicine physicians and the use of coregistered FDG-PET/CT has proved invaluable for identifying and eliminating areas of false-positive uptake from the diagnostic evaluation.[88] In some instances, background uptake can be reduced. For example, brown fat uptake can be largely eliminated by warming the patient, and, in challenging cases, premedicating the patient with fentanyl and/or benzodiazepines.[89]

Among pediatric NHL, BL most commonly presents with intra-abdominal visceral disease, and widespread extranodal involvement is often present. The initial imaging evaluation is usually directed at assessment of symptoms referable to abdominal involvement. Involvement of the peritoneum, solid abdominal organs, and bowel with complicating intussusception can be seen (**Figs. 14 and 15**).

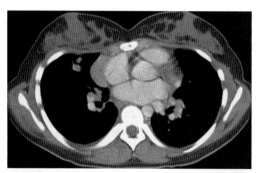
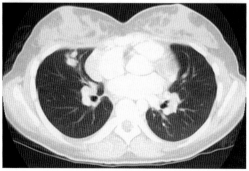

Fig. 10. A 14-year-old girl with HL. CT images show pulmonary, mediastinal, and bilateral hilar involvement.

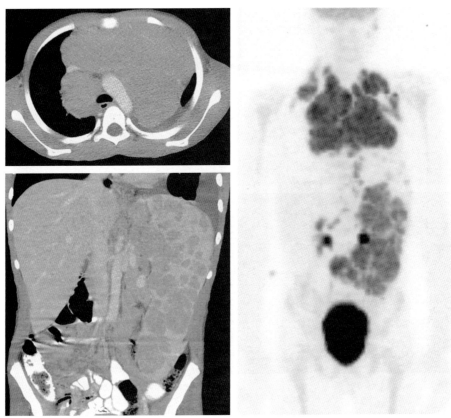

Fig. 11. Axial and coronal contrast-enhanced CT images of the chest and abdomen, respectively, show a large mediastinal mass with accompanying diffuse splenic involvement and mesenteric lymph node enlargement in this patient with HL. The accompanying FDG-PET image shows diffuse FDG uptake throughout the mass in both the chest and abdomen.

As many as 75% of patients with LL present with a mediastinal mass and dyspnea, wheezing, stridor, or dysphagia.[58] The mediastinal enlargement in LL is attributable to diffuse thymic involvement and does not show the typical nodular heterogeneous appearance more characteristic of HL and other forms of NHL (**Fig. 16**). These tumors grow rapidly and patients with LL may deteriorate quickly because of airway compression and impairment of venous return, particularly when patients are placed supine or sedated. In this population of patients, diagnostic imaging may not be possible because of the tenuous clinical status of the patient, and pleural fluid and/or bone marrow aspiration may be the only means of accurately diagnosing these patients.

ALCL is often associated with systemic symptoms and signs such as fever and weight loss, and a prolonged waxing and waning course before diagnosis. A mediastinal mass may be seen in up to 40% of patients with ALCL, and, when present, is often accompanied by large pleural and pericardial effusions. ALCL can also involve lung, skin,

and bone,[54] and often presents with extensive multifocal disease (**Figs. 17 and 18**).

DLBCL has a less characteristic clinical pattern compared with other NHL subtypes. Most patients with DLBCL present with localized disease. Anterior mediastinal and/or bulky cervical/supraclavicular lymphadenopathy are more characteristic of DLBCL than of the other NHL subtypes. Up to 70% of these patients have a mediastinal mass, which may produce airway obstruction and superior vena cava syndrome (**Fig. 19**).[54,72] In general, these tumors are more aggressive than HL and malignant pericardial effusions resulting from direct pericardial invasion, malignant pleural effusions, and pulmonary involvement may be seen (**Fig. 20**). Patients with DLBCL with disease localized to the mediastinum may be difficult to distinguish from HL based on imaging (see **Fig. 19**).[54] The presence of metachronous peripheral lymphadenopathy or bone involvement makes DLBCL the more likely diagnosis. About 20% of pediatric patients with DLBCL present with primary mediastinal disease (primary mediastinal B-cell lymphoma).[90] This presentation

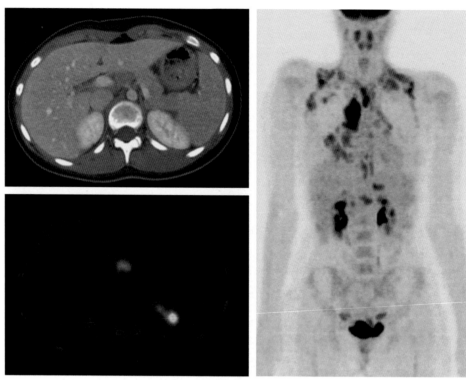

Fig. 12. Axial CT, coronal FDG-PET, and fused axial PET/CT show extensive FDG-avid HL. Retroperitoneal lymph node involvement was shown by FDG-PET and PET/CT fusion, whereas the same site shown on the CT alone could have been interpreted as unopacified bowel. This patient is the same 14 year old who is shown in **Fig. 9**, who also had extensive pulmonary nodules, confirmed as FDG-avid sites of disease.

is more common in older children and adolescents. These tumors are more aggressive and are associated with a worse outcome compared with other pediatric large B-cell lymphomas. Growth into adjacent structures is common and there is a characteristic tendency for focal involvement of the kidneys (see **Fig. 20**).

PTLD can involve multiple organs or have focal involvement. The use of FDG-PET to stage the extent of disease and assess response to therapy in PTLD is increasingly advocated (**Fig. 21**).[62,91]

Staging and Risk Stratification

The Ann Arbor system for staging of HL was developed to classify anatomic sites of disease based on a combination of clinical, surgical, and imaging findings. The Cotswold modifications of the Ann Arbor staging system incorporated the prognostic implications of tumor bulkiness and number of disease sites into the staging system.[92] The revised Ann Arbor staging system is shown in **Box 1**. Staging is largely based on identifying disease above or below the diaphragm and at identifying noncontiguous involvement of extralymphatic sites

of disease that indicate hematogenous spread. Unique to HL is the designation of extralymphatic disease that results from direct extension of an involved lymph node region, which can be challenging at the time of staging. For example, contiguous involvement of lung adjacent to a large mediastinal mass may be considered stage IIE rather than stage IV disease. However, the presence of a malignant pleural effusion that is cytologically positive for HL would be considered stage IV. For areas of questionable noncontiguous extralymphatic involvement, pathologic confirmation may be required before assignment to stage IV. The presence of B symptoms (fever, night sweats, weight loss) is included in the staging of the patient, and influences whether the patient is assigned to a low or intermediate/high-risk treatment regimen.

The posteroanterior (PA) upright chest radiograph is still used for determining the presence of bulk disease (mediastinal mass > one-third of the maximal transthoracic diameter) (see **Fig. 8**).[55] However, the Cotswolds modification of the Ann Arbor classification also defines lymph nodes greater than 10 cm in maximal dimension on CT imaging as bulky. Despite various attempts, the

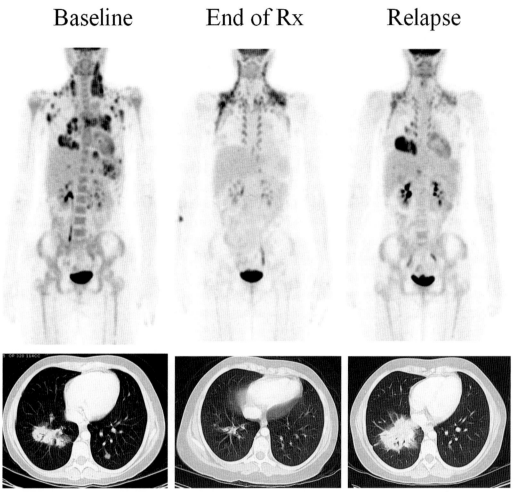

Fig. 13. A 15-year-old patient with stage IV HL. Baseline FDG-PET and CT show extensive disease, including pulmonary lesions. At the end of therapy, FDG uptake has resolved, except for presumed background brown fat uptake in the neck. Residual CT abnormalities were interpreted as scar tissue in view of the negative FDG-PET scan. By 4 months after completion of therapy the patient's pulmonary relapse was obvious by CT and confirmed by FDG-PET. Rx, treatment.

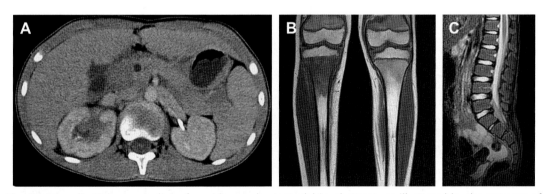

Fig. 14. Sporadic BL has a proclivity for widespread extranodal involvement, as illustrated by the presence of masses in the pancreas and right kidney on an abdominal CT image (*A*), proximal right tibial bone marrow on an T1-weighted MR image (*B*), and lumbosacral epidural space on a sagittal STIR MR image (*C*) in this 8-year-old boy.

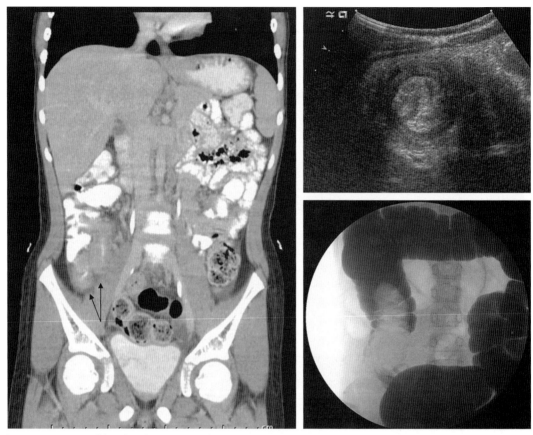

Fig. 15. An 8-year-old girl with BL. Coronal CT reconstruction shows thickening of the distal ileum and cecum (*arrows*). Two days later, the patient presented with abdominal pain. An ultrasound examination showed an intussusception. A contrast enema confirmed the intussusception, which was successfully reduced. When the intussusception recurred, she was taken to the operating room where the diagnosis of BL was established.

current definitions of bulky disease are not standardized and frequently depend on the clinical trial protocol and the cooperative group from which the protocol derives. For example, bulky disease,

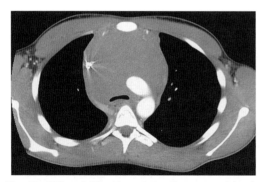

Fig. 16. Diffuse infiltration of the thymus resulting in a smoothly marginated homogeneous anterior mediastinal mass that compresses the airway and occludes the left brachiocephalic vein or superior vena cava is a common presentation of T-cell lymphoblastic lymphoma, as shown in this chest CT image.

as defined by PA chest radiograph and CT of nodal disease, is still recognized in the risk stratification of patients enrolled in Children's Oncology Group trials and St Jude Consortium trials. However, results from the German-Austrian Pediatric Multicenter trial suggest that bulk disease alone is not a prognostic factor for outcome with a risk-adapted treatment strategy.[93] Contrast-enhanced CT and FDG-PET imaging complete the contribution of imaging to staging and risk stratification. There is currently no role for bone scintigraphy in the routine staging evaluation.[94] Increasingly, particularly in Europe, the use of MR imaging, including diffusion-weighted imaging, is being advocated to reduce radiation exposure in these heavily imaged and treated patients.[95,96]

Combined FDG-PET/CT imaging provides the most sensitive and specific means of accurately staging patients with HL (see **Figs. 11–13**). For example, in one study of children and adolescents with HL, FDG-PET changed the staging in 15% of the patients, most of whom were upstaged. Most of the false negatives not detected by FDG-PET

Baseline   Post-consolidation Rx

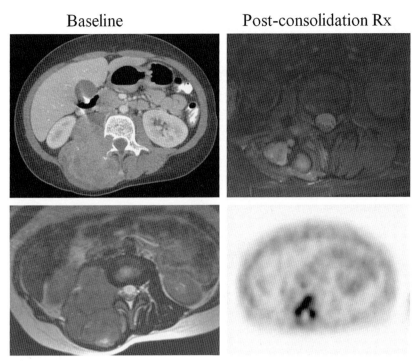

Fig. 17. An 11-year-old patient with paraspinal ALCL. CT and MR images show paraspinal mass with bone destruction and invasion of the spinal canal. An MR imaging and FDG-PET scan obtained while the patient was on therapy showed a decrease in size of the mass. Although the patient did not have a baseline FDG-PET scan, the presence of FDG uptake after completion of consolidation chemotherapy suggested residual active disease. Rx, treatment.

had tiny pulmonary nodules shown by chest CT.[97] Most discordance between CT and FDG-PET occurs at extranodal sites, such as the lung, in which CT is superior for tiny nodules, and the spleen and bone marrow, in which FDG-PET is superior.[98] The highest diagnostic accuracy is therefore achieved using a combination of FDG-PET and CT.

Despite these advances in functional imaging, staging with conventional imaging modalities (CT and/or MR imaging) alone as the standard initial staging procedure for risk and treatment stratification has historically been sufficient to achieve cure rates greater than 90% in pediatric HL. Therefore, the ultimate impact of additional whole-body imaging with either MR imaging or FDG-PET, although promising, may be modest in terms of changing overall cure rates of pediatric HL. However, the incorporation of FDG-PET/CT findings into radiation treatment planning may be significant in treatment-related toxicity, by guiding treatment dose and target treatment volume.[55,63,99] One study found that involved field radiation therapy (IFRT) volumes needed to be adjusted from FDG-PET findings in 70% of pediatric patients with HL.[98]

The St Jude (Murphy) classification is used for the staging of pediatric NHL (**Box 2**). This system is based on tumor burden, and has served clinicians well for many years. In the past, even with less effective chemotherapy, the St Jude system provided a sound basis for treatment stratification. Children with NHL, in contrast with HL, frequently present with disseminated disease. As with HL, CT scanning is most commonly used for the initial staging of NHL. For specific sites of bone or CNS disease, MR imaging is used. FDG-PET detects additional disease in a small proportion of pediatric patients with NHL (see **Figs. 17, 18** and **20**; **Figs. 22** and **23**), but it has not been shown to detect additional sites of disease that would result in frequent alterations of patient stage, nor has it been generally shown to result in any modification of treatment.[100] High cure rates result from risk-adapted intensive chemotherapy without radiation therapy, and it has not been necessary to map precisely every small site of nodal disease, because patients are being treated intensively and systemically.[58] As a result, in contrast with the adult situation, FDG-PET is not routinely included in the diagnostic staging of childhood NHL.[101] However, NHL is often disseminated at the time of initial disease presentation and, in this setting, early response assessment may be more useful in predicting ultimate patient outcome rather than

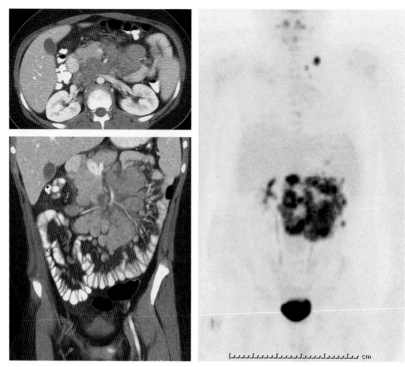

Fig. 18. A 12-year-old boy with ALCL. He initially presented with testicular pain, swelling, and left testicular enlargement. Ultrasonography (not shown) revealed heterogeneous testicular echogenicity, but no focal mass; testicular biopsy was negative for malignancy. The CT scan shown here, obtained for subsequent abdominal pain, reveals diffuse mesenteric and retroperitoneal lymphadenopathy. Occlusion of the inferior vena cava and obliteration of the left renal vein likely accounted for the initial left testicular complaints. FDG-PET scan shows uptake in the primary mass, as well as a left supraclavicular site. No uptake was present in the scrotum.

extent of disease and overall tumor burden at diagnosis (see **Fig. 23**). For these patients, diagnostic FDG-PET imaging is obtained to provide a baseline for subsequent response assessment.

ALCL is an example of disease distribution not fitting well into the St Jude NHL staging system

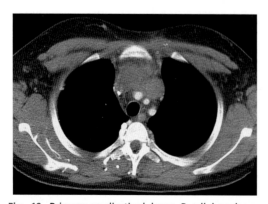

Fig. 19. Primary mediastinal large B-cell lymphoma often assumes a lobular morphology like HL and tends to occlude the superior vena cava, as shown on this chest CT image.

(see **Figs. 17** and **18**). Sites of involvement that are unusual in childhood lymphoma, such as skin, lung, and bone, are common in ALCL. LL is another example of the limitations of the NHL staging system. Most patients are stage III, with few presenting with either stage I or stage II disease. Furthermore, the outcome of patients with stage IV disease (usually the result of bone marrow involvement), differs little from those with stage III disease. Because of the overall excellent response of these patients, features such as tumor bulk, pleural effusion, and respiratory obstruction do not ultimately influence overall outcome.[54,58] As with LL, BL responds rapidly to aggressive chemotherapy.[58] Patients with localized disease have an excellent outcome after a short course of aggressive chemotherapy, and, with improvements in treatment, even patients with advanced-stage disease at diagnosis have an excellent overall outcome. Although FDG-PET scanning may be performed during staging of patients with BL, given the speed with which these tumors grow and enlarge, there is little evidence that functional imaging affects staging or outcome in this population of patients.[101]

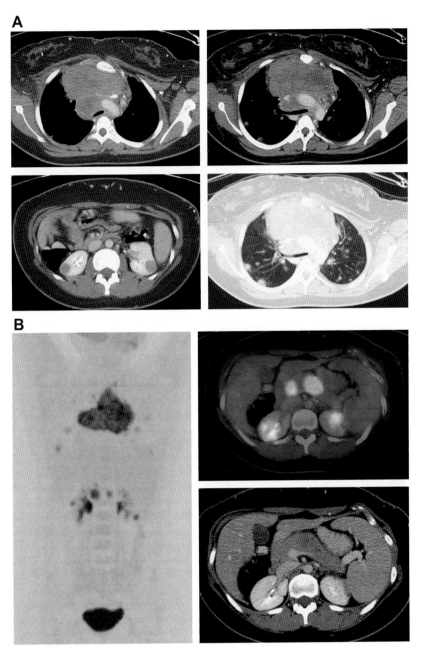

Fig. 20. (*A*) Axial CT images in a patient with mediastinal DLBCL, showing mediastinal mass, near occlusion of the brachiocephalic vein, tracheal narrowing, pulmonary metastases, and bilateral renal lesions. (*B*) FDG-PET shows uptake in the mediastinal mass, pulmonary lesions, and renal lesions. In addition, FDG-PET clearly shows 2 foci of disease in the pancreas that are difficult to resolve by CT.

Therapy Response Evaluation

Initial efforts to develop objective measurement criteria for assessing solid tumors were put forward by the WHO and used bidirectional measurement techniques.[102] These measurement techniques focused primarily on disease staging and determining initial disease bulk in an effort to stratify patients into treatment groups. Early criteria for response were also developed, and led to categories ranging from complete response (CR) to progressive disease, and included stable/ no change or partial response (PR) in the classification scheme, depending on the estimates of

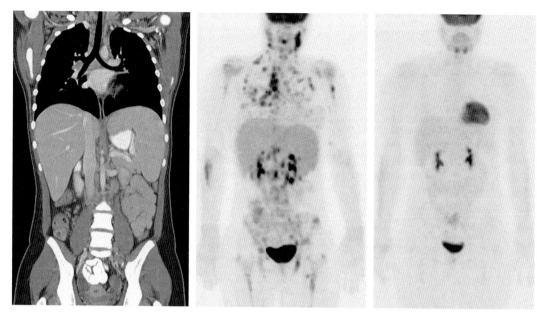

Fig. 21. A 12-year-old heart transplant recipient with fever and increased EBV titers. CT showed extensive lymph node enlargement in the retroperitoneum, supraclavicular regions, and mediastinum, as well as splenic involvement, consistent with PTLD. Disease did not respond to reduction in immunosuppression. FDG-PET confirmed extensive FDG-avid PTLD. One month after chemotherapy there is no residual disease.

change in tumor size. The WHO criteria presented many challenges, particularly for tumors such as HL, which frequently leave measurable residual posttreatment scar tissue. Minimum lesion size and numbers of lesions to be recorded were not specified and, depending on the location of tumor, size measurements of lymph nodes may have been based on physical examination estimates. In addition, these methods were devised before the advent of the multiplanar cross-sectional imaging techniques that are in common use today (CT and MR imaging), and underestimates of disease burden and the choice of measurement technique often led to errors in establishing disease progression or response.

Developing objective measures of treatment response is essential to having evaluable prospective end points in early phase clinical trials and determining whether new agents warrant further testing. The challenge is developing surrogate end points that accurately reflect the disease process and response to therapy at a time when other indicators of response (eg, change in clinical status) may not reflect treatment response. For example, a brisk response to chemotherapy is an indirect determinant of biologic homogeneity within the tumor, which, in turn, translates into more uniform chemosensitivity across the entire tumor volume. As a result, changes in FDG uptake that occur soon after the initiation of therapy serve

as an in vivo chemosensitivity test, even when significant changes in tumor volume or complete resolution of the tumor mass are not yet seen on morphologic imaging (**Fig. 24**). Studies showing that significant reductions in tumor volume and FDG-PET negativity are associated with favorable outcome in both pediatric HL and NHL suggest that rapid and homogeneous cytotoxic chemotherapy responsiveness may lead to improved disease-free survival.[103]

Several studies of FDG-PET for response assessment in pediatric lymphoma have been reported.[86,104–107] The use of FDG-PET in assessing response during therapy for tumors that are FDG avid at the time of staging is being investigated. In one study of pediatric and young adult patients with HL or NHL, the negative predictive value of FDG-PET during therapy was 96%, whereas the positive predictive value was 100%.[86] This observation, substantiated by other studies, suggests that interim FDG-PET scanning during therapy is an excellent prognostic indicator for predicting clinical outcome.

An ongoing major European study in childhood and adolescent HL is evaluating the role of interim FDG-PET in determining the need for involved field radiotherapy in patients who have a good early response to induction chemotherapy (ie, those patients who are in complete remission or in partial remission based on CT, but FDG-PET negative).[100]

Box 1
Modified Ann Arbor staging system for childhood HL

Stage I: involvement of single lymph node region (I) or localized involvement of a single extralymphatic organ or site (IE)

Stage II: involvement of 2 or more lymph node regions on the same side of the diaphragm (II) or localized contiguous involvement of a single extralymphatic organ or site and its regional lymph node(s) with involvement of 1 or more lymph node regions on the same side of the diaphragm (IIE)

Stage III: involvement of lymph node regions on both sides of the diaphragm (III), which may also be accompanied by localized contiguous involvement of an extralymphatic organ or site (IIIE), by involvement of the spleen (IIIS), or both (IIIE+S)

Stage IV: disseminated (multifocal) involvement of 1 or more extralymphatic organs or tissues, with or without associated lymph node involvement, or isolated extralymphatic organ involvement with distant (nonregional) nodal involvement

Anatomic lymph node regions for the purpose of HL staging are Waldeyer ring, cervical/supraclavicular/occipital/preauricular, infraclavicular, axillary/pectoral, epitrochlear/brachial, mediastinal, hilar, splenic/splenic hilar, mesenteric, para-aortic/celiac/periportal/retrocrural,iliac, inguinal/femoral, and popliteal.

The designation A is for asymptomatic disease and B is for the presence of unexplained fever, weight loss, or night sweats. The designation E is for minimal extra-lymphatic disease from direct extension of an involved lymph node region, originally devised to indicate extralymphatic disease limited enough to be subjected to definitive treatment by radiation therapy. The designation E is not appropriate for cases of widespread or diffuse extralymphatic disease (eg, a large pleural effusion that is cytologically positive), which should be considered stage IV.

Box 2
St Jude staging system for childhood NHL

Stage I: a single tumor (extranodal) or single anatomic site (nodal), excluding mediastinum or abdomen

Stage II: a single tumor (extranodal) with regional node involvement; 2 or more nodal sites on the same side of the diaphragm; 2 single (extranodal) tumors with or without regional node involvement on the same side of the diaphragm; a primary gastrointestinal tract tumor, with or without associated mesenteric nodes, grossly completely resected

Stage III: 2 single tumors (extranodal) on opposite sides of the diaphragm; 2 or more nodal areas above and below the diaphragm; primary intrathoracic tumors (mediastinal, pleural, thymic); extensive primary intra-abdominal disease, unresectable; paraspinal or epidural tumors

Stage IV: any of stages I–III with initial CNS or bone marrow involvement (<25%)

This represents an early effort to incorporate a response-based treatment algorithm into ongoing clinical trials of pediatric lymphoma patients. Most of the data have been obtained after 2 cycles of chemotherapy, although there is no evidence to suggest that a response evaluation after 2 or 3 cycles is either superior or inferior to that performed after 1 cycle. A very early response to therapy after 1 cycle may be more predictive than responses measured after more prolonged therapy.

As noted earlier, the use of two-dimensional measurement techniques does not account for functional and metabolic changes in the tumor. The International Harmonization Project (IHP) was convened to address this issue in adult lymphoma and issued revised criteria in 2007 for complete remission, partial remission, progressive disease, and stable disease (SD) both for HL and

NHL.[77,108] Although the focus of this project was adult lymphoma, the criteria proposed can, for the most part, be applied to pediatric lymphomas. A summary of these criteria is shown in **Table 1**. As before, measurable extranodal disease should be assessed in a manner similar to that for nodal disease. For HL, the spleen is still considered a site of nodal disease (see **Fig. 11**). Disease loci that are assessable but not measurable (eg, pleural effusions and bone lesions) are recorded as present or absent unless it is proved by biopsy to be negative. The major change to the response criteria is the emphasis placed on FDG-PET in determining response.

The most significant change of the IHP criteria from the earlier criteria used to determine response is the definition of CR. CR is defined by the IHP as disappearance of all evidence of disease, but is now primarily based on FDG-PET. In patients with typically FDG-avid lymphomas (nearly all patients with HL and most patients with NHL), a posttreatment residual mass of any size is permitted by CT or MR imaging, as long as it is FDG-PET negative (see **Fig. 24**); this is true for patients in whom the FDG-PET was positive before therapy, and even in patients with no pretreatment FDG-PET scan, provided they have typically FDG-avid lymphomas (such as HL). Variably FDG-avid lymphomas or those in which FDG avidity is unknown must have their diseased lymph nodes and nodal masses regress to normal size (not >1.5 cm in greatest transverse diameter, or not more than 1.0 cm in short axis for lymph nodes less than 1.5 cm in size at diagnosis). These

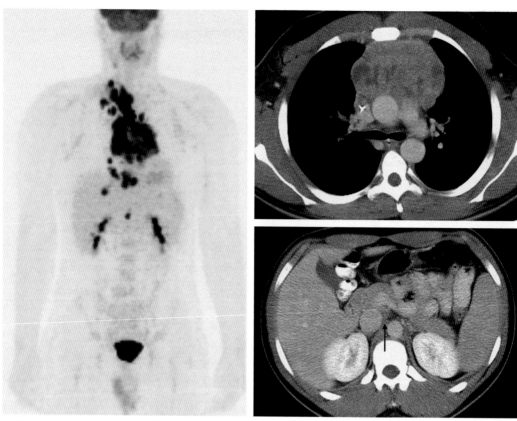

Fig. 22. A 16-year-old patient with DLBCL. Axial CT and FDG-PET show uptake in the mediastinal mass and multiple diaphragmatic lymph nodes. An additional focus of disease in a small aortocaval lymph node (*arrow*) would not have been detected without the use of FDG-PET.

criteria have been developed for adults but should be applicable for most pediatric patients, although some clinical judgment is necessary in cases with borderline enlarged lymph nodes. Splenic and/or liver involvement, either as diffuse enlargement or focal nodules, should return to normal size and nodules should disappear. However, the determination of splenic involvement may be challenging and multiple imaging modalities may be used to unequivocally establish the presence or absence of residual abdominal visceral disease (see **Fig. 24**). Bone marrow involvement, if present, must have cleared based on repeat bone marrow biopsy. Residual bone marrow abnormalities by imaging (ie, FDG-PET or MR imaging) should be confirmed by biopsy in order for a patient to be considered in CR.

PR is defined by the IHP as regression of measurable disease with no new sites of disease. There must be at least a 50% decrease in the sum of the product of the diameters of up to 6 largest dominant nodes or nodal masses, which should be clearly measurable in 2 dimensions. There should be no increase in size of other nodes, liver,

and spleen. Splenic/hepatic nodules must regress by not less than 50% in size. If bone marrow was involved before therapy and clinical CR was achieved by other criteria, but there is persistent marrow involvement, the patient is still considered a partial responder. For partial responders, posttreatment FDG-PET should be positive in at least 1 previously involved site. If FDG avidity at baseline is unknown, then the CT criteria are used.

SD is defined by the IHP as failure to attain either CR or PR, but not meeting criteria for progressive disease. For FDG-avid lymphomas, the FDG-PET scan should be positive at prior sites of disease with no new areas of involvement on the posttreatment CT or FDG-PET. If FDG-PET is not available, there must be no change in the size of the previous lesions on the posttreatment CT scan.

The appearance of any new lesion at the end of therapy should be considered relapsed (after CR) or progressive disease (after PR or SD) according to the IHP unless otherwise confirmed by histologic evaluation. Increased FDG uptake at a previously unaffected site or at a previously involved site that had responded should also be considered

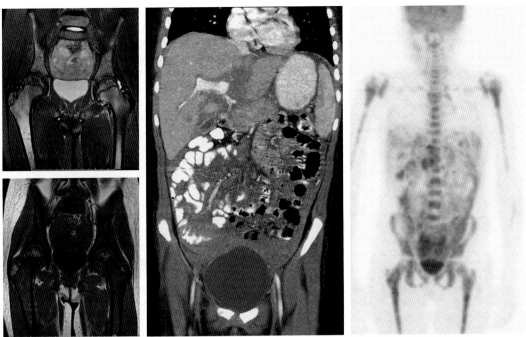

Fig. 23. An 8-year-old patient with hip pain. MR imaging shows diffuse marrow replacement on T2-weighted and T1-weighted images. CT shows extensive visceral and intra-abdominal involvement. FDG-PET confirms diffuse abnormal uptake throughout the abdomen and bone marrow. Bone marrow aspirate showed greater than 25% infiltration of the marrow by Burkitt cells, indicating Burkitt leukemia.

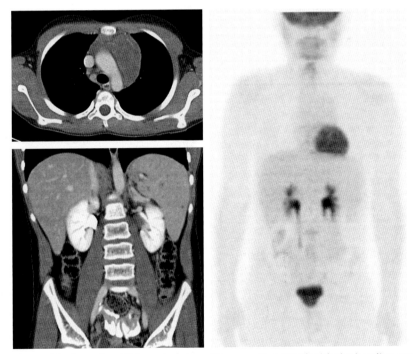

Fig. 24. This patient with HL received 2 4-week cycles of therapy. Compared with the baseline examination (see Fig. 11) there is still residual mediastinal soft tissue abnormality, although decreased from the baseline examination. The spleen is now normal in size; however, punctate hypodensities are still present in the spleen. Despite these residual CT findings, the accompanying FDG-PET shows complete resolution of abnormal FDG uptake in the mediastinal mass and in the abdomen.

Table 1
Summary of new Harmonization Project criteria for PET and CT in determining response in lymphoma[a]

Response	Criteria
CR	FDG-PET completely negative Residual lymph nodes/nodal masses allowed, if FDG negative Bone marrow biopsy negative Splenic/liver involvement must disappear No new sites of disease
PR	PDG positivity should be present in at least 1 previously involved site Regression of measurable disease; no new sites of disease ≥50% decrease in SPD of 6 dominant LNs/nodal masses ≥50% reduction in splenic/hepatic nodules, if present Even if CR by other criteria, positive bone marrow biopsy is considered PR
SD	Failure to achieve PR, but not meeting PD criteria
PD/relapse	Any lesion increased in size by ≥50% from nadir Any new lesion PET should be positive in new/progressed lesions if ≥1.5 cm

Notes: New criteria include PET in definition of CR. PET considered positive if uptake is greater than mediastinal blood pool (lesions >2 cm), or more than local background (lesions <2 cm).

Abbreviations: CR, complete response; LNs, lymph nodes; PD, progressive disease; PR, partial response; SD, stable disease; SPD.

[a] Based on work from the IHP.

Data from Juweid ME, Stroobants S, Hoekstra OS, et al. Use of positron emission tomography for response assessment of lymphoma: consensus of the Imaging Subcommittee of International Harmonization Project in Lymphoma. J Clin Oncol 2007;25:571–78; and Cheson BD, Pfistner B, Juweid ME, et al. Revised response criteria for malignant lymphoma. J Clin Oncol 2007;25:579–86.

relapsed or progressive disease (see **Fig. 13**). Lymph nodes are considered abnormal if their short axis is greater than 1.0 cm. In most patients with prior pulmonary nodules, new lung nodules identified by CT are typically benign and should be histologically confirmed to establish relapse/progressive disease. Sites of relapse or progressive disease should be FDG avid unless the lesion is too small to be detected by PET (<1.5 cm in long axis, or 1.0 cm with newer scanners).

Restaging at completion of therapy uses the same response criteria used for early interim response assessments, with CR reserved for those patients with absence of disease by clinical examination and imaging studies. As before, residual abnormalities on cross-sectional imaging are allowed, provided they remain FDG negative and no new sites of FDG activity are identified.

Currently, visual assessment is considered adequate for interpreting FDG-PET findings as positive or negative when assessing response after completion of therapy. The use of standardized uptake value (SUV) measurements is still experimental.[109] The use of mediastinal blood pool activity is currently recommended as the reference background activity to define FDG-PET positivity for residual masses,[108,109] although this can be challenging (**Fig. 25**), and a recent review emphasizes the importance of establishing standards for background activity to avoid stage migration purely as a result of improvements in technology.[110] The use of FDG-PET and functional response assessment has clearly revolutionized the response evaluation in both HD and NHL. Studies have shown that tumor responsiveness as determined by FDG-PET activity after 1 to 2 cycles of treatment can identify patients at increased risk of relapse. However, studies are still ongoing or in development in which early FDG response assessment is or will be used to dictate treatment approach.

If it is accepted that FDG-PET imaging is a valuable surrogate biomarker for assessing a response to therapy in pediatric lymphoma, then the next challenge is how to use this surrogate to effectively guide therapy. The goal is to move from a risk-adapted prediction of outcome based on staging and baseline symptoms to a response-directed treatment paradigm.[55] To validate functional imaging as a useful biomarker of response, the next era of clinical trials in pediatric lymphoma will likely require that treatment decisions be made based solely on functional imaging biomarker findings, irrespective of residual abnormalities seen on conventional cross-sectional imaging. There will be challenges. At least 1 randomized study has shown that the addition of radiation therapy in patients with bulky HL and FDG-negative postchemotherapy residual masses resulted in improved EFS compared with patients who underwent chemotherapy alone.[111] Despite development of the new harmonization criteria for adults, there are no data as yet in children to direct how to incorporate these new response assessment guidelines in pediatric treatment protocols. For example, it is

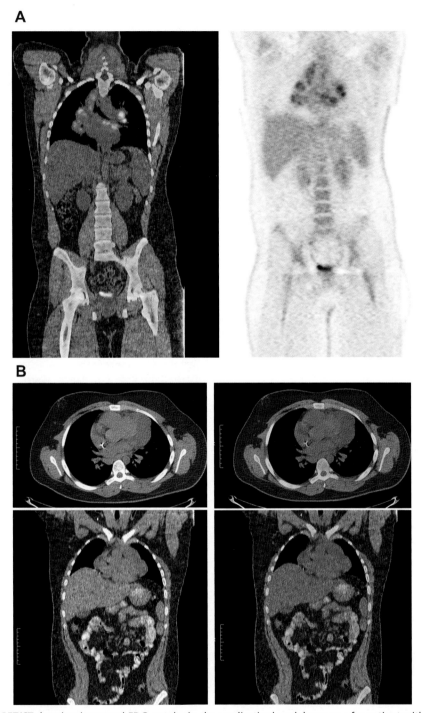

Fig. 25. (A) PET/CT showing increased FDG uptake in the mediastinal nodal masses of a patient with HL at diagnosis. The uptake is clearly greater than in the mediastinal blood pool or liver. (B) After 2 cycles of therapy, a mediastinal soft tissue mass persists. There is low-level FDG uptake in the mass, as great as in the mediastinal blood pool but less than in the liver, which emphasizes the challenge in interpreting residual FDG uptake in patients completing their up-front chemotherapy.

unclear whether radiation treatment can be reduced to initial involved sites of nodal activity or eliminated entirely for those patients with HL who have no residual nodal activity early after response to therapy.[55] One approach, for example, would be restricting radiation to sites of residual FDG uptake. The goal would be to titrate therapy using the prognostic value of early treatment response to reduce treatment intensity in those patients with rapid early responses and thereby reduce toxicity while, at the same time, intensifying treatment of those with slow early responses in an effort to improve disease control.

These approaches, all of which require confirmation in clinical trial settings, are intended to develop response-adapted therapy to identify patients with favorable chemotherapy-sensitive disease who can be treated with abbreviated chemotherapy and low-dose IFRT or no radiation therapy at all. Alternatively, rather than entirely eliminating radiation therapy, radiation therapy volumes may be restricted to lymph node regions that were initially involved with disease rather than the entire regional nodal group.[55,99] Such an approach has the potential to significantly reduce the irradiated volume of normal tissues compared with involved field radiation and, coupled with functional imaging response assessment, could produce significant reductions in radiation-related late effects.

Surveillance for Relapse

Relapse occurs in approximately 20% of pediatric patients with HL.[63] Most of these occur within the first 3 years. It has been suggested that relapses occurring beyond 1 year after the completion of therapy have a favorable prognosis relative to those occurring early after completion of therapy and therefore surveillance imaging and identification of relapse has remained an important goal of observation of therapy.

Rebound thymic hyperplasia, a potential mimic of mediastinal relapse, most characteristically presents as an enlarging thymic mass within 6 to 8 months of completion of chemotherapy (**Fig. 26**). Rebound thymic hyperplasia can show avidity for FDG, usually in a pattern of mild, diffuse uptake, in contrast with the intense, discrete uptake usually associated with lymphoma. If a child or adolescent has imaging findings compatible with rebound thymic hyperplasia, continued surveillance is advised rather than biopsy, especially if there is no other evidence of recurrence or prior neoplastic involvement of the thymus.[112]

In a recent pediatric intermediate-stage and advanced-stage HL study, relapses occurred in 10.6% of the patients, with a median time to relapse of 7 months.[113] Most of these relapses occurred within 18 months after completion of therapy and most of these relapses were local, at original sites of disease. Nearly two-thirds of these relapses were detected based on clinical symptoms, laboratory tests, or physical examination findings. Only 17% of the patients, all of whom relapsed more than 1 year after therapy, were asymptomatic and had disease detected solely from surveillance imaging. A review of the number of imaging studies performed to identify these relapses revealed that more than 400 CT scans were mandated by protocol to detect these asymptomatic relapses. Based on this, it has been suggested that CT, and imaging of any kind, is overused in the routine post-treatment surveillance of patients with HL, and modifications in surveillance protocol are indicated for routine long-term surveillance. A recent report has further emphasized the considerable increase in radiation exposure to these patients attributable to routine surveillance imaging.[114]

As has been reported in adult studies, most relapses occur in areas of initial disease and within the first year after completion of therapy, which indicates that the frequency of screening should be greatest in the early posttherapy years. The role of FDG-PET as a surveillance tool to detect relapse in asymptomatic patients has not been established. In particular, the problem of false-positive findings

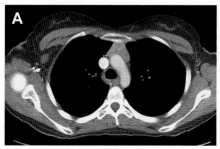 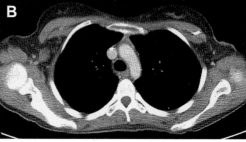

Fig. 26. A chest CT image (*A*) obtained in an asymptomatic 15-year-old patient 5 months after completion of therapy for HL shows enlargement of an anterior mediastinal soft tissue structure compared with a chest CT image (*B*) obtained at the end of therapy, representing rebound thymic hyperplasia.

remains and current recommendations do not include the use of FDG-PET for routine surveillance.[77] However, if sites of disease are detected by other imaging modalities or are suspected clinically, there may be a role for FDG-PET imaging in confirming relapse, but not as an integral part of routine surveillance in either HL or NHL.[100] In one study, the use of FDG-PET/CT to identify recurrent disease in asymptomatic patients with HL and NHL led to false-positive results in 63% and 41% of patients, respectively, for a positive predictive value of only 53%.[106] Although the negative predictive value was greater than 99% in this study, the high frequency of false positives does not allow appropriate treatment decisions to be confidently made based solely on FDG-PET surveillance imaging.

There will be understandable reluctance to reducing the intensity of surveillance imaging at a time when treatment intensity and duration of therapy are also being reduced. Nonetheless, all of the available evidence suggests that aggressive monitoring early after therapy combined with judicious imaging and close physical examination and laboratory monitoring during the surveillance period is the most effective means of following these patients.

TREATMENT-RELATED COMPLICATIONS

Overall survival rates are excellent for ALL, HL, localized low-stage NHL, and even for some advanced-stage NHL and AML. The goal of reducing toxic effects of therapy is now a focus of the next generation of treatment protocols.[55,115] Imaging plays an important role in diagnosing treatment-related complications of leukemia and lymphoma. Many of the complications associated with leukemia and lymphoma are shared because of the treatment of both with cytotoxic chemotherapy with associated marrow suppression. The complications can be acute or late in onset, and can involve virtually any organ system. Among the complications amenable to diagnosis by imaging are opportunistic infections, cerebral hemorrhage/infarction, methotrexate-induced leukoencephalopathy, venous thrombosis, anthracycline-induced cardiomyopathy, bleomycin-induced pulmonary fibrosis, bronchiolitis obliterans, radiation pneumonitis, radiation pericarditis, typhlitis, asparaginase-associated pancreatitis, hepatic veno-occlusive disease, graft-versus-host disease, hemorrhagic cystitis, posttransplant lymphoproliferative disorder, osteonecrosis, and osteoporosis. A detailed discussion of the imaging of these complications is beyond the scope of this article.

Second malignant neoplasms, including AML, NHL, and malignancies of breast, lung, and thyroid within radiation fields, are all of concern.[55] Historical treatment regimens for lymphoma, which used high radiation doses and intense chemotherapy regimens, had well-established rates of secondary malignancy.[54] The risk of secondary malignancy after low-dose radiation is not well described, because this became the standard treatment of children only in the mid 1980s and for adolescents in the early 1990s. With unknown latency periods for developing second malignancies after low-dose radiation exposure and reduced chemotherapy, there is no clear role for routine surveillance imaging in these patients.

FUTURE DIRECTIONS

With isotropic voxel acquisition of cross-sectional imaging data, the ability to generate three-dimensional tumor representations has improved and accurate tumor volume calculations are now feasible, although automated measurement techniques remain elusive. Nonetheless, changes in tumor volume, particularly with extensive multifocal sites of bulky lymphoma, may be an important variable to correlate with FDG-PET response. It seems overly simplistic to assume that all patients who become FDG negative after 2 cycles of therapy, even in the presence of large residual masses, will be uniformly free of disease progression or relapse. The ability to provide other criteria for response to develop a multivariant array of imaging criteria should allow us to best identify those patients truly manifesting a good response to chemotherapy, without overlooking those patients in whom more aggressive treatment is mandated.

In the past, MR imaging of the thoracic and abdominal cavity has been limited by motion artifact and long examination times. However, with increasing availability of faster MR imaging scanning techniques and respiratory and cardiac gating capabilities, a more routine role of MR imaging in evaluating pediatric lymphoma is becoming feasible (Fig. 27). Whole-body MR imaging has shown good agreement with FDG-PET/CT for both nodal and extranodal staging of lymphoma.[116] MR imaging false negatives occur with normal-sized involved lymph nodes and spleen, disease that is detectable by FDG-PET. MR imaging provides an alternative imaging method to CT for anatomic disease assessment at staging and restaging without ionizing radiation exposure. Furthermore, surveillance by MR imaging may be the imaging modality of choice, particularly in patients with lymphoma in whom sustained PR or CR has occurred.

Because of high tumor cellularity and high nuclear/cytoplasm ratios, most forms of lymphoma

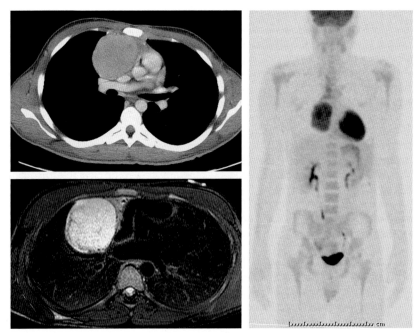

Fig. 27. A 16-year-old boy with stage IIA HL. Initial presentation with cough led to discovery of an anterior mediastinal mass, for which a broad differential diagnosis existed. Chest CT, T2-weighted chest MR imaging, and FDG-PET scan show an FDG-avid mass that abuts the pericardium, consistent with neoplasm. Gated cardiac MR imaging (not shown) sequences showed that the mass was not adherent to pericardium. The mass was subsequently excised, confirming the diagnosis of HL.

that have been studied have high signal intensity (ie, restricted diffusion) on diffusion-weighted MR images.[95,96] In one study, diffusion-weighted MR imaging matched FDG-PET/CT findings in 94% of the lymph node regions studied.[117] Furthermore, changes in diffusion characteristics may provide an additional means of evaluating residual nodal masses, because nodal apparent diffusion coefficient has been shown to increase following successful chemotherapy.[118] The use of whole-body MR imaging with diffusion-weighted imaging with background signal suppression sequences has also been shown to provide better tissue contrast in detecting malignant nodal involvement compared with conventional MR imaging sequences.[119] As these techniques are incorporated into the evaluation of pediatric lymphoma patients, it seems likely that changes in tumor characteristics as manifested by changes in diffusion or changes in enhancement may provide additional surrogates of response to help further develop a response assessment profile. Whole-body MR imaging with diffusion-weighted imaging may also serve as a more sensitive method to rapidly evaluate leukemic infiltration of the bone marrow for therapeutic response to cytotoxic chemotherapy.[120] However, widespread interindividual variation and restricted diffusion as a normal finding in the pelvis and spine of children limit the specificity of this technique, raising the risk of false-positive interpretations.[121]

SUMMARY

As the most common childhood malignancy, leukemia is frequently encountered as an underlying condition in subjects of pediatric imaging studies. The most frequent indication for imaging of children with leukemia is to evaluate for complications of treatment. Occasionally, imaging findings suggest a previously unsuspected diagnosis of leukemia, particularly in children with nonspecific musculoskeletal complaints or unexplained fever. There is no current routine role of imaging in risk stratification, therapy response assessment, or relapse surveillance for childhood leukemia.

The use of imaging in guiding diagnostic procedures, risk stratification, therapy response assessment, and relapse surveillance in childhood lymphoma has evolved in the last 20 to 30 years. From a time when nearly all patients with lymphoma were surgically staged to a time when nearly all patients have multiple imaging studies, each of which provides complimentary information, current lymphoma management requires the integration of imaging at all phases of treatment.

Current approaches should include a combination of anatomic and functional imaging techniques to predict which patients will benefit from less toxic treatment regimens and which patients will require augmented therapy. Patient-specific and disease-specific imaging biomarkers to provide specific indicators of disease activity are needed to guide the evolution from risk-adapted therapy to response-based therapy. The ongoing challenge is to optimize available imaging techniques and develop a reproducible set of validated biomarkers and image-processing tools to best accomplish these goals.

REFERENCES

1. Smith MA, Ries LAG, Gurney JG, et al. Leukemia. In: Ries LA, Smith MA, Gurney JG, editors. Cancer incidence and survival among children and adolescents: United States SEER Program 1975–1995. Bethesda (MD): National Cancer Institute; 1999. p. 17–34.

2. Greaves M. In utero origins of childhood leukaemia. Early Hum Dev 2005;81:123–9.

3. Altekruse SF, Kosary CL, Krapcho M, et al. SEER cancer statistics review, 1975–2007, National Cancer Institute. Bethesda (MD), based on November 2009 SEER data submission, posted to the SEER Web site, 2010. Available at: http://seer.cancer.gov/csr/1975_2007/. Accessed September 7, 2010.

4. Swerdlow SH, Campo E, Harris NL, et al. WHO classification of tumours of haematopoietic and lymphoid tissues. 4th edition. Lyon (France): International Agency for Research on Cancer; 2008.

5. Dainiak N. Hematologic consequences of exposure to ionizing radiation. Exp Hematol 2002;30:513–28.

6. Gaynon PS, Angiolillo AL, Carroll WL, et al. Long-term results of the Children's Cancer Group studies for childhood acute lymphoblastic leukemia 1983–2002: a Children's Oncology Group Report. Leukemia 2010;24:285–97.

7. Smith MA, Seibel NL, Altekruse SF, et al. Outcomes for children and adolescents with cancer: challenges for the twenty-first century. J Clin Oncol 2010;28:2625–34.

8. Creutzig U, Reinhardt D. Current controversies: which patients with acute myeloid leukaemia should receive a bone marrow transplantation?–A European view. Br J Haematol 2002;118:365–77.

9. Lange BJ, Smith FO, Feusner J, et al. Outcomes in CCG–2961, a children's oncology group phase 3 trial for untreated pediatric acute myeloid leukemia: a report from the children's oncology group. Blood 2008;111:1044–53.

10. Siegel MJ, Shackelford GD, McAlister WH. Pleural thickening. An unusual feature of childhood leukemia. Radiology 1981;138:367–9.

11. Abbas AA, Baker DL, Felimban SK, et al. Musculoskeletal and radiological manifestations of childhood acute leukaemia: a clinical review. Haema 2004;7:448–55.

12. Sinigaglia R, Gigante C, Bisinella G, et al. Musculoskeletal manifestations in pediatric acute leukemia. J Pediatr Orthop 2008;28:20–8.

13. Hann IM, Gupta S, Palmer MK, et al. The prognostic significance of radiological and symptomatic bone involvement in childhood acute lymphoblastic leukaemia. Med Pediatr Oncol 1979;6:51–5.

14. Melhem RE, Saber TJ. Erosion of the medial cortex of the proximal humerus. A sign of leukemia on the chest radiograph. Radiology 1980;137:77–9.

15. Bernard EJ, Nicholls WD, Howman-Giles RB, et al. Patterns of abnormality on bone scans in acute childhood leukemia. J Nucl Med 1998;39:1983–6.

16. Shalaby-Rana E, Majd M. (99m)Tc-MDP scintigraphic findings in children with leukemia: value of early and delayed whole-body imaging. J Nucl Med 2001;42:878–83.

17. Clausen N, Gotze H, Pedersen A, et al. Skeletal scintigraphy and radiography at onset of acute lymphocytic leukemia in children. Med Pediatr Oncol 1983;11:291–6.

18. Moulopoulos LA, Dimopoulos MA. Magnetic resonance imaging of the bone marrow in hematologic malignancies. Blood 1997;90:2127–47.

19. Moore SG, Gooding CA, Brasch RC, et al. Bone marrow in children with acute lymphocytic leukemia: MR relaxation times. Radiology 1986;160:237–40.

20. Babyn PS, Ranson M, McCarville ME. Normal bone marrow: signal characteristics and fatty conversion. Magn Reson Imaging Clin N Am 1998;6:473–95.

21. Ruzal-Shapiro C, Berdon WE, Cohen MD, et al. MR imaging of diffuse bone marrow replacement in pediatric patients with cancer. Radiology 1991;181:587–9.

22. Truong TH, Beyene J, Hitzler J, et al. Features at presentation predict children with acute lymphoblastic leukemia at low risk for tumor lysis syndrome. Cancer 2007;110:1832–9.

23. Niemeyer CM, Arico M, Basso G, et al. Chronic myelomonocytic leukemia in childhood: a retrospective analysis of 110 cases. European Working Group on Myelodysplastic Syndromes in Childhood (EWOG-MDS). Blood 1997;89:3534–43.

24. Murray JC, Dorfman SR, Brandt ML, et al. Renal venous thrombosis complicating acute myeloid leukemia with hyperleukocytosis. J Pediatr Hematol Oncol 1996;18:327–30.

25. Hilmes MA, Dillman JR, Mody RJ, et al. Pediatric renal leukemia: spectrum of CT imaging findings. Pediatr Radiol 2008;38:424–30.

26. Sato A, Imaizumi M, Chikaoka S, et al. Acute renal failure due to leukemic cell infiltration followed by relapse at multiple extramedullary sites in a child with acute lymphoblastic leukemia. Leuk Lymphoma 2004;45:825–8.

27. Hayek M, Srinivasan A. Acute lymphoblastic leukemia presenting with lactic acidosis and renal tubular dysfunction. J Pediatr Hematol Oncol 2003; 25:488–90.

28. Rausch DR, Norton KI, Glass RB, et al. Infantile leukemia presenting with cholestasis secondary to massive pancreatic infiltration. Pediatr Radiol 2002;32:360–1.

29. Jankovic M, Zanetto F, Conter V, et al. Cranial computed tomography findings in children with acute lymphoblastic leukemia at diagnosis. Am J Pediatr Hematol Oncol 1989;11:327–9.

30. Vazquez E, Lucaya J, Castellote A, et al. Neuroimaging in pediatric leukemia and lymphoma: differential diagnosis. Radiographics 2002;22: 1411–28.

31. Ulu EM, Tore HG, Bayrak A, et al. MRI of central nervous system abnormalities in childhood leukemia. Diagn Interv Radiol 2009;15:86–92.

32. Shackelford GD, Bloomberg G, McAlister WH. The value of roentgenography in differentiating aplastic anemia from leukemia masquerading as aplastic anemia. Am J Roentgenol Radium Ther Nucl Med 1972;116:651–4.

33. Kai T, Ishii E, Matsuzaki A, et al. Clinical and prognostic implications of bone lesions in childhood leukemia at diagnosis. Leuk Lymphoma 1996;23: 119–23.

34. Guillerman RP. Normal and abnormal bone marrow. In: Slovis T, editor. Caffey's pediatric diagnostic imaging. 11th edition. Philadelphia: Elsevier; 2008. p. 2970–96.

35. Bulas RB, Laine FJ, Das Narla L. Bilateral orbital granulocytic sarcoma (chloroma) preceding the blast phase of acute myelogenous leukemia: CT findings. Pediatr Radiol 1995;25:488–9.

36. Dusenbery KE, Howells WB, Arthur DC, et al. Extramedullary leukemia in children with newly diagnosed acute myeloid leukemia: a report from the Children's Cancer Group. J Pediatr Hematol Oncol 2003;25:760–8.

37. Schultz KR, Pullen DJ, Sather HN, et al. Risk- and response-based classification of childhood B-precursor acute lymphoblastic leukemia: a combined analysis of prognostic markers from the Pediatric Oncology Group (POG) and Children's Cancer Group (CCG). Blood 2007;109:926–35.

38. Creutzig U, Zimmermann M, Ritter J, et al. Definition of a standard-risk group in children with AML. Br J Haematol 1999;104:630–9.

39. Masera G, Carnelli V, Ferrari M, et al. Prognostic significance of radiological bone involvement in childhood acute lymphoblastic leukaemia. Arch Dis Child 1977;52:530–3.

40. Heinrich SD, Gallagher D, Warrior R, et al. The prognostic significance of the skeletal manifestations of acute lymphoblastic leukemia of childhood. J Pediatr Orthop 1994;14:105–11.

41. D'Angelo P, Mura R, Rizzari C, et al. Prognostic value of nephromegaly at diagnosis of childhood acute lymphoblastic leukemia. Acta Haematol 1995;94:84–9.

42. Yetgin S, Olgar S, Aras T, et al. Evaluation of kidney damage in patients with acute lymphoblastic leukemia in long-term follow-up: value of renal scan. Am J Hematol 2004;77:132–9.

43. Attarbaschi A, Mann G, Dworzak M, et al. Mediastinal mass in childhood T-cell acute lymphoblastic leukemia: significance and therapy response. Med Pediatr Oncol 2002;39:558–65.

44. Vande Berg BC, Lecouvet FE, Michaux L, et al. Magnetic resonance imaging of the bone marrow in hematological malignancies. Eur Radiol 1998;8: 1335–44.

45. Fletcher BD, Wall JE, Hanna SL. Effect of hematopoietic growth factors on MR images of bone marrow in children undergoing chemotherapy. Radiology 1993;189:745–51.

46. Emy PY, Levin TL, Sheth SS, et al. Iron overload in reticuloendothelial systems of pediatric oncology patients who have undergone transfusions: MR observations. AJR Am J Roentgenol 1997;168:1011–5.

47. Benz-Bohm G, Gross-Fengels W, Bohndorf K, et al. MRI of the knee region in leukemic children. Part II. Follow up: responder, non-responder, relapse. Pediatr Radiol 1990;20:272–6.

48. Gaynon PS, Qu RP, Chappell RJ, et al. Survival after relapse in childhood acute lymphoblastic leukemia: impact of site and time to first relapse—the Children's Cancer Group experience. Cancer 1998;82:1387–95.

49. Webb DK. Management of relapsed acute myeloid leukaemia. Br J Haematol 1999;106:851–9.

50. Jensen KE, Thomsen C, Henriksen O, et al. Changes in T1 relaxation processes in the bone marrow following treatment in children with acute lymphoblastic leukemia. A magnetic resonance imaging study. Pediatr Radiol 1990;20:464–8.

51. Kan JH, Hernanz-Schulman M, Frangoul HA, et al. MRI diagnosis of bone marrow relapse in children with ALL. Pediatr Radiol 2008;38:76–81.

52. Rubnitz JE, Hijiya N, Zhou Y, et al. Lack of benefit of early detection of relapse after completion of therapy for acute lymphoblastic leukemia. Pediatr Blood Cancer 2005;44:138–41.

53. Trigg ME, Steinherz PG, Chappell R, et al. Early testicular biopsy in males with acute lymphoblastic leukemia: lack of impact on subsequent event-free survival. J Pediatr Hematol Oncol 2000;22:27–33.

54. Reiter A, Ferrando AA. Malignant lymphomas and lymphadenopathies. In: Orkin SH, Fisher DE, Look AT, et al, editors. Oncology of infancy and childhood. Philadelphia: Elsevier; 2009. p. 417–508.

55. Hodgson DC, Hudson MM, Constine LS. Pediatric Hodgkin lymphoma: maximizing efficacy and minimizing toxicity. Semin Radiat Oncol 2007;17:230–42.

56. Jaffe ES, Harris NL, Stein H, et al. Pathology and genetics of tumours of hematopoietic and lymphoid tissues. World Health Organization Classification of Tumours of Haemtopoietic and Lymphoid Tissues. Lyon (France): IARC Press; 2001.

57. Claviez A, Tiemann M, Luders H, et al. Impact of latent Epstein-Barr virus infection on outcome in children and adolescents with Hodgkin's lymphoma. J Clin Oncol 2005;23:4048–56.

58. Link MP, Weinstein HJ. Malignant non-Hodgkin lymphomas in children. In: Pizzo PA, Poplack DG, editors. Principles and practice of pediatric oncology. 5th edition. Philadelphia: Lippincott Williams & Wilkins; 2006. p. 722–47.

59. Cairo MS, Raetz E, Lim MS, et al. Childhood and adolescent non-Hodgkin lymphoma: new insights in biology and critical challenges for the future. Pediatr Blood Cancer 2005;45:753–69.

60. Gottschalk S, Rooney CM, Heslop HE. Post-transplant lymphoproliferative disorders. Annu Rev Med 2005;56:29–44.

61. Shroff R, Rees L. The post-transplant lymphoproliferative disorder–a literature review. Pediatr Nephrol 2004;19:369–77.

62. Bakker NA, van Imhoff GW, Verschuuren EA, et al. Presentation and early detection of post-transplant lymphoproliferative disorder after solid organ transplantation. Transpl Int 2007;20:207–18.

63. Schwartz CL. Special issues in pediatric Hodgkin's disease. Eur J Haematol Suppl 2005;(66):55–62.

64. Punnett A, Tsang RW, Hodgson DC. Hodgkin lymphoma across the age spectrum: epidemiology, therapy, and late effects. Semin Radiat Oncol 2010;20:30–44.

65. Ruhl U, Albrecht M, Dieckmann K, et al. Response-adapted radiotherapy in the treatment of pediatric Hodgkin's disease: an interim report at 5 years of the German GPOH-HD 95 trial. Int J Radiat Oncol Biol Phys 2001;51:1209–18.

66. Nachman JB, Sposto R, Herzog P, et al. Randomized comparison of low-dose involved-field radiotherapy and no radiotherapy for children with Hodgkin's disease who achieve a complete response to chemotherapy. J Clin Oncol 2002;20:3765–71.

67. Aleman BM, Re D, Diehl V. The role of radiation therapy in patients with Hodgkin's lymphoma. Curr Hematol Malig Rep 2007;2:151–60.

68. Bradley MB, Cairo MS. Stem cell transplantation for pediatric lymphoma: past, present and future. Bone Marrow Transplant 2008;41:149–58.

69. Attarbaschi A, Dworzak M, Steiner M, et al. Outcome of children with primary resistant or relapsed non-Hodgkin lymphoma and mature B-cell leukemia after intensive first-line treatment: a population-based analysis of the Austrian Cooperative Study Group. Pediatr Blood Cancer 2005;44:70–6.

70. Abramson SJ, Price AP. Imaging of pediatric lymphomas. Radiol Clin North Am 2008;46:313–38, ix.

71. Shamberger RC. Preanesthetic evaluation of children with anterior mediastinal masses. Semin Pediatr Surg 1999;8:61–8.

72. Toma P, Granata C, Rossi A, et al. Multimodality imaging of Hodgkin disease and non-Hodgkin lymphomas in children. Radiographics 2007;27:1335–54.

73. Aygun B, Karakas SP, Leonidas J, et al. Reliability of splenic index to assess splenic involvement in pediatric Hodgkin's disease. J Pediatr Hematol Oncol 2004;26:74–6.

74. Hines-Thomas M, Kaste SC, Hudson MM, et al. Comparison of gallium and PET scans at diagnosis and follow-up of pediatric patients with Hodgkin lymphoma. Pediatr Blood Cancer 2008;51:198–203.

75. Rini JN, Nunez R, Nichols K, et al. Coincidence-detection FDG-PET versus gallium in children and young adults with newly diagnosed Hodgkin's disease. Pediatr Radiol 2005;35:169–78.

76. Mody RJ, Bui C, Hutchinson RJ, et al. Comparison of (18)F flurodeoxyglucose PET with Ga-67 scintigraphy and conventional imaging modalities in pediatric lymphoma. Leuk Lymphoma 2007;48:699–707.

77. Juweid ME, Stroobants S, Hoekstra OS, et al. Use of positron emission tomography for response assessment of lymphoma: consensus of the Imaging Subcommittee of International Harmonization Project in Lymphoma. J Clin Oncol 2007;25:571–8.

78. Hudson MM, Krasin MJ, Kaste SC. PET imaging in pediatric Hodgkin's lymphoma. Pediatr Radiol 2004;34:190–8.

79. Wickmann L, Luders H, Dorffel W. 18-FDG-PET-findings in children and adolescents with Hodgkin's disease: retrospective evaluation of the correlation to other imaging procedures in initial staging and to the predictive value of follow up examinations. Klin Padiatr 2003;215:146–50 [in German].

80. Furth C, Denecke T, Steffen I, et al. Correlative imaging strategies implementing CT, MRI, and PET for staging of childhood Hodgkin disease. J Pediatr Hematol Oncol 2006;28:501–12.

81. Hermann S, Wormanns D, Pixberg M, et al. Staging in childhood lymphoma: differences between FDG-PET and CT. Nuklearmedizin 2005;44:1–7.

82. Riad R, Omar W, Kotb M, et al. Role of PET/CT in malignant pediatric lymphoma. Eur J Nucl Med Mol Imaging 2010;37:319–29.

83. Paes FM, Kalkanis DG, Sideras PA, et al. FDG PET/CT of extranodal involvement in non-Hodgkin

lymphoma and Hodgkin disease. Radiographics 2010;30:269–91.

84. Hernandez-Pampaloni M, Takalkar A, Yu JQ, et al. F-18 FDG-PET imaging and correlation with CT in staging and follow-up of pediatric lymphomas. Pediatr Radiol 2006;36:524–31.

85. Hutchings M, Loft A, Hansen M, et al. Position emission tomography with or without computed tomography in the primary staging of Hodgkin's lymphoma. Haematologica 2006;91:482–9.

86. Miller E, Metser U, Avrahami G, et al. Role of 18F-FDG PET/CT in staging and follow-up of lymphoma in pediatric and young adult patients. J Comput Assist Tomogr 2006;30:689–94.

87. Shammas A, Lim R, Charron M. Pediatric FDG PET/CT: physiologic uptake, normal variants, and benign conditions. Radiographics 2009;29: 1467–86.

88. Kaste SC, Howard SC, McCarville EB, et al. 18F-FDG-avid sites mimicking active disease in pediatric Hodgkin's. Pediatr Radiol 2005;35:141–54.

89. Gelfand MJ, O'Hara SM, Curtwright LA, et al. Premedication to block [(18)F]FDG uptake in the brown adipose tissue of pediatric and adolescent patients. Pediatr Radiol 2005;35:984–90.

90. Bea S, Zettl A, Wright G, et al. Diffuse large B-cell lymphoma subgroups have distinct genetic profiles that influence tumor biology and improve gene-expression-based survival prediction. Blood 2005; 106:3183–90.

91. von Falck C, Maecker B, Schirg E, et al. Post transplant lymphoproliferative disease in pediatric solid organ transplant patients: a possible role for [18F]-FDG-PET(/CT) in initial staging and therapy monitoring. Eur J Radiol 2007;63:427–35.

92. Crowther D, Lister TA. The Cotswolds report on the investigation and staging of Hodgkin's disease. Br J Cancer 1990;62:551–2.

93. Dieckmann K, Potter R, Hofmann J, et al. Does bulky disease at diagnosis influence outcome in childhood Hodgkin's disease and require higher radiation doses? Results from the German-Austrian Pediatric Multicenter Trial DAL-HD-90. Int J Radiat Oncol Biol Phys 2003;56:644–52.

94. Shulkin BL, Goodin GS, McCarville MB, et al. Bone and [18F]fluorodeoxyglucose positron-emission tomography/computed tomography scanning for the assessment of osseous involvement in Hodgkin lymphoma in children and young adults. Leuk Lymphoma 2009;50:1794–802.

95. Kwee TC, Takahara T, Vermoolen MA, et al. Whole-body diffusion-weighted imaging for staging malignant lymphoma in children. Pediatr Radiol 2010; 40(10):1592–602.

96. Kwee TC, Fijnheer R, Ludwig I, et al. Whole-body magnetic resonance imaging, including diffusion-weighted imaging, for diagnosing bone marrow involvement in malignant lymphoma. Br J Haematol 2010;149:628–30.

97. Kabickova E, Sumerauer D, Cumlivska E, et al. Comparison of 18F-FDG-PET and standard procedures for the pretreatment staging of children and adolescents with Hodgkin's disease. Eur J Nucl Med Mol Imaging 2006;33:1025–31.

98. Robertson VL, Anderson CS, Keller FG, et al. Role of FDG-PET in the definition of involved-field radiation therapy and management for pediatric Hodgkin's lymphoma. Int J Radiat Oncol Biol Phys 2011;80(2):324–32.

99. Krasin MJ, Hudson MM, Kaste SC. Positron emission tomography in pediatric radiation oncology: integration in the treatment-planning process. Pediatr Radiol 2004;34:214–21.

100. Shankar A, Fiumara F, Pinkerton R. Role of FDG PET in the management of childhood lymphomas-case proven or is the jury still out? Eur J Cancer 2008;44:663–73.

101. Pinkerton R. Continuing challenges in childhood non-Hodgkin's lymphoma. Br J Haematol 2005; 130:480–8.

102. Miller AB, Hoogstraten B, Staquet M, et al. Reporting results of cancer treatment. Cancer 1981;47:207–14.

103. Hutchings M, Barrington SF. PET/CT for therapy response assessment in lymphoma. J Nucl Med 2009;50(Suppl 1):21S–30S.

104. Meany HJ, Gidvani VK, Minniti CP. Utility of PET scans to predict disease relapse in pediatric patients with Hodgkin lymphoma. Pediatr Blood Cancer 2007;48:399–402.

105. Montravers F, McNamara D, Landman-Parker J, et al. [(18)F]FDG in childhood lymphoma: clinical utility and impact on management. Eur J Nucl Med Mol Imaging 2002;29:1155–65.

106. Rhodes MM, Delbeke D, Whitlock JA, et al. Utility of FDG-PET/CT in follow-up of children treated for Hodgkin and non-Hodgkin lymphoma. J Pediatr Hematol Oncol 2006;28:300–6.

107. Furth C, Steffen IG, Amthauer H, et al. Early and late therapy response assessment with [18F]fluoro-deoxyglucose positron emission tomography in pediatric Hodgkin's lymphoma: analysis of a prospective multicenter trial. J Clin Oncol 2009; 27:4385–91.

108. Cheson BD, Pfistner B, Juweid ME, et al. Revised response criteria for malignant lymphoma. J Clin Oncol 2007;25:579–86.

109. Delbeke D, Stroobants S, de Kerviler E, et al. Expert opinions on positron emission tomography and computed tomography imaging in lymphoma. Oncologist 2009;14(Suppl 2):30–40.

110. Gallamini A, Fiore F, Sorasio R, et al. Interim positron emission tomography scan in Hodgkin lymphoma: definitions, interpretation rules, and clinical validation. Leuk Lymphoma 2009;50:1761–4.

111. Picardi M, De Renzo A, Pane F, et al. Randomized comparison of consolidation radiation versus observation in bulky Hodgkin's lymphoma with post-chemotherapy negative positron emission tomography scans. Leuk Lymphoma 2007;48:1721–7.

112. Guillerman RP, Parker BR. Pediatric lymphoma. In: Guermazi A, editor. Radiological imaging in hematological malignancies. Berlin; Heidelberg: Springer-Verlag; 2004. p. 247–88.

113. Voss SD, Constine LS, London WB, et al. Evaluation of surveillance CT imaging for the detection of relapse in Hodgkin lymphoma. Pediatr Radiol 2010;40:590.

114. Chong AL, Grant RM, Ahmed BA, et al. Imaging in pediatric patients: time to think again about surveillance. Pediatr Blood Cancer 2010;55:407–13.

115. Metzger ML, Hudson MM. Balancing efficacy and safety in the treatment of adolescents with Hodgkin's lymphoma. J Clin Oncol 2009;27:6071–3.

116. Punwani S, Taylor SA, Bainbridge A, et al. Pediatric and adolescent lymphoma: comparison of whole-body STIR half-Fourier RARE MR imaging with an enhanced PET/CT reference for initial staging. Radiology 2010;255:182–90.

117. Lin C, Luciani A, Itti E, et al. Whole-body diffusion-weighted magnetic resonance imaging with apparent diffusion coefficient mapping for staging patients with diffuse large B-cell lymphoma. Eur Radiol 2010;20:2027–38.

118. Punwani S, Shankar A, Daw S, et al. Derivation of histographic apparent diffusion coefficient changes associated with successful response to first line chemotherapy of adolescent and childhood lymphoma. Pediatr Radiol 2010;40:1098.

119. Savelli S, Maurizio MD, Mortilla M, et al. Whole-body MRI with diffusion-weighted whole-body imaging with background signal suppression sequences for disease detection and staging of pediatric oncological patients. Pediatr Radiol 2010;40:1097.

120. Ballon D, Watts R, Dyke JP, et al. Imaging therapeutic response in human bone marrow using rapid whole-body MRI. Magn Reson Med 2004;52:1234–8.

121. Ording Muller LS, Avenarius D, Olsen OE. High signal in bone marrow at diffusion-weighted imaging with body background suppression (DWIBS) in healthy children. Pediatr Radiol 2011;41(2):221–6.

Index

Note: Page numbers of article titles are in **boldface** type.

Radiol Clin N Am 49 (2011) 799–804
doi:10.1016/S0033-8389(11)00105-9
0033-8389/11/$ – see front matter © 2011 Elsevier Inc. All rights reserved.

Moving?

Make sure your subscription moves with you!

To notify us of your new address, find your **Clinics Account Number** (located on your mailing label above your name), and contact customer service at:

Email: journalscustomerservice-usa@elsevier.com

800-654-2452 (subscribers in the U.S. & Canada)
314-447-8871 (subscribers outside of the U.S. & Canada)

Fax number: 314-447-8029

Elsevier Health Sciences Division
Subscription Customer Service
3251 Riverport Lane
Maryland Heights, MO 63043

*To ensure uninterrupted delivery of your subscription, please notify us at least 4 weeks in advance of move.